Geriatric Otorhinolaryngology

THE AMERICAN ACADEMY OF OTOLARYNGOLOGY — HEAD AND NECK SURGERY, INC.

COMMITTEE ON GERIATRIC OTOLARYNGOLOGY

Haskins Kashima, M.D., *Chairman*
Charles I. Berlin, Ph.D.
Robert M. Conlon, M.D.
Orel Friedman, M.D.
Richard Hawkins, D.D.S.
Fred S. Herzon, M.D.
Hueston King, M.D.
Charles F. Koopmann, M.D.
Yosef Krespi, M.D.
Charles Long, M.D.
Frank Lucente, M.D.
Michael Papsidero, M.D.
Harold F. Schuknecht, M.D.
George A. Sisson, M.D.
Fred Stucker, M.D.

Geriatric Otorhinolaryngology

Editors

JEROME C. GOLDSTEIN, M.D.
Executive Vice-President
American Academy of Otolaryngology–Head and Neck Surgery, Inc.
Washington, DC
Visiting Professor
Department of Otolaryngology–Head and Neck Surgery
The Johns Hopkins University School of Medicine
Baltimore, Maryland

HASKINS K. KASHIMA, M.D.
Professor
Department of Otolaryngology–Head and Neck Surgery
The Johns Hopkins University School of Medicine
Baltimore, Maryland

CHARLES F. KOOPMANN Jr., M.D.
Associate Professor
Department of Otolaryngology–Head and Neck Surgery
University of Michigan Medical School
Ann Arbor, Michigan

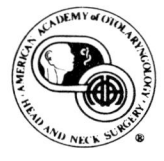

American Academy of Otolaryngology–
Head and Neck Surgery, Inc.

1989
B.C. Decker Inc • Toronto • Philadelphia

Publisher	**B.C. Decker Inc** 3228 South Service Road Burlington, Ontario L7N 3H8		**B.C. Decker Inc** 320 Walnut Street Suite 400 Philadelphia, Pennsylvania 19106
Sales and Distribution			
United States and Possessions	**The C.V. Mosby Company** 11830 Westline Industrial Drive Saint Louis, Missouri 63146		
Canada	**The C.V. Mosby Company, Ltd.** 5240 Finch Avenue East, Unit No. 1 Scarborough, Ontario M1S 5P2	Asia	**Info-Med Ltd.** 802-3 Ruttonjee House 11 Duddell Street Central Hong Kong
United Kingdom, Europe and the Middle East	**Blackwell Scientific Publications, Ltd.** Osney Mead, Oxford OX2 OEL, England	South Africa	**Libriger Book Distributors** Warehouse Number 8 "Die Ou Looiery" Tannery Road Hamilton, Bloemfontein 9300
Australia and New Zealand	**Harcourt Brace Jovanovich Group (Australia) Pty Limited** 30-52 Smidmore Street Marrickville, N.S.W. 2204 Australia	South America	**Inter-Book Marketing Services** Rua das Palmeriras, 32 Apto. 701 222-70 Rio de Janeiro RJ, Brazil
Japan	**Igaku-Shoin Ltd.** Tokyo International P.O. Box 5063 1-28-36 Hongo, Bunkyo-ku, Tokyo 113, Japan		

NOTICE

The authors and publisher have made every effort to ensure that the patient care recommended herein, including choice of drugs and drug dosages, is in accord with the accepted standards and practice at the time of publication. However, since research and regulation constantly change clinical standards, the reader is urged to check the product information sheet included in the package of each drug, which includes recommended doses, warnings, and contraindications. This is particularly important with new or infrequently used drugs.

Geriatric Otorhinolaryngology   ISBN 1-55664-104-4

© 1989 by B.C. Decker Incorporated under the International Copyright Union. All rights reserved. No part of this publication may be reused or republished in any form without written permission of the publisher, with the exception of Chapter 2 (Cell Biology of Human Aging).

Library of Congress catalog card number: 88-71653   10 9 8 7 6 5 4 3 2 1

CONTRIBUTORS

DANIEL AMSTERDAM, Ph.D.

Professor of Microbiology and Associate Professor of Medicine, SUNY at Buffalo; Director, Clinical Microbiology Laboratories, Erie County Medical Center, Buffalo, New York
Histocompatibility Antigens, Sensorineural Hearing Disorders, and Senescence

BYRON J. BAILEY, M.D., F.A.C.S.

Wiess Professor and Chairman, University of Texas Medical Branch, Galveston, Texas
Summary: Perspectives on Health Care for the Elderly

HUGH O. BARBER, M.D., F.R.C.S.C.

Professor of Otolaryngology, University of Toronto Faculty of Medicine; Director, Dizziness Unit, Sunnybrook Medical Centre, Toronto, Ontario
Ataxia of the Elderly

GEORGE BERCI, M.D.

Clinical Professor of Surgery, UCLA School of Medicine; Associate Chief of Surgery, Cedars-Sinai Hospital, Los Angeles, California
Diagnosis of Neuromuscular Voice Impairment

GERALD S. BERKE, M.D.

Assistant Professor of Surgery, UCLA School of Medicine, Los Angeles, California
Diagnosis of Neuromuscular Voice Impairment

JOEL M. BERNSTEIN, M.D., Ph.D.

Assistant Clinical Professor of Otolaryngology and Pediatrics, SUNY at Buffalo and Adjunct Professor, Division of Speech-Language Pathology and Audiology, State College of New York at Buffalo, Buffalo, New York
Histocompatibility Antigens, Sensorineural Hearing Disorders, and Senescence

BRIAN W. BLAKLEY, M.D., Ph.D., F.R.C.S.C.

Assistant Professor, Department of Otolaryngology and Director, Cochlear Implant Program, Dizziness Clinic, Wayne State University School of Medicine, Detroit, Michigan
Ataxia of the Elderly

ANDREW BLITZER, D.D.S., M.D.

Professor of Clinical Otolaryngology and Vice Chairman; Director, Division of Head and Neck Surgery, Columbia University College of Physicians and Surgeons; Attending Otolaryngologist and Director, Head and Neck Surgery, Columbia-Presbyterian Medical Center, New York, New York
Swallowing Disorders and Aspiration in the Elderly

DERALD E. BRACKMANN, M.D.

Clinical Professor of Otolaryngology, University of Southern California School of Medicine; Staff, Otologic Medical Group Inc. and House Ear Institute, Los Angeles, California
Communication Assistive Devices

DAVID BROADWAY, M.D.

Fellow, Facial Plastic and Reconstructive Surgery, University of Illinois Medical Center, Chicago, Illinois
Facial Plastic and Reconstructive Surgery in an Aging Population: A Critical Overview

ROBERT W. CANTRELL, M.D., F.A.C.S.

Fitz-Hugh Professor and Chairman, Department of Otolaryngology-Head and Neck Surgery, University of Virginia Medical Center; Otolaryngology-Head and Neck Surgeon-in-Chief, University of Virginia Hospital, Charlottesville, Virginia
Etiologic Factors in the Development of Cancer

RAYMOND H. COLTON, Ph.D

Associate Professor, Department of Otorhinolaryngology and Communication Sciences, SUNY Health Science Center at Syracuse, Syracuse, New York
Objective Evaluation of Voice Dysfunction in the Elderly

JOHN CONLEY, M.D.

Professor of Otolaryngology (Emeritus), Columbia-Presbyterian Medical Center, New York, New York
Oncology and Aging: Introduction

ROBERT A. DOBIE, M.D.

Professor of Otolaryngology-Head and Neck Surgery, University of Washington School of Medicine, Seattle, Washington
Tinnitus, Depression, and Aging

RICHARD L. DOTY, Ph.D.

Assistant Professor, Department of Otorhinolaryngology and Human Communication, University of Pennsylvania School of Medicine; Director, Smell and Taste Center, Hospital of the University of Pennsylvania, Philadelphia, Pennsylvania
Age-Related Alterations in Taste and Smell Function

BRUCE R. GERRATT, Ph.D.

Assistant Professor of Surgery, UCLA School of Medicine, Los Angeles; Chief, Section of Speech Pathology and Director of Speech Research, VA Medical Center, West Los Angeles, California
Diagnosis of Neuromuscular Voice Impairment

ARAM GLORIG, M.D.

Otologic Medical Group, Los Angeles, California
Presbyastasis: The Dysequilibrium of Aging: Introduction

DAVID G. HANSON, M.D., F.A.C.S.

Associate Professor of Surgery, UCLA School of Medicine, Los Angeles; Vice-Chief, Division of Head and Neck Surgery, UCLA Hospital and Chief, Section of Head and Neck Surgery, VA Medical Center, West Los Angeles, California
Diagnosis of Neuromuscular Voice Impairment

LEONARD HAYFLICK, Ph.D.
Professor of Anatomy, University of California, School of Medicine, San Francisco, California
Cell Biology of Human Aging

LEONARD F. JAKUBCZAK, Ph.D.
Program Director, Neuropsychology of Aging, Neuroscience and Neuropsychology of Aging Program, National Institute on Aging, National Institutes of Health, Bethesda, Maryland
Hearing, Voice, and Swallowing Disorders in Aging: A Report to Congress

FRANK JOHNSON, M.D.
Chairman, Department of Chemical Pathology, Armed Forces Institute of Pathology, Washington, D.C.
Pathology of the Skin in Aging

FRANK M. KAMER, M.D., F.A.C.S.
Associate Clinical Professor, UCLA School of Medicine; Attending Surgeon, UCLA Medical Center, Los Angeles, California
Rhinoplasty, Blepharoplasty, and Rhytidectomy in the Aging Patient

HASKINS K. KASHIMA, M.D.
Professor, Department of Otolaryngology–Head and Neck Surgery, The Johns Hopkins University School of Medicine, Baltimore, Maryland
Presbyphagia: Introduction

WAYNE J. KATON, M.D.
Associate Professor and Chief, Consultation-Liaison Services, Department of Psychiatry and Behavioral Sciences, University of Washington School of Medicine, Seattle, Washington
Tinnitus, Depression, and Aging

SAMUEL P. KORPER, Ph.D, M.P.H.
Associate Director, National Institute on Aging, Bethesda, Maryland
Epidemiologic and Demographic Characteristics of the Aging

FRED H. LINTHICUM Jr., M.D.
Associate Clinical Professor of Otolaryngology, University of Southern California School of Medicine; Director, Morphology Laboratories, House Ear Institute, Los Angeles, California
Presbyastasis

LESLIE T. MALMGREN, Ph.D.
Professor, Department of Otolaryngology, Head and Neck Morphology Laboratory, SUNY Health Science Center at Syracuse, Syracuse, New York
Aging-Related Changes in Peripheral Nerves in the Head and Neck

RICHARD A. MILLER, M.D., Ph.D.
Associate Professor of Pathology, Boston University School of Medicine, Boston, Massachusetts
Age-Related Immune Deficiency

ANDREW A. MONJAN, Ph.D., M.P.H.
Chief, Neurobiology and Neuropsychology Units, Neuroscience and Neuropsychology of Aging Program, National Institute on Aging, National Institutes of Health, Bethesda, Maryland
Hearing, Voice, and Swallowing Disorders in Aging: A Report to Congress

RUE MOORE, A.B., M.Div.
Associate Professor, History of Medicine, Albany Medical College of Union University, Albany, New York
Medical/Surgical Care: Should Age be a Variable?

MURRAY D. MORRISON, M.D., F.R.C.S.C.
Professor of Surgery, University of British Columbia Faculty of Medicine; Head, Division of Otolaryngology, Vancouver General Hospital, Vancouver, British Columbia, Canada
Evaluation and Management of Voice Disorders in the Elderly

HAMISH NICHOL, M.B., F.R.C.P.C.
Associate Professor of Psychiatry, University of British Columbia, Vancouver, British Columbia, Canada
Evaluation and Management of Voice Disorders in the Elderly

JEFFREY B. PALMER, M.D.
Assistant Professor, Division of Rehabilitation Medicine, The Johns Hopkins University School of Medicine; Active Staff, The Good Samaritan Hospital and The Johns Hopkins Hospital, and Consultant, The Johns Hopkins Swallowing Center, Baltimore, Maryland
Techniques for Examining Pharyngeal Swallowing

LINDA A. RAMMAGE, B.A., M.Sc., S–LP(C)
Clinical Instructor, University of British Columbia Faculty of Medicine; Speech/Language Pathologist, Vancouver General Hospital Voice Clinic, Vancouver, British Columbia
Evaluation and Management of Voice Disorders in the Elderly

CONNIE S. SAKAI, M.S.P.A.
Audiologist, Department of Otolaryngology–Head and Neck Surgery, University of Washington School of Medicine, Seattle, Washington
Tinnitus, Depression, and Aging

HAROLD F. SCHUKNECHT, M.D.
Walter Augustus LeCompte Professor (Emeritus), Department of Otology and Laryngology, Harvard Medical School; Chief of Otolaryngology (Emeritus), Massachusetts Eye and Ear Infirmary, Boston, Massachusetts
Pathology of Presbycusis

THOMAS C. SHANAHAN, Ph.D.
Research Associate Professor of Microbiology, SUNY at Buffalo; Chief Histocompatibility Laboratory, Erie County Medical Center, Buffalo, New York
Histocompatibility Antigens, Sensorineural Hearing Disorders, and Senescence

JAMES B. SNOW Jr., M.D.
Professor and Chairman, Department of Otorhinolaryngology and Human Communication, University of Pennsylvania School of Medicine; Staff, Hospital of the University of Pennsylvania, Philadelphia, Pennsylvania
Clinical Disorders of Olfaction and Gustation in the Aged

MARK SULLIVAN, M.D., Ph.D.
Acting Assistant Professor, Department of Psychiatry and Behavioral Sciences, University of Washington School of Medicine, Seattle, Washington
Tinnitus, Depression, and Aging

M. EUGENE TARDY Jr., M.D., F.A.C.S.
Professor of Clinical Otolaryngology–Head and Neck Surgery and Director, Division of Plastic and Reconstructive Surgery, Department of Otolaryngology, University of Illinois Medical Center, Chicago, Illinois
Facial Plastic and Reconstructive Surgery in an Aging Population: A Critical Overview

JERRY V. TOBIAS, Ph.D., F.A.S.H.A., F.A.S.A.

Professor, Communication Sciences Department, University of Connecticut, Farmington, Connecticut and Professor, Program in Speech and Hearing Sciences, Graduate Center, Mount Sinai School of Medicine of the City University of New York, New York, New York
Speech Understanding and Aging

DEAN TORIUMI, M.D.

Resident in Otolaryngology–Head and Neck Surgery, Northwestern University, Chicago, Illinois
Facial Plastic and Reconstructive Surgery in an Aging Population: A Critical Overview

PAUL H. WARD, M.D., F.A.C.S.

Professor and Chief, Division of Head and Neck Surgery, UCLA School of Medicine, Los Angeles, California
Diagnosis of Neuromuscular Voice Impairment

T. FRANKLIN WILLIAMS, M.D.

Clinical Rank Director, National Institute on Aging, National Institutes of Health, Bethesda, Maryland
Future Training and Research in Aging

GREGORY T. WOLF, M.D., F.A.C.S.

Associate Professor, Department of Otolaryngology–Head and Neck Surgery, University of Michigan Medical School; Chief, Head and Neck Surgery Division, Veterans Administration Medical Center, Ann Arbor, Michigan
Aging, the Immune System, and Head and Neck Cancer

PREFACE

Today one can only be impressed with the graying of America. Twelve percent of our population now is over the age of 65. This equals 28 million people, which is more than the population of Canada, and will increase to 18% in the next decade. We are all aware that the fastest growing segment of our population is the over-85 group, which now equals 2.7 million. By the year 2000, this number will almost double. There are now 35,000 Americans over 100 years old, and in 12 years this number will triple. Interestingly, this is the opposite of what is happening in the medical profession where some 50 percent of United States physicians now are under the age of 40. Articles have recently appeared that cite the lack of physicians trained to treat this age group. The first board examination for a certificate of added competence in geriatric medicine (to be given by the American Board of Internal Medicine and American Board of Family Practice) will be offered this spring. To quote from the National Institutes of Health (NIH) consensus development conference held last October: "The population of elderly persons is growing with extraordinary rapidity. Although the majority are well, many of these persons suffer from multiple illnesses and significant disability."

One of the benefits of my position is the opportunity to travel and to learn. I recently was exposed to a fascinating exhibit in the San Francisco airport that introduced me to the book, "Growing Old Is Not for Sissies," authored by Etta Clark. This is a study of 65 vigorous older Americans. The photo exhibit in San Francisco included the likes of:

Ada Thomas, a 72-year-old Black female who started jogging at age 65, ran her first marathon at age 68, and now runs 5 miles each day.

Eleanor Hyndman, age 80, who took up karate 5 years ago and now has a purple belt.

Helen Zechmeister, age 81, a power lifter who deadlifts 245 pounds, squatlifts 148 pounds, and works out daily with running, swimming, and lifting.

Walter Stack who, at age 76, bikes 15 miles a day. He combines this with a run across the Golden Gate Bridge to Sausalito and back and a mile swim in the Bay. At age 74 he was the oldest man to complete Hawaii's Iron Man Triathalon.

The NIH consensus statement refers to those individuals you see in the office and hospital who tend to exhibit great medical complexity and vulnerability. They have illnesses with atypical and obscure presentations; they suffer major cognitive, affective, and functional deficits; they are especially vulnerable to iatrogenesis; they are often socially isolated and economically deprived; and they are at high risk for institutionalization.

Our realization of these facts, combined with appreciation of the number of otolaryngologic problems that affect this population, instigated this meeting. These problems are represented in the diversity of our program: ethical issues, hearing and balance disorders, voice problems, swallowing disorders, cancer, cosmetic concerns, and taste and smell disturbances.

The logical progression from the "meeting" was to publish the proceedings, hence this book, *Geriatric Otorhinolaryngology*. Future meetings and editions of the book will broaden the scope of the topics to include sleep apnea and additional subjects of clinical importance.

Jerome C. Goldstein, M.D.

CONTENTS

Opening Remarks xv
    Congressman Edward Roybal

Introduction 1
    Victor Hurst

GENERAL CONSIDERATIONS

Chapter One
Future Training and Research in Aging 4
    T. Franklin Williams

Chapter Two
Cell Biology of Human Aging 8
    Leonard Hayflick

Chapter Three
Epidemiologic and Demographic Characteristics of the Aging Population 19
    Samuel P. Korper

Chapter Four
Hearing, Voice, and Swallowing Disorders in Aging: A Report to Congress 29
    Andrew A. Monjan
    Leonard F. Jakubczak

Chapter Five
Speech Understanding and Aging 32
    Jerry V. Tobias

Chapter Six
Medical/Surgical Care: Should Age be a Variable? 36
    Rue Moore

PRESBYCUSIS: THE HEARING LOSS OF AGING

Chapter Seven
Pathology of Presbycusis 40
    Harold F. Schuknecht

Chapter Eight
Tinnitus, Depression, and Aging 45
    Robert A. Dobie
    Wayne J. Katon
    Mark Sullivan
    Connie S. Sakai

Chapter Nine
Communication Assistive Devices 49
    Derald E. Brackmann

PRESBYASTASIS: THE DYSEQUILIBRIUM OF AGING

Introduction 54
    Aram Glorig

Chapter Ten
Presbyastasis 55
    Fred H. Linthicum Jr.

Chapter Eleven
Ataxia of the Elderly 58
    Hugh O. Barber
    Brian W. Blakley

THE AGING VOICE

Chapter Twelve
Evaluation and Management of Voice Disorders in the Elderly 64
    Murray D. Morrison
    Linda A. Rammage
    Hamish Nichol

Chapter Thirteen
Diagnosis of Neuromuscular Voice Impairment 71
    David G. Hanson
    Paul H. Ward
    Bruce R. Gerratt
    George Berci
    Gerald S. Berke

Chapter Fourteen
Objective Evaluation of Voice Dysfunction in the Elderly 79
    Raymond H. Colton

SMELL, TASTE, AND AGING

Chapter Fifteen
Clinical Disorders of Olfaction and Gustation in the Aged 92
James B. Snow Jr.

Chapter Sixteen
Age-Related Alterations in Taste and Smell Function 97
Richard L. Doty

IMMUNOLOGY

Chapter Seventeen
Age-Related Immune Deficiency 106
Richard A. Miller

Chapter Eighteen
Histocompatibility Antigens, Sensorineural Hearing Disorders, and Senescence 112
Joel M. Bernstein
Thomas C. Shanahan
Daniel Amsterdam

PRESBYPHAGIA

Introduction 122
Haskins K. Kashima

Chapter Nineteen
Swallowing Disorders and Aspiration in the Elderly 124
Andrew Blitzer

Chapter Twenty
Techniques for Examining Pharyngeal Swallowing 134
Jeffrey B. Palmer

Chapter Twenty-One
Aging-Related Changes in Peripheral Nerves in the Head and Neck 138
Leslie T. Malmgren

ONCOLOGY AND AGING

Introduction 146
  John Conley

Chapter Twenty-Two
Etiologic Factors in the Development of Cancer 148
  Robert W. Cantrell

Chapter Twenty-Three
Aging, the Immune System, and Head and Neck Cancer 158
  Gregory T. Wolf

FACIAL PLASTIC AND RECONSTRUCTIVE SURGERY IN AN AGING POPULATION: A CRITICAL OVERVIEW

Chapter Twenty-Four
Facial Plastic and Reconstructive Surgery in an Aging Population: A Critical Overview 168
  M. Eugene Tardy Jr.
  Dean Toriumi
  David Broadway

Chapter Twenty-Five
Pathology of the Skin in Aging 184
  Frank Johnson

Chapter Twenty-Six
Rhinoplasty, Blepharoplasty, and Rhytidectomy in the Aging Patient 186
  Frank M. Kamer

Summary
Summary: Perspectives on Health Care for the Elderly 189
  Byron J. Bailey

Index 193

OPENING REMARKS

First of all, I want to welcome each and every one of you to the nation's capital. I also wish to thank the Academy for their kind invitation for requesting that I speak to this distinguished group, but I never thought it was going to be this soon. I just came in and immediately find myself here at this podium. In what I say today, I will be making some requests. If the answers to my questions are as fast as your action today, then I believe we will see some progress in days to come. It is true that my deep personal interest in health care spans several decades. This interest goes back to the time when I was just a young man, when I was working in the field of public health education in the city of Los Angeles. I became interested in what was then a major catastrophe: the field of tuberculosis control. I entered that field, not because I had any training (I received training later), but simply because I was interested in doing something about the situation. I saw that there was a great problem in the area in which I lived, particularly in the various ethnic groups that were not being taken care of. For that reason I entered that field and got interested; so interested that today many times I even take credit for the eradication of tuberculosis! But then, you know, when I actually look at reality, I know for a fact that we did not eradicate tuberculosis; it is still a problem today. It is a problem today primarily because of neglect.

We will be talking about those matters of neglect, as we call them, today. However, my remarks today will be on the need to develop and to fund programs to provide quality training for those interested in entering geriatrics, as well as for those already established and professionally offering health care to the elderly. I will also be discussing the financial accessibility of health care and the vital role that can be played by you and your peers. I must emphasize to you who are specialists in the field of head and neck surgery the increasing importance of your field to the nation's ever-increasing elderly population. Hearing impairments, cancer of the head and neck, voice disorders, and swallowing difficulties are common ailments in the aging community of the United States. At present, 30 percent of adults age 65 to 74, and over 50 percent of adults age 75 or older, suffer some degree of hearing loss. More than 50,000 Americans will develop cancer of the head and neck this year alone. Fifteen thousand of these Americans will die from neglect, mostly from a preventable condition.

Now, why are we concerned? Are we really concerned about the future? Yes, we are. We must be concerned simply by looking at the numbers. The portion of adults age 65 and older constitutes 12 percent of the population of the United States today. By the year 2020, one in five Americans will be over 65 years of age. They too will experience the same ailments, as well as many other health concerns. As the elderly population increases, so does the great need for trained individuals to provide services to meet those special needs.

In recent years, and even now, the need for qualified individuals in the field of geriatrics and gerontology has been and is growing faster than has the supply. As a result, a troubling situation is emerging. There will continue to be too few health professionals trained in geriatrics and gerontology to meet the growing needs of an aging America. Already we are behind in our effort to create a core of health professionals who specialize in the care of the senior citizen community of the United States. We are also behind, ladies and gentlemen, in our efforts to upgrade the skill of those who may not specialize in geriatrics, but who provide the bulk of day-to-day care of older Americans.

Unfortunately, just at the time in history when we are finally beginning to understand the health care problems of our elderly population, we have an administration that wants to virtually stop federal funding of training programs for health professions. As compared to 1988, it has been proposed to cut training funding from $110 million to $40 million. Now I ask you, what impact will this policy have on the elderly? What impact will it have on the health problems of the American community? More than that, what impact will it have on our children, yours and mine, the young people of America who want to become professionals in your field. Well, unfortunately, the impact will be negative, and both the young and the old will just have to suffer the consequences. Now I believe, and I'm sure we all believe, that there are young people who decided to enter the health care field that provides services to the elderly. However, many of these young people face several obstacles when they try to enter the health profession training programs. Many of the children of underserved populations, i.e., racial and ethnic minorities, the poor, and rural residents, have much greater difficulty getting into training programs and, of course, much greater difficulty in paying for those programs. Now, in spite of our best efforts, major cutbacks in federal health profession training funds have the greatest impact on the children of the poor and of the racial and ethnic minorities. Special training programs to help address the need of central city and rural residents never even got off the ground. I believe that one of the saddest legacies that this administration will have is its failure to understand these special problems of the underserved and of those who want to be trained to serve them.

While the training of our young people is a way to care for the growing number of the elderly, we clearly need to work on health care professionals who already are in the field. Here the thrust of training is somewhat different. Our job here is to convince practitioners that caring for the elderly presents different challenges and requires special training to meet those challenges. We need to give them incentives to upgrade their skill in caring for the elderly. For some practitioners, the decision will be to become full-fledged geriatricians, specializing in the field. For most practitioners, they will decide to upgrade their skills so that they are better able to care for the elderly. Whichever is the case, we need the help of health professional organizations like the Academy. We need to launch an aggressive, private and public sector recruitment effort to bring more people into the health professions, especially into geriatrics and gerontology.

You are probably thinking at this moment that it is easy to say, "Bring more people into these health professions," that it is a simplistic solution to an extremely complex problem, and you are correct. To give an analogy, to see a population starving and to say, "Bring them food," is also too simplistic a solution to a complex problem of hunger. The same is true of health care today. Training more health professionals in geriatrics and gerontology is an indisputable necessity for adequate health care for aging populations in this country. There is no doubt about that.

Now here, and just for a moment, I would like to speak to you on an issue that I believe is of great importance to the Academy. That is the issue of the availability and the training of clinical investigators. I, of course, share your concern that we lack sufficient number of clinical investigators to support the training programs I have just discussed and to support the development of your specialty and the clinicians who will care for the aging. With your help and through that of the National Institutes of Health, (NIH), it is my hope that we can develop and fund programs that will recruit more young investigators and provide them with badly needed training. I learned of your concern, concern in this area of clinical research, just last year. That was when Dr. Robert Ruben was testifying before my Committee on Appropriations. At that particular time, I took interest in what he was saying. I requested a report of the National Institutes of Health, a report on the scientific opportunities and the research manpower requirements for this specific field. The report stated, "Critical to any expansion of this research endeavor is the recruitment of qualified investigators," *the recruitment of qualified investigators*. "There is a need," the report went on to say, "for an appropriate professional, clinical organization to stimulate the development of the specialty." I wonder who they had in mind. I think they had in mind your Academy. Also, the NIH study stated, "There is a profound lack of such clinical research expertise at the present time." Do you agree? Yes, you do, because that is the truth. Now, these assuagements were also supported recently by an article in your own *Bulletin*, an article written by Dr. Byron Bailey. It makes some extremely interesting observations. For example, it says that, "Less than 1 percent of the physicians in your specialty, probably less than 50 throughout the nation, are currently trained and funded for active, ongoing clinical investigation." *Less than 50* ! The doctor went on to say, "Most of the funded clinical investigators are older." In other words, what is happening to the young men in your profession? Where are they? Why aren't they given the opportunity? Then he goes on to say, "A few of our academics are being drawn towards an investigative career, only very few." Then came the shocker: there is an attitude of pessimism regarding the attraction of sustained funding of clinical investigation. Now these are facts that come from the National Institutes of Health, that come from one of your own colleagues, it no doubt comes from your own organization. We see one thing for sure: clearly, we need a well-defined program to produce such young clinical researchers, but that well-defined program is not going to come from the Congress of the United States. If it is going to come from any place, it is going to come from you. If something is going to be done, you must define that program.

During the time of the appearance and question before my committee, I asked the following question of the Director of the National Institute of Neurology and Communicative Diseases, and now I'm going to ask you the same question. I asked him, "It has been asserted that the field of head and neck surgery faces a crisis in terms of shortage of clinical investigations. Is this assertion true?" You know what the answer is? "Yes, it is true." Then I also asked him to please explain the nature of the problem in detail, to outline a strategic plan to deal with it. I asked him to indicate what training programs now exist with the Institute or might be created that could be utilized to help solve this problem, and what resources would be required to increase the emphasis on clinical investigator manpower. Also, I asked the bureau, "Please indicate if there is a way that the current clinical research center program of the Institute could be assisted or modified to help increase a supply of these clinical investigators, and what resources and methods would be required to accomplish this." I am going to leave this question with you. I am going to compare the two answers. I want to know if you are really an organization that can stimulate the development of your specialty. I also want to assure you that, if you in your specialty don't move, don't expect we who are in the Congress of the United States to do anything. I believe that a great deal can be done, but it can be done only if we work together. Without the active support of health care professionals such as yourselves, we will not succeed. Without a strong and concerted effort by your members and by the rest of your profession, I and other members of Congress who are supportive of your cause will not be able to overcome those who favor the funding of Star Wars over the funding of Health Wars. I think that the future of America depends on what you do today, on the training you make available to young people, because the need is there. More than 37 million Americans have no health insurance whatsoever. More than 200 million Americans are underinsured. There is a need, not only for your expertise, but for good medicine in this country. We are the only industrial nation in the world outside of South Africa that does not have a national system of health care. That can be in the future. What we are interested in today is the training of individuals, of young men and women, giving them the opportunity to obtain this training so that they can serve the elderly of tomorrow, because in the year 2000, or a little bit after that, one out of every five individuals in the United States will be 65 years of age or older. Those who look at the problem as it is know that the need will increase, and I sincerely hope that we can work together to remedy the situation.

Now ladies and gentlemen, I really don't know why I stand here and make this offer, but I will. I am interested in your work and interested in the health of America. I sit on the Committee that can move, and that does move on occasion, but it does so only when someone is on our back. This is the function of the Congress, really, for if the American people don't care, the Congress does not move. I make this offer to you. Why don't you get together and define such a program, and then I will do everything I possibly can to see that the funding is made available. Now I cannot promise that this is going to be done, but one thing I can promise you is that I will try to do the best I possibly can. The only thing I am requesting of you today is that you do likewise. Devise a plan and let's get together and implement it. If we don't do that now, your profession will ultimately suffer, but above all, it will be the American people who will suffer the most.

Edward Roybal
Congressman, California

INTRODUCTION

I am pleased to represent the 28-million-member American Association of Retired Persons (AARP). Before I begin, I promised our new executive director, Horace Deets, that I would pass on to you a message from him. Mr. Deets wanted to express his special thanks to his good friend Dr. Goldstein for having the keen foresight to organize this, the first conference your group has held, to focus on the geriatric area of your profession. We commend you for that. I know, Dr. Goldstein, that you and Mr. Deets have met several times in recent years in an effort to strengthen what is a natural relationship between our associations. Both associations are concerned with making certain that quality health care is accessible to all Americans, including the elderly.

AARP's members are extremely interested in the work you are doing, especially in the field of research on aging. It is particularly gratifying to see that your group has recognized the rapid aging of the country and is attempting to address the unique needs of the older population. Conferences such as this one are essential to improving the quality of necessary health care. I commend The American Academy of Otolaryngology, Head and Neck Surgery, and The National Institute on Aging for giving all of us this opportunity to discuss these critical health care issues.

Alan Greenspan, chairman of the Federal Reserve, recently noted in the *Wall Street Journal* that America as a nation pays proportionately more out of its gross national product and more per capita for health care than any other industrialized country, and probably gets less for its dollar than anyone else. He was puzzled by that. So am I. I think part of the problem is that we do not have a national policy for health care. Health care costs have outpaced the consumer price index for years and continue to do so. This means that access to health care—quality health care—is not available to everyone on an equal basis. Some 37 million Americans lack health insurance of any kind. Many of those with insurance still have high out-of-pocket costs for uncovered bills. As many of you know, much needs to be done to develop a health care system that provides accessible quality care for all Americans, including the 30 million who are 65 and older. That group, which includes 3 million people 85 and older, is the fastest growing segment of the United States population. By the year 2000, people 65 and older are expected to represent 13 percent of the population. That percentage may climb to 21.2 percent by the year 2030 as the baby boom generation ages. I might add here, because I think it is a fact we need to be concerned with, that it is also predicted that, by the year 2000, the population of this country will be approximately 60 percent white, 20 percent black, and 20 percent Hispanic. Where the other nationalities come in I'm not sure, but I would say they probably will be carved out of the white 60 percent.

While people are living longer and, for the most part, healthier, most older persons have at least one chronic condition and many have multiple conditions, as most of you know far better than I. The most frequently occurring conditions for the elderly in 1986 were arthritis (48 percent), hypertension (39 percent), hearing impairments (29 percent), heart disease (30 percent), orthopaedic impairments (29 percent), sinusitis (17 percent), cataracts (14 percent), and diabetes and visual impairments (10 percent each).

In 1984, benefits from government programs, including Medicare ($59 billion) and Medicaid ($15 billion), were projected to cover about two-thirds, or 67 percent, of the health expenditures of older persons. Medicare also contributes, on average, about one-quarter of the incomes of physicians. Indeed, Medicare payment to physicians is the fastest growing component of the United States budget and has increased on average nearly 16 percent annually over the past decade. In 1984, Medicare's allowed amount for otolaryngology was $196 million. However, despite the fact that the elderly need more health services because of their increased incidence of chronic and acute illness, only a tiny number of physicians have received any training in geriatrics.

The elderly face heavy direct and indirect out-of-pocket costs for their medical care. Medicare covers only about half of the cost of physician services. Beneficiaries are liable for:

1. Medicare part B premium, which must cover 25 percent of the total part B costs. The 1988 premium is 38.5 percent higher than last year—nearly $300.
2. A $75 deductible fee, and I know you've read a lot about that.
3. Copayments equal to 20 percent of Medicare's allowed amount. This is the fastest growing component of beneficiary liability and totalled nearly $6 billion in 1987.
4. Balances billed above Medicare's allowed amount for unassigned claims. This liability amounted to nearly $3 billion last year, despite rapidly rising assignment rates.

Although about 70 percent of Medicare's allowed amounts are paid on the basis of assignment, beneficiary liability for extra bills has remained stable because growth in the number of claims far exceeds growth in the assignment rate. The assignment rate also continues to vary sharply by geography and by physician specialty. For example, in 1985 the assignment rate for your specialty was 51 percent, compared with a national average of 60 percent. In 1986, only 25 percent of otologists, laryngologists, and rhinologists were Medicare-participating physicians. That number increased to 27 percent in January, 1987, compared with a national average of 30.1 percent.

Clearly, payments to physicians must be reformed as soon as possible. These reforms should increase equity among physicians, make payments rational and predictable, and increase financial protection for beneficiaries and taxpayers, who pay 75 percent of part B. AARP endorses a resource-based relative value scale, as does the Physician Payment Review Commission. Our members want some of the savings that are achieved from reduced payments for overpriced procedures to be reinvested in underpaid primary care services. Once a rational and fair payment system is devised, AARP wants that payment to be payment in full.

In the interim, our association supports limits on balance billing and on state mandatory laws, provided they are not regulated by means-testing and do not create access problems for beneficiaries. Reform of the payment system, however, will not moderate expenditures unless controls are placed on the volume of services ordered by physicians. All government studies done in this area have found that the rapid rise in part B outlays is due to a combination of higher unit prices plus a vastly increased volume of billed services for each enrollee. The aging of the population plays a minimal role in rising outlays, and the demand for services by patients has also not been found to be a factor.

Your association and AARP share a common purpose in our attempts to improve the quality of health care and to increase access to the health care system for the nation's growing older population. For our part, AARP pledges to continue its efforts to reform Medicare's payments to physicians so that the system works equitably for everyone—beneficiaries, physicians, and taxpayers. AARP will also work to ensure that the elderly have access to quality medical care and to make certain that care is provided efficiently. For your part, ladies and gentlemen, AARP asks for your help and cooperation to ensure that the vital care you provide meets the otolaryngic needs of the elderly. Together, we can make the health care system in this country the best and most accessible in the world.

Victor Hurst

Victor Hurst is a member of the Board of Directors of the AARP, and was a luncheon speaker on the second day of the conference. This speech provides a fitting introduction to *Geriatric Otorhinolaryngology*.

GENERAL CONSIDERATIONS

Chapter One

FUTURE TRAINING AND RESEARCH IN AGING

T. FRANKLIN WILLIAMS, M.D.

I am glad to see such interest in the fields of hearing, speech, and swallowing in relation to aging. National Institute on Aging (NIA) program staff are eager to talk with anyone interested in pursuing investigative aspects related to aging. They can work with you in advisory ways to try to fit individual needs into the options that exist at the National Institutes of Health (NIH), as well as work with grantees as they carry on with their awards. I believe you will find real friends and colleagues among our staff who are interested in encouraging those things you may wish to pursue.

NIA has the broad mission to conduct research and research training in biomedical, behavioral, and social aspects of aging and in the common problems of older people. Within that mission we continually try to consider what our priorities should be and what we should be encouraging at any given point in time. These priorities grow out of essentially two streams of thought. One stream is scientific readiness. Where is science ready, because of the development of a scientific field, to tackle new problems, or new aspects of a problem, related to aging? The other stream is the public view, public importance, or public significance of issues affecting health for older people. Fortunately, these two streams usually intermesh, although not always. Public concern may be ahead of the science, or at times, the science may be thriving, but may not be an issue that is seen as quite that pressing from the public point of view. However, for the most part, these two forces interact to affect our priorities.

In arriving at priorities we rely heavily on experts in the fields with which we are working. Small workshops help us to define the research agenda. We are eager to take part in meetings like this where we can find direction for our research. It is from this kind of scientific exchange that we draw guidance for the establishment of priorities.

On the side of public concern, Congress, speaking for the public it represents, ultimately defines our final agenda through the appropriations it makes. Congress is sensitive and responsive to the public, including the lay public, the professional and scientific public, and the practicing public. It is important that you make your own views about priorities in the fields of hearing, speech, and swallowing disorders known to Congress and to the Administration. Each administration has views about priorities, but in the last analysis, Congress is the deciding force.

By law, the National Advisory Council on Aging, a body of distinguished professional and lay people appointed by the Secretary of Health and Human Services, must approve any area of research and any specific application we receive before the application is granted. Members of the Council also serve as policy advisors with regard to our priorities.

I would like now to describe the research priorities that lead our list at present. A basic priority is that of understanding aging itself, that is, the fundamental biological, behavioral, and social aspects of aging. To try to understand the basic processes of aging is a continuing priority of NIA, and aspects of it relate to your fields. Basic research on changes with age in the auditory system, in speech understanding, and in voice and swallowing are all legitimate and important areas for research.

A second general area is that of health maintenance, or maintaining good health and effective functioning—preventive strategies, if you will. This is one of the most important areas in thinking about old age. Old age is a time when it is possible to be quite healthy and functional provided one pursues good health habits and is fortunate enough to be spared many of the devastating diseases that do strike some of us. But this means learning everything we possibly can about preventive practices.

In relation to maintaining effective function in your area, I want to touch on the issue of noise contamination in our society. The question of how much noise is a public health hazard, and thus a specific problem affecting increased deafness, is an issue that needs to be addressed further from the point of view of good preventive practices in the fields of hearing, speech, and swallowing disorders.

There are other preventive health practices that would benefit from more attention. Earlier detection and intervention of hearing losses need to be examined from the point of view of good health maintenance in relation to your fields. Good nutrition, obviously, is also relevant here.

When we turn to the common disorders that affect older people, our main interests from the NIA point of view are disorders that threaten loss of function. The goal is to try to help maintain independence to the maximum extent possible. The diseases and disorders that threaten loss of function are our highest priorities.

By contrast, our institute has not been much involved in some of the killers of older people—for example, cancer, heart disease, or stroke. To a large extent this is reasonable because other institutes at NIH are involved heavily in these fields. They are the big killers and that is certainly of great concern to all of us. However, the focus at NIA is on conditions that threaten independence. This includes, first of all, dementia as one of the most common and devastating problems. High on the list, too, are sensory losses that limit independence. Obviously, this bears directly on hearing, vision, and smell and on other areas that threaten loss of function and loss of mobility, such as disequilibrium with the risk or fear of falling and the symptoms of vertigo. Our overall concerns about threats to mobility also include problems of osteoporosis, osteoarthritis, muscular weakness, poor lifestyles, and lack of regular exercise.

What can we offer in the way of support for research in these high priority areas? Let me discuss briefly the various mechanisms that are available. Basically, most of our direct research support is through the regular NIH research grant mechanism where formal applications are filed. Our staff will advise any applicant as to how to make the application as strong as possible and how to satisfy the necessary ground rules. All the applications are reviewed by nonfederal scientific peer review committees and rated for scientific excellence. We then take these to our Council, which considers the program or priority relevance of the applications. Depending finally on the priority scores (the scores for relative excellence of the applications and the money available to us), we make awards for approximately 3 to 5 years. This is a well-established procedure and the fundamental way in which we work with potentially interested researchers.

Up to now, so few research-oriented people have entered the field of aging that NIA has established other mechanisms to develop scientists in this area. We are seeing an increasing number of researchers in the aging fields each year, and the future looks promising; but we still need many more researchers. In a study conducted by NIA a few years ago, it was found that there exists only about 10 percent of the academic leadership needed in the fields of gerontology and geriatrics. We have a long way to go, but fortunately things are changing.

We have a number of mechanisms for the support of people who come into the area of research related to aging. The basic mechanism for people starting out is the postdoctoral fellowship, or an individual fellowship. This means working out, with a mentor, a plan for a research program that will help the researcher move on to be a more independent investigator after 2 to 3 years as a postdoctoral fellow.

Beyond that type of support, but at that same level, we also have institutional training grants. These are grants that we award to academic institutions. We issue a training grant to a leading investigator and teacher, who in turn may select his or her own fellows. The stipends awarded to these fellows would be similar to individual fellowships, but the institutional training grant officer would choose his or her own fellows—however many the available money allows—to work around a general area of concentration. I would encourage senior academic people in the otolaryngology field to consider the possibility of institutional training grants in aging-related issues.

Another rather imaginative program that NIA has instituted at this level is the addition of some training and fellowship slots to training grants supported by other institutes at NIH. This program is possible when the training would be oriented towards research related to aging. For example, if there were an otolaryngology training grant, perhaps from the National Institute of Neurological and Communicative Disorders and Stroke (NINCDS), and if the training officer wanted to add one or two slots to train people with a goal towards research in aging, we have mechanisms for arranging this. If there were a person in the ENT field who wanted to apply immunologic research skills to issues in immune changes in aging as they affect the ear, nose, and throat, we could certainly consider and, very likely, add on a training slot to an immunology training grant at some academic institution. So we can provide postdoctoral fellowship support for people who want to enter this field as beginning investigators and training grants to the more senior staff in order for them to develop their own trainees.

Beyond the fellowship level, we have what we refer to as Career Development Awards. These awards come into effect beyond the fellowship level. For people who have already had some background in research, this award may be the first received from NIA. Career Development Awards go under various names. We have a 3 to 5 year Clinical Investigator Award at a junior faculty level. The money is to be used essentially as salary and research support to help a person to spend at least half of their time on research while they are developing their clinical and academic skills. We also have a Physician-Investigator Award that is a somewhat more senior type of award.

I am told by Drs. Monjan and Jakubczak that NIA will be issuing a special announcement regarding the Special Emphasis Research Career Award, which is pointed explicitly toward the field of otolaryngology. It will be targeted specifically to this field so that applications that come in will receive special attention, will get special review, and in effect, will draw from a designated amount of money. The basic idea is that these are all awards at the junior faculty level—at the career development level. We are prepared to discuss the opportunities in this field with any of you, whether you are at this stage or if you are a more senior faculty member and have junior colleagues who really would like to invest their efforts into developing academic careers oriented towards otolaryngology and aging.

A few areas in the field of epidemiology of hearing, smell, swallowing, and speech disorders in older people have not been stressed yet. We could use much more data about the general nature or the prevalence of these conditions and about their association with other conditions. I told one of your colleagues earlier of an intriguing observation in one of the epidemiology studies we are doing. People aged 65 years and older who had high blood pressure as well as visual and hearing disorders were found to have much higher mortality rates than people who did not have these three conditions. It is not surprising that the survival rate of a severely hypertensive person is shorter, but how do you factor in the hearing correlate? Why would a hearing impairment add to the risk of mortality in somebody who has high blood pressure and some visual impairment? All we have is the observation and the questions. I simply offer this example as the type of clue that comes out of epidemiologic studies and associations of conditions, one with another.

What are the clues that these studies give us? Are there differences in racial, cultural, or ethnic groups? Are there differences around the world? The question of noise levels in parts of the world has come up several times. Where noise levels are excessively low, hearing disorders or deafness may be far less prevalent than in our country and in other developed countries. Is that a fact or a fantasy? How much difference does it make? It is a challenge for worldwide epidemiologic studies. I mention this to illustrate that there are epidemiologic questions of importance that are directly related to your fields of interest.

Earlier in this conference, you heard a report from the National Academy of Sciences on speech comprehension. The whole realm of brain function in relation to speech comprehension and speech understanding is an extremely important area, from hearing, to interpretation, and to use of the knowledge that is transmitted. We have heard presentations on swallowing disorders and on peripheral nerve function changes in aging. These fields are areas of interest to our institute and we would be very much interested in talking to potential applicants in order to consider support. I cannot guarantee support, as I have already said. Applications are peer reviewed, and we fund the best based on their judgment. We are not able to fund nearly as many as we would like. Overall, we can fund only about 30 percent of the approved applications after peer review and, in our judgment, at least 50 or 60 percent would be well worth funding as high quality research. Our funding depends ultimately on the amount of money available. We go as far as our money will take us.

I believe that about half of the applications we do fund are second submissions. People apply, they get a good priority score and a good rating, but not suitable enough to get funded. They then receive a detailed review of their application. Most applicants take advantage of this critical review and resubmit an application. A much higher proportion of applicants are funded after the second application than after the first. I bring this fact up as something for those of you who are directly interested in this to keep in mind, that the funding rate for second submissions is considerably higher than for first submissions and a second application is well worth considering if the first does not produce grant support.

There are other areas that provide research support in relation to your interests. You are all probably familiar with the Deafness Research Foundation. There are other foundations that are taking much more interest in aging research, including research in your fields.

Finally, I would just like to mention, for any who may want to consider it, that this year NIA will have a second, one-week-long Summer Institute for new or potential investigators. At least one of your members, Dr. Long, attended the first of these summer institutes last year. Recent Ph.Ds. or M.Ds. just beyond their residency who are interested in a career in aging research might consider applying for this program. An announcement about this will be available shortly, but I would be interested in hearing from any of you directly, as would any of our staff members. Entrance to the program is highly competitive. Last summer, for example, we had 40 positions to fill from 120 applications. This summer we will fill about 35 slots. The admission cost is paid by a grant from the Brookdale Foundation. Those who participated last summer found it a useful introduction to the area of research in aging, so much so that it seemed well worth repeating and we hope to do so every year.

I would like to thank NIA staff people for their participation in this conference—Dr. Sam Korper, Dr. Andy Monjan, and Dr. Len Jakubczak. They are available to meet and to talk with you or to assist you should you have any questions regarding your specific plans in the area of research on aging.

Chapter Two

CELL BIOLOGY OF HUMAN AGING

LEONARD HAYFLICK, Ph.D.

The phenomenon of biological aging is generally believed to be a universal property of all living things. It is a manifestation of the sum of a multitude of biological decrements that occur after sexual maturation. Yet this concept cannot be accepted without qualification.

There are animals in which aging is rare or has never been demonstrated. Some fish and amphibians that have an indeterminate size may also have an indeterminate life span.[1] Thus the universality of aging, even in vertebrates, remains unproven. These animals are not immortal. Although normal age changes may not occur, they die eventually of disease, predation, or accidents at an actuarily-determined annual rate, which is not true aging.

In fact, the occurrence of aging arguably is restricted to humans and to the domestic and zoo animals that we choose to protect. The extreme manifestations of old age that are found to occur in humans simply do not occur in feral animals. If aging occurs at all in wild animals, its expression is brief because the physiologic decrements of aging quickly make these animals vulnerable to disease and predation. Few feral animals live long enough after sexual maturation to experience old age. As soon as they incur even slight decrements in, say, running speed or jumping ability, they are culled by predators. Similarly, as soon as their immune system becomes less capable, they may die of disease or, what is more likely, they are culled by predators when disease has reduced their ability to elude capture. As a result, the likelihood is remote that evolution could have selected for the aging process. There are simply too few feral animals on which selective pressure could have been applied. Thus, aging cannot be viewed as an adaptation.

In developed countries, humans have been so successful in resolving causes of death attributable to acute diseases that their aging is expressed to an extreme unattainable by wild animals. Civilization has produced life expectations that were unknown in prehistoric times, thereby revealing a plethora of physiologic decrements that perhaps, teleologically, never were intended to be revealed. Aging may be an artifact of civilization or of domestication because these "unnatural" circumstances have permitted the expression of aging, which otherwise would not have occurred.

AGING AND DISEASE

Aging must be distinguished from disease. Biological changes attributable to aging are frequently referred to as "normal age changes," as if there was a category of "abnormal age changes." Age changes are not diseases, they are natural losses of function. Loss and greying of the hair, reduced exercise capacity and stamina, wrinkled skin, menopause, presbyopia, loss of short-term memory, and hundreds of other similar decrements of old age are not diseases. They do not increase our vulnerability to death. Other "normal" decrements in vital organs do produce increased vulnerability to pathologic change. For example, normal age-related decrements in immune system functions increase vulnerability to diseases that, in youth, would be easily resolved. Or, antigens recognized as self in youth might be recognized by an aging immune system as non-self, thus producing many of the chronic autoimmune diseases of old age.

ETIOLOGY OF AGING

What is the cause of the aging phenomenon? This question, which is fundamental in the science of gerontology, might well be analogous to asking: What is the cause of development? Similarly, the frequently-asked question: How can aging be stopped or slowed? is equivalent to asking: How can development be stopped or slowed?

There is no good reason why aging has to happen. August Weismann believed that aging occurs to benefit the species by removing less fit animals from an environment where limited space and other resources should be conserved for the young.[2] This is an illogical argument because, if chronologically-older animals continued to remain fit, their deaths would not benefit younger members. Thus there would be no basis for an aging process to evolve in the first place. Weismann's notion also can be discredited because, with few or no old feral animals surviving, there is little possibility that evolution could have selected for the aging process.

Furthermore, there is no selective advantage for a species to have its members live much beyond the age of sexual maturity and of child rearing. For example, from the standpoint of simple survival of the species, there is no advantage for humans to live much beyond the age of, say, 30. This would permit sufficient time for production of new progeny and for rearing of that progeny to sexual maturation. Since life expectation at birth in prehistoric times was about 18 years, it is apparent that the human species has survived for a much longer period of time with an 18-year life expectation than it has with the current 75-year life expectation. Thus the human species has survived for a much longer period of time with rare, or no, old members than it has with many old members.

Weismann, however, was prescient on one major point. He surmised correctly that the ability of normal somatic cells to replicate and function was limited. Despite the fact that the opposite was believed for decades, this dogma was finally upset by Hayflick and Moorhead in 1961.[3] Thus the limited ability for normal human and animal cells to replicate and function may represent a fundamental reason why the lives of individual animals are finite. In fact, many of the multitude of functional decrements reported to occur in cultured normal human cells as they reach the end of their life span are identical to the changes that occur in humans as they age.

FOUNDATIONS OF CYTOGERONTOLOGY

The origin of age changes in multicellular organisms can be attributed to only three possibilities that are not mutually exclusive. Aging in metazoans can only result from (1) perturbations within individual cells, (2) changes in the extracellular matrix, or (3) influences of more highly-organized cell hierarchies on other tissues or organs.

An essential element in considering the role of the cell as the origin of age changes is whether or not those cells are capable of normal function, including division, for an indefinite period of time. That is, are normal somatic cells immortal?

Centennial of the Controversy

The controversy that arose in efforts to answer this fundamental question actually began about 100 years ago. However, even this fact has been brought to light only recently.[4] In 1881 the great German biologist August Weismann proposed that the somatic cells of higher animals would be found to have a limited doubling potential. Although he provided no experimental evidence for his surmise, Weismann stated, "... death takes place because a worn-out tissue cannot forever renew itself, and because a capacity for increase by means of cell division is not everlasting but finite."[5]

There are at least two ways in which the immortality of normal cells can be determined. First, vertebrate cells can be serially cultured in laboratory glassware, and second, similar cells containing specific markers that allow them to be distinguished from host cells can be serially transplanted in isogenic laboratory animals. The transplanted tissue is regrafted to a younger host when the previous host becomes old. The goal of such studies has been to answer this fundamental question: Can normal vertebrate cells that function and replicate under ideal conditions escape from the inevitability of aging and death that is obligatory for the animal from which they were derived?

Immortal Heart Cells?

In respect to studies undertaken in cell culture, one investigation stood out as the classic response to this question before 1960. In the early part of this century, Alexis Carrel, a noted cell culturist, surgeon, and Nobel Laureate, described experiments purporting to show that fibroblasts derived from chick heart tissue could be serially cultured indefinitely. The culture was voluntarily terminated after 34 years.[6] This finding created world-wide interest, not only in the scientific community, but in the lay press as well.

Its importance to gerontologists was clear. If true, it strongly implied that cells released from in vivo control could divide and function normally for a period of time in excess of the life span of the species. Thus, either the types of cells cultured play no role in the aging phenomenon or aging results from changes in the intracellular matrix or at higher levels of cell organization. That is, aging could result from physiologic interactions between cells only when they are organized as tissues or organs. In any case, Carrel's results and their interpretation were of vital concern to biogerontologists because they strongly suggested that aging is not the result of events occurring within individual cells.

In the years that followed Carrel's observations, support for his experimental results seemed to be forthcoming from many laboratories where it was observed that several cell populations seemed to have the striking ability to replicate apparently indefinitely. Immortal cell populations derived from a variety of human and animal tissues were reported to occur spontaneously in dozens of laboratories in the 20-year period from the early 1940s to the early 1960s. These cell populations, numbering in the hundreds, are best known by the prototype cell lines HeLa (derived from a human cervical carcinoma in 1952) and L cells (derived from mouse mesenchyme in 1943). They continue to flourish even to this day in cell culture laboratories throughout the world.

Immortal cell populations still arise spontaneously from normal cell cultures by a mysterious process. However, now they can be created, albeit at low efficiency, by exposure to radiation, chemical carcinogens, or certain oncogenic viruses. More recently, this process of "immortalization," as it has come to be called, can be accomplished routinely by fusing mortal antibody-producing lymphocytes to immortal myeloma cells. The resulting hybrid, known as a hybridoma, will continue to express specific antibody indefinitely.[7] Use of this technique is one important cause of the current revolution in biotechnology.

Nevertheless, what seemed to be incontrovertible evidence for the existence of immortal cells soon fell to new insights and a preponderance of opposing information.

AGING UNDER GLASS

Of central importance to the question of cell immortality as it relates to biogerontology is whether the cell populations studied in vitro are composed of normal or abnormal cells. Clearly the aging of animals occurs in normal cell populations. If we are to equate the behavior of normal cells in vivo with that of similar cells in vitro, then the latter must be shown to be normal as well. Twenty-seven years ago Moorhead and I postulated that all immortal cell populations are abnormal in one or more important property.[3] As such, they are not proper subjects for the study of aging and, indeed, are not proper subjects for the study of many other biological phenomena for which they are frequently wrongly used. All immortal cell lines vary in chromosome number, morphology, or banding pattern from the original animal or human cells from which they were derived. Most, but not all, produce tumors when inoculated into experimental animals.

Aging is Inevitable

Moorhead and I described the finite replicative capacity of normal human fibroblasts and interpreted the phenomenon as aging at the cellular level.[3] We demonstrated that, when normal human embryonic cells are grown under the most favorable conditions, aging and death is the inevitable consequence after about 50 population doublings. We called this the Phase III phenomenon. We also showed that the death of our cultured normal human cells was not attributable to some trivial cause involving medium components or culture conditions, but was an inherent property of the cells themselves.[3,8] This observation now has been confirmed in hundreds of laboratories where variations in medium components and culture conditions have been as numerous as the laboratories themselves.

Since our observation and interpretation was made in 1961, no normal human or animal cell population has been shown to be immortal. Immortality is defined as continuous serial cultivation in vitro or in vivo in which at least 100 population doublings occur over a minimum of at least 2 years. Cultured or transplanted normal cells are defined as those having properties identical to the cells that compose the tissue of origin.

All Immortal Cells are Abnormal

The widespread use of immortal, abnormal cell populations for a variety of research purposes has created enormous problems in the interpretation of experiments in which these cells are used. It is virtually impossible to extrapolate results obtained with these abnormal cell populations to the behavior of normal cells in vivo. The failure to recognize this fundamental distinction is the reason why much of the effort in modern cancer biology is seriously flawed. The current widespread use of such abnormal cell lines as C3H, 3T3, and BHK 21 in efforts to understand the conversion of normal cells to cancer cells is indefensible. These cells are widely used as normal cells in order to determine whether various treatments will convert them to cancer cells. There is little regard for the fact that these cells already have been proven to produce tumors when inoculated into laboratory animals.[9,10] Even if they did not produce tumors, the fact that they are chromosomally abnormal and are immortal should be sufficient reason not to use them for studies in which the use of normal cells is mandated.

This fundamental flaw in the conduct of much research in modern cancer biology can be circumvented by appreciation of the fact that entirely normal cell populations can be cultured in vitro. Such cultures are normal in every respect if they are derived from normal tissue and, of course, have a finite capacity to replicate.

Conceptual Origins

Although there were many reports prior to ours that described the failure of most cultured cells to proliferate indefinitely, none characterized the cells as normal, ruled out artifacts as the cause, or suggested that the phenomenon might be associated with aging.[11-13] In fact, the observation that cultured cells frequently failed to replicate indefinitely was probably made hundreds of times from the genesis of cell culture techniques in the early 1900s to our report 60 years later.

Those prior failures were unreported because the existing dogma insisted that the failure of cells to proliferate indefinitely in vitro must be attributable to errors in the "art" required to keep cells dividing forever. That dogma was so well entrenched that our original manuscript[3] was rejected by The Journal of Experimental Medicine with the statement that "The largest fact to have come out from tissue culture in the last 50 years is that cells inherently capable of multiplying will do so indefinitely if supplied with the right milieu in vitro." That belief was tantamount to the belief that, given the right milieu in vivo, human beings also will live forever.

The finding that cultured normal cells have a finite capacity to replicate has had important implications in gerontologic theory. However, before these implications are considered, it will be necessary to discuss how Carrel was misled into believing that he had successfully cultured chick fibroblasts for 34 years.

ALEXIS CARREL AND THE MYTH OF HIS IMMORTAL CHICK CELLS

By the late 1960s, it became apparent to myself and to others that Carrel's claim to have cultured chick fibroblast cells for 34 years was spurious.[14,15] It had to be assumed that Carrel's chick cultures consisted of normal cells. This is so because, until quite recently, no one has ever found an immortal chick fibroblast population.[16] One of these immortal cell lines was produced by exposure of the chick cells to the carcinogen N'-methyl-N'-nitro-N'-nitrosoguanidine, and the other cell line arose spontaneously. In both cases, the immortal cells were shown to be abnormal and to produce retroviruses.

It has been 50 years since the voluntary termination of Carrel's alleged immortal chick fibroblasts, and this is the first authentic report of a spontaneous transformation of normal chick fibroblasts. The rarity of this event can be appreciated when one considers that chick tissue has been one of the most frequently cultured tissues in the past 50 years. Thus, the likelihood that Carrel had found such a population is remote, especially since, until now, all attempts to repeat his findings have been negative.[16-19] Furthermore, even if his observation was legitimate, the immortal cells must have been abnormal. Therefore, they cannot be used as evidence that normal cells had escaped the inevitability of the Phase III phenomenon.

I have proposed one explanation for Carrel's findings in which the method of preparation of chick embryo extract, used as a source of nutrients for his culture, allowed for the introduction of new, viable fibroblasts into the so-called "immortal" culture at each feeding.[15] Although I believe that Carrel was unaware of this artifact, Witkowski, in a lengthy study of Carrel's immortal cells, suggests otherwise.[20-22]

INVERSE RELATIONSHIP BETWEEN DONOR AGE AND CELL POPULATION DOUBLINGS

In the decade that followed our first report,[3] further evidence appeared from studies in cytogerontology[4,5] that provided important new insights into cellular aging. In 1965 we reported that cultured fibroblasts derived from older humans replicated fewer times than those derived from embryos.[8] Because the technique for determining population doublings was crude at that time, we were unable to establish a direct relationship between donor age and population-doubling potential. Subsequently, studies done by others not only confirmed the principle that we had observed, but extended it significantly.

Martin and his colleagues derived cultures from human donors ranging from fetal age to 90 years of age.[23] Although the data reveals considerable scatter, they observed a regression coefficient from the first to the ninth decade of -0.2 population doublings per year of life with a standard deviation of 0.05 and a correlation coefficient of -0.50. The scatter found is not unlike that reported to occur with virtually any age-related change that is measured cross-sectionally and not longitudinally. Nevertheless at least nine more studies have confirmed the finding that the number of population doublings of cultured human cells is inversely proportional to donor age. This inverse relationship has now been shown to occur in normal human cells derived from such diverse tissue as lung,[8] skin,[23-26] liver,[27] arterial smooth muscle,[28] lens,[29] and T lymphocytes.[30,31]

DIRECT RELATIONSHIP BETWEEN MAXIMUM SPECIES LIFE SPAN AND POPULATION DOUBLINGS OF THEIR CULTURED CELLS

Several years ago we suggested that the population-doubling potential of cultured fibroblasts from several animal species revealed a surprisingly good direct correlation with maximum species life span.[32] In the years that followed, several other reports have appeared that have added substantially to this idea, especially the work of Rohme.[33] One report in which several marsupial species were studied does not support this finding. However, the authors did not determine population doublings by conventional means, nor are the maximum life spans of the species they studied known.[34] Figure 2-1 shows the direct proportionality between the maximum life spans of different species and the population-doubling potential of their cultured fibroblasts. Embryonic fibroblasts were used in nine of the 10 species studied. Juvenile tissue was used in the study on the Galapagos tortoise.

If this relationship can be extended and confirmed, it suggests the presence of a chronometer or pacemaker within all normal cells that is characteristic for each species and that dictates maximum cell doubling or functional capacity with an apparent evolutionary basis. The postulated chronometer may or may not be the same one that we suggest might control the inverse relationship between donor age and population-doubling potential.

THE MEMORY OF CULTURED NORMAL HUMAN CELLS

When we first established human diploid cell strains almost 25 years ago, it became apparent that their finite lifetime imposed a serious limit on the capacity to work with any single strain. We found that a strain derived from fetal tissue underwent 50 ± 10 population doublings over a period of about 1 year and was then lost.[5,8] In order to circumvent this important limitation, we succeeded in freezing viable normal human cells at sub-zero temperatures.[3] In this way it was possible to fully characterize a single human diploid cell strain and have it available for study for long periods of time. The potential yield of cells from a population capable of 50 population doublings is about 20 million metric tons.[8]

In 1962 we developed and placed into liquid nitrogen storage several hundred ampules of our normal human diploid cell strain WI-38, which subsequently became the most completely characterized normal human cell population in the world. Today it is the archtype normal human fibroblast and is used worldwide for applications in biological research, in virus isolation and identification, and in the production of several human virus vaccines.

WI-38 has been in cryogenic storage for 26 years, which represents the longest period of time that a viable normal human cell population has ever been stored. The ability to preserve normal cell strains has permitted experimentation directed toward answering a fundamental question in cytogerontology: If cells are frozen at various population-doubling levels up to Phase III, how many population doublings will the cells undergo when they are thawed or reconstituted? Do they have a "clock" that is arrested in the cold at the

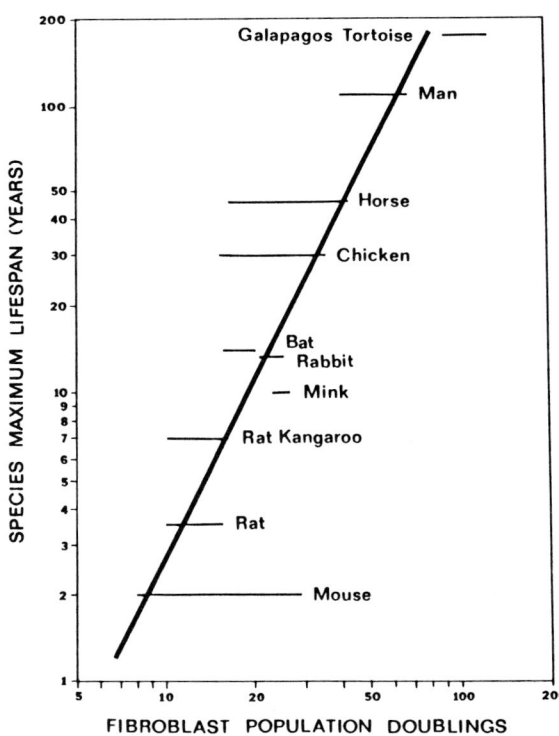

Figure 2–1 Fibroblasts from the embryos of 10 different species multiply in culture to a maximum number of population doublings that is roughly proportional to the life span for that species. Galapagos tortoise cells were derived from a juvenile animal.

population-doubling level at which they were frozen? If so, then the total cumulative number of doublings both before and after freezing would be about 50 in the case of a fetal strain. Or does freezing reset the clock to zero or to some random number?

In the 26 years since 1962 we have shown that WI-38 and other human cell strains have remarkable memories. Even after 26 years, WI-38 cells remember at which population-doubling level they were frozen and, on reconstitution, undergo the number of population doublings that remain from the time they were frozen to make a total of 50 population doublings. More than 130 ampules have been reconstituted by us in the past 26 years, and the memory of the cells is as accurate today as it was in 1962.

FUNCTIONAL FAILURE AS CULTURED NORMAL HUMAN CELLS REACH PHASE III

The probability that animals age because one or more cell type loses its ability to proliferate is unlikely. It is more likely that decrements in physiologic function that appear before cells lose their capacity to replicate are the true causes of age changes. In 1971 we reported the first functional decrement in a normal human cell population before its loss of proliferative capacity.[35] We found that WI-38 cells lost much of their ability to synthesize collagen and to induce collagenolytic activity after almost 40 population doublings.

In the next decade, almost 200 functional changes have been found to occur in cultured normal human cells prior to their loss of replicative capacity. A full tabulation is presented in a review.[36] The reported changes cover virtually all aspects of cell biochemistry, morphology, and behavior. They include changes in lipids, carbohydrates, amino acids, proteins, RNA, DNA, enzymes, cell cycle dynamics, cell size and morphology, synthesis, incorporation, and stimulation.

Mitotic Failure Does Not Cause Aging

These changes, which herald the approaching loss of division capacity, likely play the central role in the expression of aging and result in the death of the individual animal well before its cells fail to divide.

Of great importance is the realization that many of these same changes that have been reported to occur in cultured normal human cells as they age in vitro are identical to changes that are known to occur in cells in vivo as humans age.[36] This finding adds considerable weight to our contention that the Phase III phenomenon is indeed an expression of aging at the cellular level.

Clearly, there are several classes of cells that are incapable of division in mature animals, and it is just as likely, if not even more likely, that these cells play a greater role in the expression of age changes than those cells that are capable of dividing. Examples of nondividing cells are neurons and muscle cells. It is important to emphasize that the cessation of mitotic activity is only one functional decrement with a genetic basis that may be similar to those functional decrements known to occur in aging nondividing cells. We have proposed, therefore, that the same kind of gene action that results in physiologic decrements in aging nondividing cells also occurs in aging cells that can still divide. It is not our belief that age changes result necessarily from loss of the function to divide, but simply from the loss of any function characteristic of an aging cell. The basis for loss of any of these functions is thought to be similar.

If these conclusions are accurate, an understanding of the mechanism by which normal cells lose their capacity to replicate could provide insights into the causes of decrements in other functional properties, such as those that occur in aging neurons or muscle cells.

THE FINITE LIFETIME OF NORMAL CELLS IN VIVO

As indicated at the outset of this discussion, there are two ways in which a determination of cell immortality can be made. The first method is to grow normal cells in culture. That has been discussed, and the conclusion is that under these conditions normal cells do have a finite capacity to replicate and function. The second method by which cell immortality can be determined is to ascertain whether normal cells can proliferate indefinitely in vivo.

If all cell types were continually renewed without loss of function or capacity for self-renewal, organs composed of such cells would be expected to function normally indefinitely and their host would live forever. Regrettably, renewal cell populations do not occur in most tissues, and when they do, cell proliferation is not indefinite.

Is it possible, then, to circumvent the death of normal animal cells that results from the death of the "host" by transferring marked cells to younger animals seriatim? Such experiments would provide an in vivo counterpart to the in vitro experiments previously described. If the analogy is accurate, we would predict that normal cells transplanted serially to proper inbred hosts would, like their in vitro counterparts, age. Such experiments would largely rule out objections to in vitro studies that are based on the artificiality of the in vitro environment. The question could be answered by serial orthotopic transplantation of normal somatic tissue to new, young, inbred hosts each time the recipient approaches old age.

Data reported from many different laboratories in which rodent mammary tissue,[37] skin,[38] and hematopoietic cells,[39-44] were employed demonstrate that normal cells serially transplanted to inbred hosts do not survive indefinitely. Studies done with hematopoietic cells to investigate this point actually number in the dozens.[36]

The trauma of transplantation does not appear to influence the results and, in heterochronic transplants, survival time is related to the age of the grafted tissue.[38] Cancer cells, on the other hand, frequently can be transplanted indefinitely. Thus, the immortality of cancer cells in vitro is precisely mimicked in vivo.

Many grafts transplanted in vivo have been found to survive much longer than the life span of the host or the donor species before aging and dying. This fact has been erroneously interpreted by some to mean that normal cells can replicate continuously for periods of time in excess of the species' known lifespan. However, grafted tissue behaves quite differently from cultured cells. The latter are usually kept in a state of continuous proliferation. The cells in grafted tissue are not dividing continuously, nor are the number of cells in the dividing pool as great as in cell cultures. If fibroblasts in grafted tissue replicated to the extent that comparable cells do in vitro, the graft would quickly weigh more than its host. Thus, it is important to appreciate that long survival time is not equivalent to proliferation time or to rounds of division. Cells in grafts have an extremely low reproductive turnover rate. This is analogous to holding normal cell cultures at room temperature, which extends calendar time for cell survival, but does not result in increased population doublings.

THEORIES OF BIOLOGICAL AGING

What then are the most likely causes of biological aging? The relative newness of the field of gerontology as a seriously studied science and the consequent lack of an extensive and reliable data base has encouraged speculations on the theoretic underpinnings of the field. An additional cause of the plethora of biogerontologic theories is that manifestations of biological changes over time affect virtually all components of living systems from the molecular level up to that of the whole organism. These hierarchical changes have made it possible to construct theories of aging based on events that occur over time at the level of molecules, cell organelles, cells, tissues, organs, or the whole animal.

Depending more on the bias of the theorist than on actual fact, a selected age-associated change within this hierarchy is often defended with great vigor and emotion. Nevertheless, most current theories of biological aging suffer from the criticism that they are, or may be, mere expressions of the effect of some more fundamental change. There is common failure to realize that changes more fundamental to the one observed may induce the effect that was chosen for study.

Since all fundamental life processes depend on genetic events, theories of aging that depend on these events have attracted the most attention.

The Somatic Mutation Theory

This theory of aging enjoyed its greatest popularity in the late 1950s and early 1960s as a derivative of burgeoning developments in the field of radiobiology. The central concept is that the accumulation of a sufficient level of mutations in somatic cells will produce physiologic decrements characteristic of aging. If mutations are the fundamental cause of age changes, they must occur randomly in time and location.[46] Early champions of this idea were Szilard[47] and Failla.[48] Failla postulated dominant mutations as causes of aging. Szilard argued that aging was caused by genes ("targets") being "hit" or "struck" by a mutational event that, unlike Failla, he regarded as recessive. Thus, a pair of homologous genes must be hit at a particular rate and in a sufficient number of cells in order to achieve phenotypic expression.

Maynard-Smith[46] pointed out that, if Szilard was correct, inbred animals, homologous at most gene loci, would display the maximum species life span since homozygous faults would be lethal and heterozygous faults would be few or nonexistent. Yet, inbreeding reduces life span in mice and *Drosophila*. Furthermore, Szilard's hypothesis would predict that diploid organisms would live longer than their haploid counterparts, which contain only one chromosome set. In the hymenopteran wasp, *Habrobracon*, haploid and diploid males have identical life spans. Haploid males are more sensitive to ionizing radiation than are diploid male wasps, yet irradiation shortens the life span of diploids far more than that of haploids. These observations are inconsistent with the mutation theory. Although reduced life spans do occur in irradiated animals, extended life spans have also been observed.[49] Also, irradiated old animals should show accelerated age changes as should animals treated with mutagenic agents, but they do not.[50]

Curtis and Miller,[51] the last major advocates of the somatic mutation theory, based their conclusions on the frequency of abnormalities observed in the chromosomes of dividing cells in the livers of old mice. They found a higher frequency of abnormalities in the cells of a short-lived strain when compared with those found in long-lived strains. Curtis made similar findings in guinea pigs and dogs. Nevertheless, other comparisons between short- and long-lived strains were inconsistent with these findings, and hybrids between short- and long-lived strains did not yield the expected results. Neutron irradiation of dividing cells was found by Curtis to yield aberrations in up to 90 percent of the cells, yet life span was unaffected.

In the past decade, few significant studies have been conducted on the role of somatic mutations in aging. In spite of the contrary evidence, there is an expectation that the critical experiments should be redesigned using the technology of modern molecular biology.

The Error Theory

This theory, to some extent derivative of the somatic mutation theory, was first postulated by Medvedev[52] and elaborated by Orgel.[53]

It has been suggested that the repeated DNA nucleotide sequences in the genome of eukaryotic organisms may be (1) a reserve of information for evolutionary change, (2) a means of increasing functional expression, and (3) a reserve mechanism for protecting vital information from random errors that may occur in functioning DNA sequences. Medvedev proposed that the loss of unique, nonrepeated DNA sequences could produce age decrements and that selected reiterated sequences may be an evolved means for delaying the inevitability of the event by providing redundancy necessary for the maintenance of vital information.

Derivative of error accumulation in reiterated DNA sequences is the notion of Orgel.[53] He postulates the occurrence of inaccuracy in protein synthesis as the essential source of age-associated decrements in cell function. This hypothesis resulted in a flurry of experiments designed to learn whether an incorrect amino acid incorporated in a protein molecule could accelerate aging phenomena or whether misspecified proteins accumulated in old cells. Errors in enzyme molecules that processed information-containing molecules were thought to be the most important potential sources of important damage. A misspecified enzyme could produce a cascade of faulty molecules with presumably profound effects, called an "error catastrophe." One group has claimed to have obtained evidence for the error catastrophe theory, but most other studies have failed to provide evidence for its support. The idea is now in general disfavor despite the fact that altered proteins are frequently found in the cells of old organisms.

A correlate of error accumulation as a cause of age changes is the effectiveness of those systems that repair genome damage. Evidence from the cultured cells of several different species revealed that the efficiency of repair of ultraviolet damage to DNA was directly correlated to species' life span.[54] Again, contrary evidence has also been reported, and the original finding remains equivocal.[50]

The Program Theory of Aging

Adherents of this theory, unlike advocates of such stochastically-based theories as error accumulation, postulate a purposeful sequence of events written into the genome. This leads to age changes much as similar instructions written into the genetic message leads to the orderly expression of developmental sequences.

The conceptual simplicity of this idea is part of its attractiveness, but the attempts to test it experimentally have met with little success. The finding that cultured normal human and animal cells have a finite ability to replicate and function has provided the best evidence in support of the theory, but so does the fundamental fact that aging occurs naturally in intact animals.[3] Programming assumes an orderly sequence of events with which few would disagree, but it does not provide mechanistic details.

On the other hand, it has been argued effectively that, although events occurring from conception to the full expression of adulthood may be programmed, postreproductive events or aging may not be purposely determined by the genome. That is, age changes may be produced by a kind of free-wheeling, non-genome-dependent continuation of the inertia developed from previously determined developmental events. Therefore, function declines or terminates in a more or less random fashion like the eventual demise of a new automobile that is poorly repaired or maintained.

To complete the analogy, the manufacture of an automobile, like the growth of an individual animal, is predicated on the presence of accurate blueprints and their proper execution. What happens after the automobile is built or after the individual reaches sexual maturation is not governed by blueprints, but occurs in most systems randomly and inevitably. Which system fails first and leads to the demise of the automobile or the individual is, therefore, a random process with, nevertheless, a narrowly expressed "mean time to failure." This would be characteristic of the specific brand of automobile or the particular animal species.

Entropy and Aging

In terms of modern physics, a genetic program should succumb to the second law of thermodynamics, which states that a closed system tends to a state of equilibrium or of maximum entropy in which nothing more happens. That is, ordered systems tend to move to greater disorder. The initially well-organized genetic program, by increasing entropy, thus becomes disordered and produces those changes recognized as aging. Our mortality may, in this way, be decreed by the second law of thermodynamics. Although this may be a tenable hypothesis as it pertains to somatic cells or to individual members of a species, it seems to fly in the face of the enormous amount of evidence for biological evolution that superficially appears to be in conflict with the second law. Moreover, it seems to be in conflict with the apparent immortality of the germ plasm and of certain immortal, abnormal, cancer cell populations.

Delayed Expression of Deleterious Genes

Medawar[55] has argued persuasively that the presence of deleterious genes in a species might be thwarted by a selection process that would postpone their manifestions if it were not possible to eliminate them. This strategy would result in the piling up of deleterious genes in the postreproductive period when their expression would do less harm.

A variation of this theme is expressed by Williams,[56] who postulates pleiotropic genes that have both favorable and unfavorable actions. If the favorable gene expression is able to increase fecundity, that gene might be selected even though it might express a deleterious action later in life. Deleterious age changes then would be the penalty paid by individuals for the expression of beneficial genes early in life. An accumulation of such late-acting genes in various organ systems would behave like late-programmed events and would give rise to the entire constellation of age changes.

Longevity Assurance Genes

Sacher[57] is critical of the program theory of aging for what he believes to be errors in logic. He illustrates his point by comparing the life histories of annual plants and of mammals. Annual plants are semelparous; that is, they are characterized by a single reproductive effort that is completed at the end of the life span and frequently not until somatic cell death. The final step of the reproductive process, seed dispersal, depends on the death of the plant, and this requires that senescence be closely integrated with prior stages. The stages are known to be under the specific control of hormones and end with formation of specific hydrolytic enzymes.

Sacher restricts programmed aging to cases such as this where there is specific control of onset by either internal or external signals, there is a specific enzyme mechanism present, and, finally, there is a functional role for senescence and/or death in a specific temporal relationship with other life processes. The rapid aging and death of the Pacific salmon after spawning is a good example of this event occurring in animals.

Mammals, on the other hand, are examples of iteroparous reproduction where reproductive success depends on producing a number of litters over an extended reproductive span. Sacher argues that this offers no functional role for senescence and death. On the contrary, he maintains that this would place a premium on the maintenance of physiologic vigor and survival. Long life in mammals, therefore, is the result of selection for an extended period of assured physiologic performance. A great whale that lives 30 times longer than a mouse has a million times more cells at risk for age changes. Nevertheless, a comparable whale cell is orders of magnitude more stable than a mouse cell.

"It would be expected," says Sacher, "that the selective process acts on mechanisms for *increasing* the stability of the organism at all levels, from the molecular to the systemic." Sacher emphasizes the more evolutionary logical role of genetic systems that maintain life, rather than theories that these systems might program age changes. Until it can be shown that evolution selects for greater longevity, at least in mammals, the study of life maintenance systems or "longevity-assurance genes" may be more productive than the current emphasis on a search for the causes of age-associated physiologic decrements.[57]

The postulated longevity-assurance genes may be simply sets of genes that have evolved to express themselves at later times during the development of an animal in order to increase its survivability. These genes would not per se be directly involved with aging, but, by their later expression, would serve to delay age changes. Aging then would be a secondary manifestation of earlier-occurring developmental events. For example, natural selection in a species may favor individuals capable of reaching sexual maturity at a later time in order to provide better opportunities for survival of progeny. A secondary effect of this, and not directly selected for, would be a concommitant delay in the expression of aging.

"Why do we age?" may be the wrong question. The right question could be: "Why do we live as long as we do?"

Adapted from Hayflick L. The cell biology and theoretical basis of human aging. In: Carstensen LL, Edelstein BL, Oxford: Pergamon Press, 1987:3.

References

1. Comfort A. The biology of senescence. 3rd ed. New York: Elsevier, 1979.
2. Weismann A. Aufsatze uber vererbung und verwandte biologische fragen. Jena: Verlag von Gustav Fischer, 1892.
3. Hayflick L, Moorhead PS. The serial cultivation of human diploid cell strains. Exp Cell Res 1961; 25:585-621.
4. Kirkwood TBL, Cremer T. Cytogerontology since 1881: a reappraisal of August Weismann and a review of modern progress. Hum Genet 1982; 60:101-121.
5. Weismann A. Essays upon heredity and kindred biological problems. 2nd ed. Oxford: Clarendon Press, 1891.
6. Parker RC. Methods of tissue culture. New York: Harper and Row, 1961.
7. Kohler G, Milstein C. Continuous cultures of fused cells secreting antibody of predefined specificity. Nature 1975; 256:495-497.
8. Hayflick L. The limited in vitro lifetime of human diploid cell strains. Exp Cell Res 1965; 37:614-636.
9. Boone CW. Malignant hemangioendotheliomas produced by subcutaneous inoculation of Balb/3T3 cells attached to glass beads. Science 1975; 188:68-70.
10. Boone CW, Takeichi N, Paranjpe M. Vasoformative sarcomas arising from Balb/3T3 cells attached to solid substrates. Cancer Res 1976; 36:1626-1633.
11. Puck TT, Cieciura SJ, Fisher HW. Clonal growth in vitro of human cells with fibroblastic morphology. J Exp Med 1957; 106:145-158.
12. Puck TT, Cieciura SJ, Robinson A. Genetics of somatic mammalian cells. III. Long-term cultivation of euploid cells from human and animal subjects. J Exp Med 1958; 108:945-956.
13. Swim HE, Parker RF. Culture characteristics of human fibroblasts propagated serially. Am J Hygiene 1957; 66:235-243.
14. Hayflick L. Aging under glass. Exp Gerontol 1970; 5:291-303.
15. Hayflick L. Cell senescence and cell differentiation in vitro. In: Academy of Science and Literature, Mainz, Germany. Aging and development. Stuttgart: F. K. Schattauer Verlag, 1972.
16. Harris M. Quantitative growth studies with chick myoblasts in glass substrate cultures. Growth 1957; 21:149-166.
17. Hay RJ, Strehler BL. The limited growth span of cell strains isolated from the chick embryo. Exp Gerontol 1967; 2:123-135.
18. Lima L, Macieira-Coelho A. Parameters of aging in chicken embryo fibroblasts cultivated in vitro. Exp Cell Res 1972; 70:279-284.
19. Ponten J. The growth capacity of normal and Rous-virus-transformed chicken fibroblasts in vitro. Int J Cancer 1970; 6:323-332.
20. Witkowski JA. Alexis Carrel and the mysticism of tissue culture. Med Hist 1979; 23:279-296.
21. Witkoswki JA. Dr. Carrel's immortal cells. Med Hist 1980; 24:129-142.
22. Witkowski JA. The myth of cell immortality. Trends in Biochemical Sciences 1985; 10:258-260.
23. Martin GM, Sprague CA, Epstein CJ. Replicative lifespan of cultivated human cells. Effect of donor's age, tissue, and genotype. Lab Invest 1970; 23:86-92.
24. Goldstein S, Moerman EJ, Soeldner JS, Gleason RE, Barnett DM. Chronologic and physiologic age effect replicative life-span of fibroblasts from diabetics, prediabetics and normal donors. Science 1978; 199:781-782.
25. Schneider EL, Mitsui Y. The relationship between in vitro cellular aging and in vivo human aging. Proc Natl Acad Sci USA 1976; 73:3584-3588.
26. Vracko R, McFarland BM. Lifespan of diabetic and nondiabetic fibroblasts in vitro. Exp Cell Res 1980; 129:345-350.
27. LeGuilly Y, Simon M, Lenoir P, Bourel M. Long-term culture of human adult liver cells: morphological changes related to in vitro senescence and effect of donor's age on growth potential. Gerontologia 1973; 19:303-313.
28. Bierman EL. The effect of donor age on the in vitro lifespan of cultured human arterial smooth-muscle cells. In Vitro 1978; 14:951-955.
29. Tassin J, Malaise E, Courtois Y. Human lens cells have an in vitro proliferative capacity inversely proportional to the donor age. Exp Cell Res 1979; 123:388-392.
30. Walford RL. Studies in immunogerontology. J Am Geriatr Soc 1982; 30:617-625.
31. Walford RL, Jawaid SQ, Naeim F. Evidence for in vitro senescence of T-lymphocytes cultured from normal human peripheral blood. Age 1981; 4:67-70.
32. Hayflick L. The biology of human aging. Am J Med Sci 1973; 265:433-445.
33. Rohme D. Evidence for a relationship between longevity of mammalian species and life spans of normal fibroblasts in vitro and erythrocytes in vivo. Proc Natl Acad Sci USA 1981; 78:5009-5013.
34. Stanley JF, Pye D, MacGregor A. Comparison of doubling numbers attained by cultured animal cells with the life span of species. Nature 1975; 255:158-159.
35. Houck JC, Sharma VK, Hayflick L. Functional failures of cultured human diploid fibroblasts after continued population doublings. Proc Soc Exp Biol Med 1971; 137:331-333.
36. Hayflick L. Cell aging. In: Eisdorfer C, ed. Annual review of gerontology and geriatrics. New York: Springer Publishing Co, 1980:26.
37. Daniel CW, deOme KB, Young JT, Blair PB, Faulkin LJ Jr. The in vivo lifespan of normal and preneoplastic mouse mammary glands: a serial transplantation study. Proc Natl Acad Sci USA 1968; 61:53-60.

38. Krohn PL. Review lectures on senescence. II: Heterochronic transplantation in the study of aging. Proc R Soc Lond (Biol) 1962; 157:128-147.
39. Cudkowicz G, Upton AC, Shearer GM, Hughes WL. Lymphocyte content and proliferative capacity of serially transplanted mouse bone marrow. Nature 1964; 201:165-167.
40. Ford CE, Micklem HS, Gray SM. Evidence of selective proliferation of reticular cell-clones in heavily irradiated mice. Br J Radiol 1959; 32:280.
41. Harrison DE. Normal production of erythrocytes by mouse marrow continuous for 73 months. Proc Natl Acad Sci USA 1973; 70:3184-3188.
42. Harrison DE. Normal function of transplanted marrow cell lines from aged mice. J Gerontol 1975; 30:279-285.
43. Hellman S, Botnick LE, Hannon EC, Vigneulle RM. Proliferative capacity of murine hematopoietic stem cells. Proc Natl Acad Sci USA 1978; 75:490-494.
44. Siminovitch L, Till JE, McCulloch EA. Decline in colony-forming ability of marrow cells subjected to serial transplantation into irradiated mice. J Cell Compar Physiol 1964; 64:23-31.
45. Hayflick L. Cytogerontology. In: Rockstein M, ed. Theoretical aspects of aging. New York: Academic Press, 1974:83.
46. Maynard-Smith J. Review lectures on senescence. I. The causes of aging. Proc R Soc Lond (Biol) 1962; 157:115-127.
47. Szilard L. On the nature of the aging process. Proc Natl Acad Sci USA 1959; 45:30-45.
48. Failla G. The aging process and somatic mutations. In: Strehler BL, ed. The biology of aging. Publication No. 6. Washington, DC: American Institute of Biological Sciences, 1960:170.
49. Sacher GA. Effects of x-rays on the survival of *Drosophila melanogaster*. Physiological Zoology 1963; 36:295-311.
50. Hayflick L. Theories of biological aging. Exp Gerontol 1985; 20:145-159.
51. Curtis HJ, Miller K. Chromosome aberrations in liver cells of guinea pigs. J Gerontol 1971; 26:292-293.
52. Medvedev ZA. Repetition of molecular-genetic information as a possible factor in evolutionary changes of life-span. Exp Gerontol 1972; 7:227-234.
53. Orgel LE. The maintenance of the accuracy of protein synthesis and its relevance to aging. Proc Natl Acad Sci USA 1963; 49:517-521.
54. Hart RW, Setlow RB. Correlation between DNA excision repair and life-span in a number of mammalian species. Proc Natl Acad Sci USA 1974; 71:2169-2173.
55. Medawar PB. The uniqueness of the individual. London: Methuen, 1957.
56. Williams GC. Pleiotropy, natural selection, and the evolution of senescence. Evolution 1957; 11:398-411.
57. Sacher GA. Molecular versus systemic theories on the genesis of aging. Exp Gerontol 1968; 3:265-271.

Chapter Three

EPIDEMIOLOGIC AND DEMOGRAPHIC CHARACTERISTICS OF THE AGING POPULATION

SAMUEL P. KORPER, Ph.D., M.P.H.

The program announcing this conference on Geriatric Otolaryngology states that the Academy has determined that... "the time is appropriate for indepth consideration of the needs of this growing segment of our population... to review current issues and challenges in research on aging and... to clarify the geriatric dimension of clinical practice." It is my task to integrate the methods and perspectives of several disciplines in an attempt to put forward an initial response to that statement of purpose.

Let me begin by combining the definition of otorhinolaryngology as the "sum of knowledge regarding the ear, nose, and larynx and their diseases" with that of epidemiology as... "that field of science dealing with the relationships of the various factors which determine the frequencies and distributions of an infectious process, a disease or a physiologic state." Adding to these the study of the characteristics of human populations, such as their size, growth, density, and distribution, which is demography, we have available the scope of the challenge and, ostensibly, the means to gain insight into the use, patterns, risks, and costs associated with geriatric otorhinolaryngology. Referring to generally available morbidity and mortality data, Jacob Brody and Dwight Brock, in their chapter in the *Handbook of the Biology of Aging*[1], state:

> "except for demographic trends, none of these sources of data can be considered robust, hence, critical information is lacking or only partially reliable... Data concerning morbidity and disability are even more suspect on a national level, although we do believe that these data are useful for trend analysis and perhaps, in some specific conditions... extremely valuable information is currently available which is not being linked or utilized at present."

The next two speakers each describe reports and studies, Dr. Jakubczak in the area of hearing, voice, and swallowing, and Dr. Tobias discussing speech, which provide estimates of disability and impairment in aging persons. I will leave those estimates to them. However, in the 1987 National Institutes of Health Report to Congress, in reference to the clinical impression of increased incidence of voice and swallowing disorders among older persons, it is stated that..."it is unclear whether such problems are normal age-related changes or whether they reflect diseases or iatrogenic causes which also occur with increasing frequency in older populations."[2] This is clinical impression, but limited data. With that, let me now turn to the first of my responsibilities, establishing the demographic context for our discussions.

DEMOGRAPHICS

Like most countries of the world, the United States is experiencing unparalleled growth in the number of older people (Table 3–1). This growth shows every indication of continuing well into the 21st century. There are today about 29 million people, or about 12 percent of the American population, who are over the age of 65. During the 35-year period between 1985 and 2020, the proportion of the total population that is 65 years and older is expected to increase by about 50 percent, from about 12 percent to about 18 percent of the total population, some 54 million persons (Table 3–2).

The rate of growth of the elderly population is expected to be somewhat greater after the year 2000 than during the next decade or so. The fastest-growing age group also changes. Between 1985 and 2000 the group 85 years and older will increase most rapidly at an average rate of about 4 percent a year (Fig. 3–1). Subsequently, between the years 2000 and 2020, the group aged 65 to 74 years will increase most rapidly as the post-World War II baby boom generation enters the elderly category. The proportion age 85 years and older is likely to double—from 1.2 percent to 2.4 percent—and to continue to increase sharply thereafter.

These population projections may be conservative. In actuality, the elderly population may grow at an even faster rate. The projections cited here are based on the assumption that future death rates will decrease at about half the average rate of reduction that occurred between 1980 and 1983 (Fig. 3–2). A more optimistic assumption—that death rates will

TABLE 3-1 Countries With More Than 2 Million Elderly in 1985 (Numbers in Thousands)

Country	Population Aged 65 and Over	Country	Population Aged 65 and Over
China	52,889	Poland	3,484
India	32,698	Bangladesh	3,119
United States	28,609	Pakistan	2,818
Soviet Union	25,974	Mexico	2,797
Japan	12,125	Canada	2,651
Germany (Fed Rep.)	8,812	Argentina	2,610
United Kingdom	8,466	Vietnam	2,393
Italy	7,443	Nigeria	2,307
France	6,748	Germany (Dem. Rep.)	2,217
Indonesia	5,901	Romania	2,155
Brazil	5,828	Turkey	2,093
Spain	4,274		

Source: United Nations, 1986, unpublished data from the 1984 assessment of world population prospects; and United States Bureau of the Census, Center for International Research.

TABLE 3-2 Projected Population (in Millions)

	1985		2000		2020	
	Number	%	Number	%	Number	%
Grand Total	247.4	100.0	277.1	100.0	307.7	100.0
Total 65+	29.1	11.8	36.4	13.1	54.5	17.7
65–74	17.0	6.9	18.5	6.7	31.7	10.3
75–84	9.2	3.7	12.7	4.6	15.4	5.0
85+	2.9	1.2	5.2	1.9	7.3	2.4

Source: Social Security Administration, 1985.

decline at about the same average rate as in the past—would result in an additional 4 million elderly persons in 2020, of which about half would be over 85 years of age.

Reductions of such killers as heart disease, cancer, stroke, and infectious diseases, in addition to improved health care and healthier lifestyles, have contributed to the large number of older people in our society today. In 1984, life expectancy at birth for men was 71 years and 78 years for women—an additional generation longer than for people born in 1900 when life expectancy was only 47 years (Fig. 3–3). Perhaps more truly astounding is that, at age 65, men today can expect to live another 14½ years, while women can expect to live nearly 19 additional years.

There are other observations to be made from current life expectancy figures. It is not surprising, for example, that there are many more older women than men who are living without spouses. While most older men are married, most older women are likely to become widowed as they grow older. In 1984, nearly 78 percent of the men over 65 were married, compared to nearly 40 percent of the

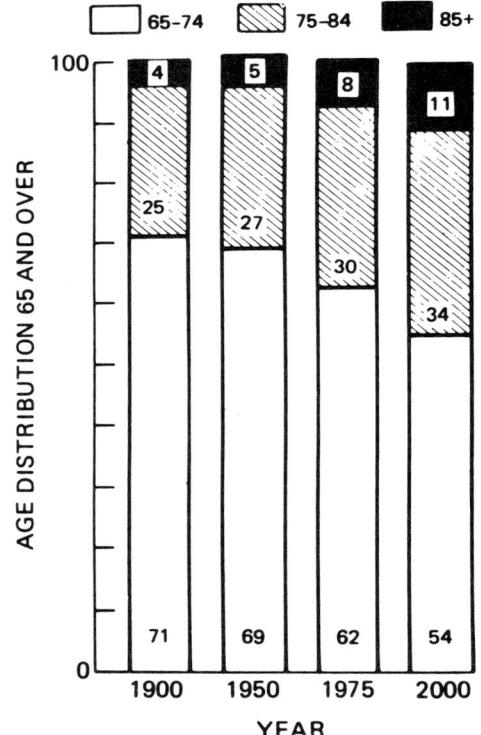

Figure 3-1 The percentage of the very old among the elderly is increasing. Source: United States Bureau of the Census.

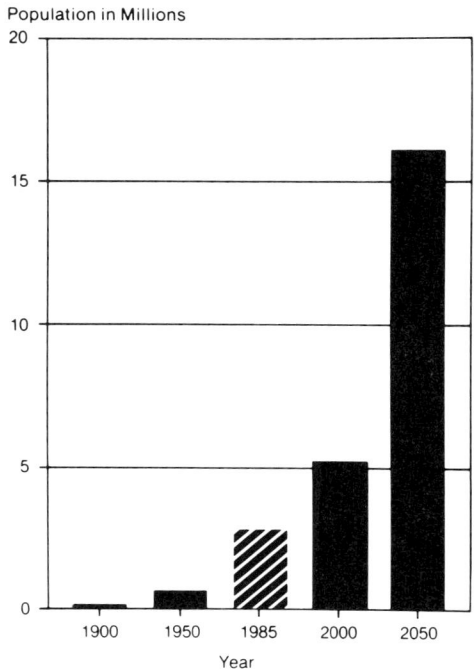

Figure 3-2 United States population 85 years and over. Source: United States Bureau of the Census.

women in the same age group. Another implication of this sex ratio gap is that more noninstitutionalized older women than men live alone. Again in 1984, 41 percent of the older women and only 15 percent of the older men live alone. Older women living alone are at the greatest risk for poverty. In 1984 for example, the median income for elderly women was $6,020, while unmarried men realized an income of $10,450.

A central theme voiced by those interested in older populations concerns the quality of life experienced by people as they grow very old. Four out of five older persons suffer at least one chronic and disabling condition. Many of these people suffer from more than one (Fig. 3-4). The incidence of arthritis, for example, is 80 percent higher for persons aged 65 and over than for persons aged 45 to 64. Osteoarthritis affects 16 million Americans. In 1983, 388 of every 1,000 older people suffered from hypertension. Hearing impairment was ranked high among the 10 leading chronic conditions of older people; the rate per 1,000 persons was nearly 300 for people 65 and over. It is important for health professionals to note that, though heart conditions and cancer are common killers among the aged, close attention must be given to those conditions that affect a person's ability to function independently. These include diabetes, dementia, depression, osteoporosis and osteoarthritis, and incontinence.

Chronic disease or physical or mental impairment limit many older people in their ability to function independently or to maintain the lifestyle to which they became accustomed. In 1981, the National Health Interview Survey reported that 47 percent of persons aged 65 or over were limited in some way in their daily activities, compared to 11 percent of those under 65 (Fig. 3-5). After age 75, over 53 percent of the people surveyed were limited in their daily activities.[3]

The 1984 National Health Interview Survey included a special questionnaire, the Supplement on Aging (SOA), aimed at older persons living in the community. Results indicate that about 2.5 million persons, or 10 percent of all noninstitutionalized Americans 85 years and over, had difficulty and received help with personal care activities such as

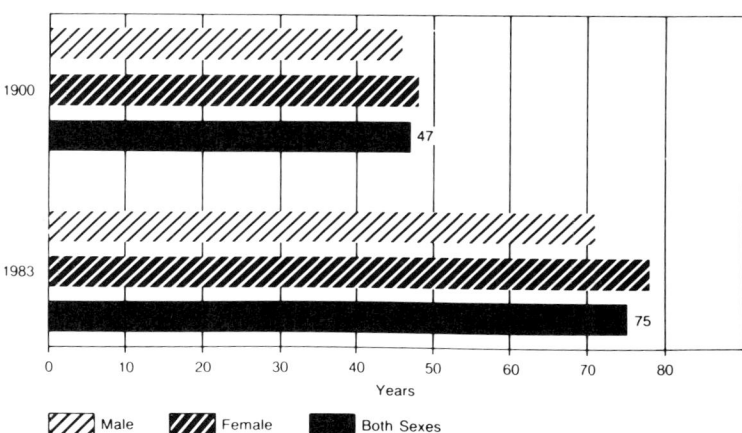

Figure 3-3 United States life expectancy at birth. Source: National Center for Health Statistics.

22 / Geriatric Otorhinolaryngology

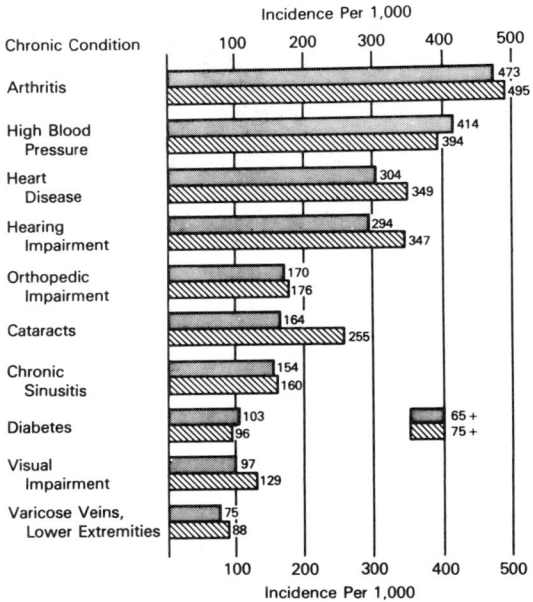

Figure 3–4 Major chronic conditions among persons 65+ and 75+, 1984. Source: National Center for Health Statistics, 1984.

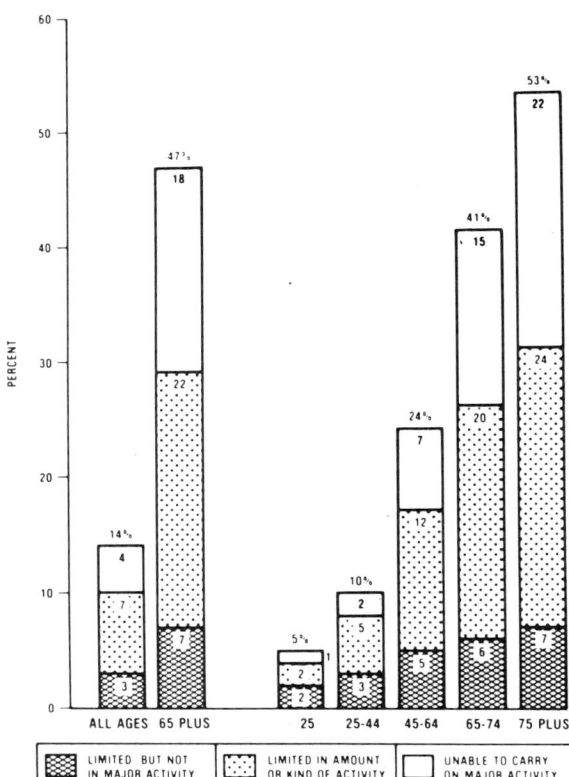

Figure 3–5 Limitation of activity due to chronic conditions by type of limitations and age, 1981. Source: National Center for Health Statistics, 1981. Health Interview Survey, unpublished.

bathing, dressing, and toileting (Fig. 3–6). If the prevalence of functional limitations is measured by the proportion of persons who experience any difficulty in performing home management activities such as housework, shopping, preparing meals, etc., about 27 percent of those over 65 were functionally limited (Fig. 3–7).[4,5]

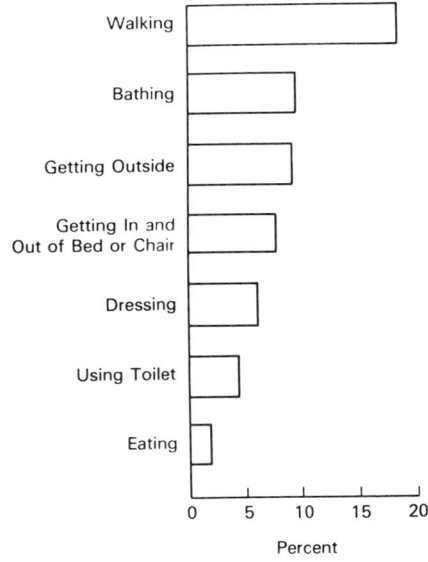

Figure 3–6 Noninstitutionalized population 65 years of age and over who have difficulty with activities of daily living. Source: Division of Health Interview Statistics, National Center for Health Statistics: Data from the National Health Interview Survey 1984 Supplement on Aging.

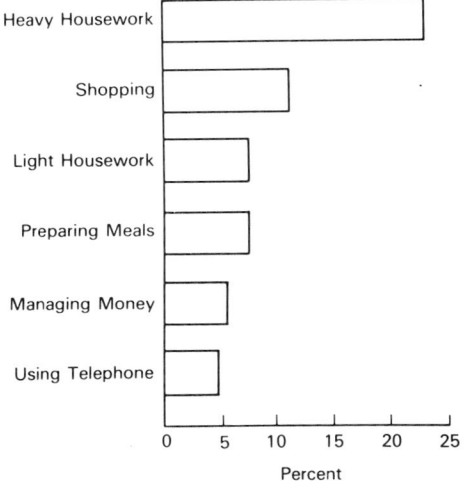

Figure 3–7 Noninstitutionalized population 65 years of age and over who have difficulty with instrumental activities of daily living. Source: Division of Health Interview Statistics, National Center for Health Statistics: Data from the National Health Interview Survey 1984 Supplement on Aging.

Because of the high prevalence of chronic conditions and illnesses, the older population utilizes more health services than any other age group. Though representing about 12 percent of the total population, older persons account for about 33 percent of hospital discharges and over 40 percent of total days of hospital care (Fig. 3-8). Additionally, older people account for one in every six physician visits. Older people also use more medication, accounting for 25 percent of all prescription drug use. (Seventy-five percent of the older population are reported to take at least one prescription drug annually as compared to 58 percent of the total population.)

Based on these figures, one can readily see that health professionals will be required to spend an increasingly larger proportion of their time with older patients. Figure 3-9 depicts the magnitude of the projected increase, ranging from 100 percent to over 200 percent in the use of services such as physician visits, hospitals, and nursing homes by the population over age 65 between now and the year 2020. We must accept the reality of it, plan for it, and become more knowledgeable about the needs of older people as they relate to our respective disciplines.[6]

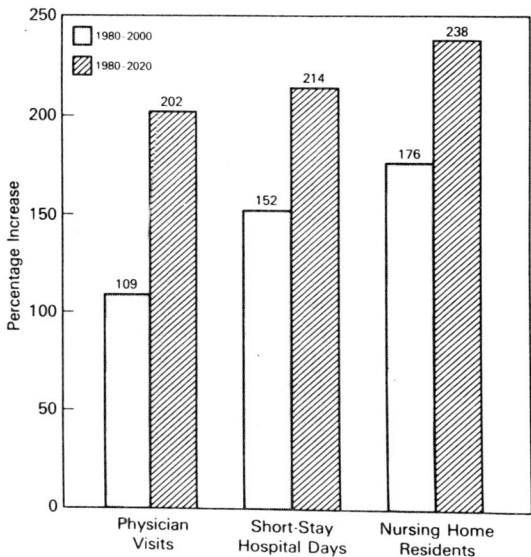

Figure 3-9 Projected percentage increase in use of health services in persons 65 years and older, 1980-2000 and 1980-2020. Source: Rice D, Feldman H. Living longer in the United States: demographic changes and health needs of the elderly. Milbank Memorial Fund Quarterly, Health and Society 1983; 61(3): 362-396.

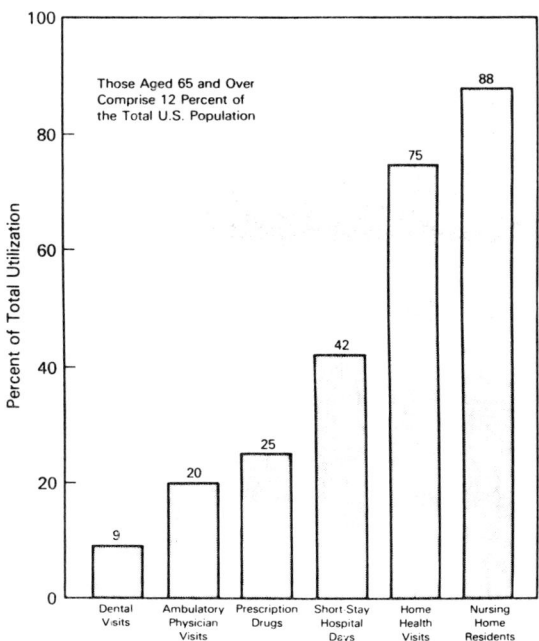

Figure 3-8 Utilization of health services by persons 65 years and older in recent years. Source: National Center for Health Statistics, Health Care Financing Administration.

EPIDEMIOLOGY AND UTILIZATION

Moving now to my second assignment, let me simply say that I had at first thought this would entail a fairly straightforward review and discussion of findings from the literature on otolaryngologic diagnostic and utilization patterns of older populations. It quickly became apparent that the supposed literature is almost nonexistent. A review conducted through a National Library of Medicine MEDLARS bibliographic search revealed only a handful of articles published on this general subject during the past decade, and almost *none* that considered these issues for populations over 65. Despite much anecdotal evidence, apparently no systematic study has been undertaken to provide a picture of otolaryngology utilization in this segment of the population. Thus, it was decided to undertake an experiment in data linkage and analysis to determine the feasibility of addressing the research issues posed by this conference: presbycusis, disequilibrium, voice, smell, and taste, swallowing, plastic and reconstructive surgery, and so forth.

To that end, I am briefly going to present selected results of the linkage and analysis of six diverse data sources in an effort to demonstrate the vast and largely untapped potential of these resources in learning more about the older population and their experience with otolaryngology—its diagnoses and procedures (Table 3-3).

The analysis focuses on Major Diagnostic Category (MDC) 3, Diseases and Disorders of the Ear, Nose, and Throat, which are derived from aggregating the data for separate diagnosis-related groupings (DRGs) (ranging from DRG 49 to 74), themselves composed of more than 1,300 ICD-9-CM codes for a wide range of diagnoses and procedures.

The data reviewed for each of these sources were limited to only *populations over age 65* for each diagnosis or procedure considered. Further, except as noted, they focus primarily on inpatient utilization. As several others have suggested, many procedures are increasingly shifting to ambulatory settings, so these results likely represent only a partial picture for many of the procedures discussed.

The six data sources reviewed for this brief analysis included the following.

The National Hospital Discharge Survey (NHDS). Sponsored by the National Center for Health Statistics (NCHS) since 1965, this continuous voluntary survey of a national sample of general and specialty short-stay hospitals in the United States is based on discharge summaries from a sample of inpatient records (Table 3-4).

The Medicare Short-Stay Hospital Inpatient Record File. Sponsored by the Health Care Financing Administration (HCFA), this 20 percent sample inpatient stay record file yields information on the patient, the hospital, and the hospitalization (Table 3-5).

The Hospital Cost and Utilization Project (HCUP) Survey. Sponsored by the National Center for Health Services Research, this is a national sample survey that includes American Hospital Association (AHA) data on some 388 United States hospitals for the years 1980 to 1985 (Table 3-6). The sampled dimensions include geographic region, urban and rural differences, teaching status, bed size, and ownership.

The Supplement on Aging to the 1984 National Health Interview Survey (SOA—NHIS). Sponsored by the NCHS, this is a nationwide survey of the noninstitutionalized United States population (some 40,000 households) and provides reliable national estimates for people over age 65 for a variety of health and social characteristics (Table 3-7).

The National Ambulatory Medical Care Survey (NAMCS). Sponsored by the NCHS, this survey sampled over 5,000 nonfederal, office-based physicians in the United States, thus characterizing the physicians, patients, and visits (Table 3-8).

TABLE 3-3 Data Sources Reviewed, MDC 3*, Population >65 Years

National Hospital Discharge Survey
Medicare Short-Stay Hospital Inpatient Record File
Hospital Cost and Utilization Project Survey
National Health Interview Survey—Supplement on Aging
National Ambulatory Medical Care Survey
Baltimore Longitudinal Study on Aging

* DRG Major Diagnostic Category 3 = Diseases and Disorders of Ear, Nose, and Throat

TABLE 3-4 National Hospital Discharge Survey

National Center for Health Statistics
Continuous voluntary survey since 1965
National sample of United States short-stay general and specialty hospitals (194,800 records from 414 hospitals in 1985)
Discharge summaries of a sample of inpatient medical records

TABLE 3-5 Medicare Short-Stay Hospital Inpatient Record File

Health Care Financing Administration
20 percent inpatient stay record file yielding information on patient, hospital, and hospitalization
Combines utilization bill file, health insurance entitlement file, provider services file

TABLE 3-6 Hospital Cost and Utilization Project Survey

National Center for Health Services Research (NCHSR and HCTA)
Hospital data base includes AHA survey data on national sample of hospitals for 1980-1985
Probability of 2,018 hospitals; 388 in sample
Dimensions: geographic region, urban and rural, teaching status, bed size, ownership, extent of state regulation

TABLE 3-7 Supplement on Aging to the 1984 National Health Interview Survey

National Center for Health Statistics
Continuing nationwide survey of noninstitutionalized United States population (97% response rate from people in 40,000 households = 16,697 interviewed)
Reliable national estimates for people over age 65
Items comparable to many other surveys
Characterize health and social status of older population

TABLE 3-8 National Ambulatory Medical Care Survey

National Center for Health Statistics
In 1985, a sample of 5,032 nonfederal, office-based physicians in United States (71,594 patient records)
Physician, patient, visit characteristics

The Baltimore Longitudinal Study on Aging (BLSA). Sponsored by the Gerontology Research Center of the National Institute on Aging, this is a long-term panel study of over 1,000 male and female volunteers that seeks to differentiate between changes in the subjects owing to aging and those attributable to disease or environmental influences (Table 3-9).

RANK ORDER OF THE DIAGNOSIS-RELATED GROUPINGS

Several initial analyses were conducted to ascertain the extent of agreement, congruence, and communality among and between the several procedures and diagnoses for each data source. The level of agreement was found to be high (Table 3-10). For example, the National Hospital Discharge Survey ranked the top six procedures (those shown on the top half of the table), which, in this survey, accounted for 90 percent of the procedures in MDC 3. Similarly, the top seven diagnoses (shown in the lower half of the table) accounted for some 75 percent of all diagnoses in MDC 3 for the population over age 65. With reference to the Medicare short-stay hospital records, basically the same procedures and diagnoses were included in the top five in each category (Table 3-11). For the Hospital Cost and Utilization Project Survey, again the same procedures and diagnoses were ranked in the top five, in identical order to those of the Medicare file (Table 3-12).

The overall comparison is displayed in Table 3-13. The top five ranked diagnoses and procedures for all three data sources are largely in alignment. The identical alignment of the Medicare and HCUP files is apparent, while the third set, the NHDS, is strikingly similar, though not exact. It is of note that these two surveys and the 20 percent sample of Medicare records, while employing such different approaches and methodologies, yielded such similar initial results.

TABLE 3-9 Baltimore Longitudinal Study on Aging

Gerontology Research Center of the National Institute on Aging (NIA)
Long-term study of over 1,000 male and female volunteers
Differentiate between changes caused by aging and those attributable to disease or environmental influences

AVERAGE LENGTH OF STAY

Similar comparisons were carried out for a variety of characteristics such as average charges, total

TABLE 3-10 National Hospital Discharge Survey (MDC 3, >65 Years)

Rank	DRG	
Top six procedures (90%)		
1	53	Sinus and mastoid procedures
2	55	Miscellaneous ENT procedures
3	50	Sialoadenectomy
4	49	Major head and neck procedures
5	63	Other ENT surgical procedures
6	56	Rhinoplasty
Top seven diagnoses (75%)		
1	68	Otitis media and URI and/or CC
2	65	Dysequilibrium
3	64	ENT malignancy
4	73	Other ENT diagnoses
5	69	Otitis media and URI w/o CC
6	66	Epistaxis
7	72	Nasal trauma and deformity

ENT = ear, nose, and throat; URI = upper respiratory infection; CC = complication or comorbidity; w/o = without

TABLE 3-11 Medicare Short-Stay Hospital Record File (MDC 3, >65 Years)

Rank	DRG	
Top five procedures		
1	55	Miscellaneous ENT procedures
2	53	Sinus and mastoid procedures
3	50	Sialoadenectomy
4	49	Major head and neck procedures
5	63	Other ENT surgical procedures
Top five diagnoses		
1	65	Dysequilibrium
2	68	Otitis media and URI and/or CC
3	66	Epistaxis
4	73	Other ENT diagnoses
5	64	ENT malignancy

ENT = ear, nose, and throat; URI = upper respiratory infection; CC = complication or comorbidity

TABLE 3-12 Hospital Cost and Utilization Project Survey (MDC 3, >65 Years)

Rank	DRG	
Top five procedures		
1	55	Miscellaneous ENT procedures
2	53	Sinus and mastoid procedures
3	50	Sialoadenectomy
4	49	Major head and neck procedures
5	63	Other ENT surgical procedures
Top five diagnoses (65%)		
1	65	Dysequilibrium
2	68	Otitis media and URI and/or CC
3	66	Epistaxis
4	73	Other ENT diagnoses
5	64	ENT malignancy

ENT = ear, nose, and throat; URI = upper respiratory infection; CC = complication or comorbidity

TABLE 3-13 Comparison of Data Sources by Leading DRGs (MDC 3, > 65 Years)

Rank	DRG		
	Medicare (HCFA)	NHDS (NCHS)	HCUP (NCHSR)
Diagnoses			
1	65	68	65
2	68	65	68
3	66	64	66
4	73	73	73
5	64	69	64
Procedures			
1	55	53	55
2	53	55	53
3	50	50	50
4	49	49	49
5	63	63	63

days of hospitalization, and number of discharges. Table 3-14 shows the average length of a patient hospital stay (ALOS) for each of the top five DRGs. As can be seen, for two data sets for which this characteristic was compared, the Medicare sample and the National Hospital Discharge Survey, the lengths of stay, particularly for diagnoses, are quite similar. While there is some overlap in the hospitals from which the data are drawn, the general trend and comparability of the findings are noteworthy.

TRACKING SPECIFIC DIAGNOSIS

Another approach taken to exploit the possibilities afforded by the data sets was to track findings for several of the specific dimensions of geriatric otolaryngology examined by the conference. From

TABLE 3-14 Comparison of Data Sources for Top Five DRGs, Average Length of Stay (MDC 3, >65 Years)

	DRG	Medicare	NHDS
Diagnoses			
64	ENT malignancy	8.4	11.8
65	Dysequilibrium	4.3	4.4
66	Epistaxis	4.4	4.1
68	Otitis media and URI and/or CC	5.9	5.8
69	Otitis media and URI w/o CC	4.4	4.1
Procedures			
49	Major head and neck procedures	16.9	24.7
50	Sialoadenectomy	3.7	7.2
53	Sinus and mastoid procedures	3.5	4.7
55	Miscellaneous ENT procedures	2.6	2.8
63	Other ENT surgical procedures	7.7	6.7

ENT = ear, nose, and throat; URI = upper respiratory infection; CC = complication or comorbidity

the eight separate issues, all of which offered extensive opportunities for indepth analysis, I will present only the findings for "dysequilibrium" as an example. The diagnosis of dysequilibrium, DRG 65, includes 28 ICD-9-CM codes including dizziness. You will recall that dysequilibrium was the first or second most common diagnosis in each of the short-stay hospital data sets, and it accounted for, on average, some 4.3 days of care. To demonstrate further the potential of data linkage and the relationship of a symptom of relevance to a major health problem for older persons, the National Health Interview Survey Supplement on Aging, which includes a section on "conditions and impairments," was reviewed. The SOA contains specific questions on a topic of continuing concern—falls (Table 3-15). Falls occur at a high rate in the population over 65. As a result, each year approximately 200,000 elderly Americans break a hip, mostly as a result of a fall. Of those 200,000, some 15 percent die of complications from the injury.[7] Many others become disabled for a prolonged period of time or permanently. The SOA to the NHIS reveals that over 18 percent of persons over age 65 and over 25 percent of those over 75 have fallen in the past year. Related to the question of dizziness, in response to the question, "Did you fall because you felt dizzy?", 15 to 23 percent responded, "Yes." And beyond the question of falls, in response to the general question, "Does dizziness prevent you from doing things you otherwise could do?", a startling 34 percent of those 65 to 74 years of age and over 37 percent of those over age 75 answered in the affirmative. That is an estimated total of some 12,500,000 persons over age 65 in this country for whom dizziness appears to represent a significant deterrent to their normal pursuits.

Finally, in confirmation of this pervasive problem, the National Ambulatory Medical Care Survey offers the following finding: of the 25 symptoms most frequently presented at visits for patients older than 75 years of age (some 82 million visits for the 1 year survey period) the top ranked symptom was dizziness.[8] It was mentioned over 38 times

TABLE 3-15 National Health Interview Survey Supplement on Aging

Answered "Yes" to Question	Ages		Total
	65 to 74	>75	
Have you fallen in the past 12 months?	18%	25%	21.5%
Did you fall because you felt dizzy?	15%	23%	19%
Does dizziness prevent you you from doing things you otherwise could do?	34.4%	37.3%	35.7%

per each 1,000 visits. It was followed by vision dysfunctions, back pains, and leg pain all the way down to skin irritation at number 25. For further research, it is noteworthy that the symptom "dizziness" does not permit easy linkage to diagnosis as might be the case for most of the other symptoms on the list. Transient cerebral ischemias, for example, were associated with fewer than 5 percent of dizziness visits. An obvious area for further research is the possible interaction and effect of the multiple drugs often administered to older persons. Indeed, overall one is struck by the multifactorial, interrelated nature of disease and disability in older populations, a phenomenon clearly requiring further analysis (and one not limited to DRG 49-74).

CONCLUSION

The brief epidemiologic exploration has demonstrated that record linkage to explicate otolaryngologic issues is entirely feasible. Coupled with the demographic imperatives described earlier, which revealed that the 12 percent of our population over age 65 currently accounts for over a third of the use of physician time, 25 percent of medications, and 40 percent of hospital admissions, the *quality* of medical care for this segment of the population will be of ever increasing concern.

Quality of care assessment is being undertaken whether or not refinements in methods or the accuracy of data bases keeps pace. Clinical impression is being replaced by cynical reexamination. Recently published and hotly contested comparisons of hospital mortality rates by Medicare and Medicaid (HCFA) are soon to be followed by a consumer guide to the nation's 16,000 nursing homes. Consumers, the Congress, and special task forces will continue to focus on the quality of care given to older persons. Indeed, it is to be noted that during the recent debate on legislative changes affecting Peer Review Organizations (PROs), among those most closely involved were the Congressional Special Committees on Aging. Individual practitioners, the several separate disciplines, and the American Academy of Otolaryngology—Head and Neck Surgery have, through this conference, recognized the importance of these issues. In the *Handbook of the Biology of Aging,* Brody and Brock have set the challenge:

"...with such data in hand, one can start making some of the critical associations that would almost surely be highly insightful and beneficial to the individual and to society. In the short run, we cannot afford to deny the physician and his patient access to... health information. In the longer run, we cannot deny these data to researchers."[9]

Clearly, opportunities for research in this area abound. This presentation has demonstrated that there are many data sources (and resources) that lend themselves well to learning more about the otolaryngologic needs of older persons.

Among the charges developed for the Academy's new Committee on Geriatric Otolaryngology was the following: "Compile and maintain data concerning the otolaryngic needs of the geriatric population." It appears that with a reasonable effort this charge can be met.

References

1. Finch CE, Schneider EL, eds. Handbook of the biology of aging. 2nd ed. New York: Van Nostrand Reinhold Co., 1985:3.
2. National Institutes of Health, U.S. Public Health Service. Report on hearing, voice and swallowing disorders in aging. Bethesda, MD: U.S. Department of Health and Human Services.
3. National Center for Health Statistics. Collins JG. Prevalence of selected chronic conditions, United States, 1979-1981. Vital and Health Statistics. Series 10, No. 155. OHHS Pub. No. (PHS) 86-1583. Public Health Service. Washington: U.S. Government Printing Office, July 1986.
4. National Center for Health Statistics. Dawson D, Hendershot G, Fulton J. Aging in the eighties, functional limitations of individuals age 65 years and over. Advance data From Vital and Health Statistics. No. 133. DHHS Pub. No. (PHS) 87-1250. Hyattsville, MD: Public Health Service, June 10, 1987.
5. National Center for Health Statistics. Havlik RJ. Aging in the eighties, impaired senses for sound and light in persons age 65 years and over. Preliminary data from the Supplement on Aging to the National Health Interview Survey, United States, January-June 1984. Advance data from Vital and Health Statistics. No. 125. DHHS Pub. No. (PHS) 86-1250. Hyattsville, MD: Public Health Service, Sept. 19, 1986.
6. National Institute on Aging. Personnel for health needs of the elderly through the year 2020. Bethesda, MD: Public Health Service, U.S. Department of Health and Human Services.
7. National Center for Health Statistics. Havlik RJ, Liu BM, Kovar MG, et al. Health statistics on older persons, United States 1986. Vital and Health Statistics. Series 3, No. 25. Pub. No. (PHS) 87-1409. Washington, D.C.: U.S. Government Printing Office, June 1987:66.
8. National Center for Health Statistics. Koch H, Smith MC. Office-based ambulatory care for patients 75 years old and over, National Ambulatory Medical Care Survey, 1980 and 1981. Advance data from Vital and Health Statistics. No. 110. DHHS Pub. No. (PHS) 85-1250. Hyattsville, MD: Public Health Service, Aug. 21, 1985.
9. Finch CE, Schneider EL, eds. Handbook of the biology of aging. 2nd ed. New York: Van Nostrand Reinhold Co., 1985:3-25.

Chapter Four

HEARING, VOICE, AND SWALLOWING DISORDERS IN AGING: A REPORT TO CONGRESS

ANDREW A. MONJAN, Ph.D., M.P.H.
LEONARD F. JAKUBCZAK, Ph.D.

About 2 years ago, Congress asked the National Institute on Aging (NIA) to report on what the National Institutes of Health (NIH) is doing in the support of research in hearing, voice, and swallowing disorders among the elderly. This report was a collaborative effort by staff from the NIA, the National Institute of Neurological and Communicative Disorders and Stroke (NINCDS), and the National Institute of Dental Research (NIDR). Segments from that report are presented here.

BACKGROUND

At present, it is estimated that over 20 million persons in this country have some degree of hearing impairment. The National Health Interview Survey of 1984 found that, among noninstitutionalized men and women aged 65 years and older, 9.2 million reported hearing problems. This survey did not include the estimated 5 percent of elderly in nursing homes, of whom about 50 percent have hearing difficulties. Thus, hearing losses associated with the process of aging (termed presbycusis) affect over a third of the elderly population in this country. In other terms, approximately 30 percent of adults aged 65 through 74 years and more than 50 percent of those over age 75 bear some degree of hearing loss.

Similar national data do not exist for voice and swallowing difficulties in the elderly. Such problems can appear secondary to neurodegenerative diseases and cancers that occur more frequently among the aged. Although there is a clinical impression of an increased incidence of serious voice and swallowing disorders among aged persons, especially those in nursing homes, it is unclear whether such problems are normal age-related changes or whether they reflect diseases or iatrogenic causes (e.g., medications, surgical procedures) that also occur with increased frequency in older populations. Inadequate salivary gland performance can result in marked oropharyngeal swallowing difficulties. The best known pathologic entity associated with salivary dysfunctions is Sjögren's syndrome, an autoimmune disease of the exocrine glands. In the United States, this condition affects an estimated 4 million persons, almost all of whom are postmenopausal women. Furthermore, over 400 common medications, including diuretics, antihypertensives, antidepressants, and antihistamines, are considered to affect salivary function. It is estimated that 25 percent of persons aged 65 years or older are taking one or more of such medications.

NATIONAL INSTITUTE ON AGING

Extramural scientists supported by the NIA are investigating a variety of behavioral, anatomical, electrophysiologic, and biochemical changes of the auditory system that occur during normal aging and are studying the potential of the aging nervous system to compensate for these changes. From this research, we will learn how the auditory system ages, what is to be expected as normal hearing and speech perception, and where interventions can be applied to correct age-related deficits.

What are the structural changes that occur with age? NIA-supported studies in rats have shown specific age-related changes along the auditory pathway. At the periphery, there are losses of auditory hair cells in the ear. Within the lower brain, it appears that the numbers of auditory cells are not reduced. Rather, there is a reduction in the number of contacts between cells. Thus, aging results in a reduced ability of cells to communicate with each other in these brain areas. Researchers are now studying higher brain areas in the auditory pathway to see if these phenomena exist at these levels. Such changes may be the basis for the impaired speech perception and the interference of auditory processing introduced by other noise sources that commonly are observed in the elderly. Studies similar to those done on rodents are beginning to be performed on aging monkeys in which the anatomy and physiology more closely approximate those of elderly humans. To facilitate such research, the NIA is assisting investigators in the maintenance of colonies of aged primates.

NIA-funded scientists also are studying hearing losses in elderly humans. One such project is a multidisciplinary study of auditory processing problems in the elderly, involving neuropsychology, neurology, audiology, and otolaryngology. The aim is to determine whether the auditory processing problems of the elderly are primarily a manifestation of an auditory-specific disorder, a broader cognitive disorder, or a complex disorder involving interactive senescent changes in both the auditory and cognitive domains. This project should lead to a better characterization of the various contributing factors in presbycusis. We may be able to define the precise ways in which cognitive factors are linked to specific variations in the auditory processing abilities of the elderly. Understanding the relation between auditory and cognitive factors may provide important information for rehabilitation and for hearing aid prescription.

As part of the NIA's Small Business Innovative Research (SBIR) program, an electronic means of transmitting several channels of information through a single electrode that would be implanted in the ear is being developed. This could lead to a new generation of hearing aids. Another SBIR investigator has developed and field tested a high resolution tactile aid for the deaf and the deaf-blind. It is ready for mass production by the private sector.

NATIONAL INSTITUTE OF NEUROLOGICAL AND COMMUNICATIVE DISORDERS AND STROKE

Neuroscientists supported by the NINCDS are studying normal and abnormal conditions of the ear, larynx, swallowing mechanisms, and central nervous system in the aging population.

Studies on the effects of aging on communication are concerned with otologic, epidemiologic, audiologic, neurophysiologic, morphologic, histochemical, and laryngologic aspects of age-related communication disorders, chiefly clinical hearing and laryngeal dysfunctions in the elderly. From this research we hope to better understand the pathophysiology of these disorders, develop new diagnostic tests, establish better defined hypotheses for future studies, and thus add to our ability to prevent, modify, and eventually treat age-related communication dysfunction.

An NINCDS study underway will assess speech perception difficulties experienced by elderly and hearing-impaired listeners because of environmental reverberations in a variety of settings. Information gained can be used in counseling, auditory rehabilitation, and the development of clinical procedures. Other studies on hearing loss and speech perception are examining the listener's age as a factor in hearing impairment and the dynamics of speech recognition.

One of the most ambitious aids to hearing is the cochlear implant for the sensory deaf. The implant uses tiny electrodes to apply electrical stimulation to auditory nerve fibers. Two different cochlear implants were given premarket approval by the Food and Drug Administration and are now available to the deaf. These implants utilized research results and technology developed by the NINCDS neural prostheses program.

Recognition of speech has been achieved by the profoundly deaf by using electronic cochlear implants. Speech recognition is an important step toward hearing of conversational speech. A clinical comparison of single and multichannel electronic cochlear implants for the deaf will provide information concerning the optimum design of implants as well as information on the types of persons who can benefit from the use of these devices.

Voice disorders become more frequent with aging. Voice loss can occur for many reasons, including the removal of the larynx or radiotherapy to treat cancer of the larynx. With aging, muscle tremor may affect the larynx, thus resulting in a weak, tremorous voice that is difficult for others to hear. The loudness of voice may also be reduced because of structural changes that occur in the larynx with aging. Cartilage may shrink in size, the lubricating cells of the mucosa can become dry, and muscle strength may be reduced. These changes can alter the delicate vibratory mechanism of the larynx. The voice may also be affected by almost all of the degenerative neurologic disorders, thereby leaving people speechless at the same time that they become physically disabled and dependent on others. Diseases such as Parkinson's disease, Huntington's disease, and amyotrophic lateral sclerosis, although not limited to the aged, can have a particularly devastating effect on the voice. All of these disorders affect swallowing and thus rob people of both speech and eating functions in their later years. NINCDS research in voice disorders is aimed at several aspects of these problems of the elderly.

The morphologic changes in the larynx with aging and, in particular, alterations in tissue tension, pliability, muscle contractions and the mucosa are being quantified. How these tissue changes affect voice production in older people is now better understood. Change in respiratory function in the aged also alters voice production. NINCDS research is addressing the critical need of the aged to produce vocal sounds despite reduced lung capacity.

NATIONAL INSTITUTE ON DENTAL RESEARCH

NIDR intramural scientists, in collaboration with their colleagues from the NIA and the Department of Rehabilitative Medicine at the NIH Clinical Center, are among the few in this country investigating normal age-related changes in swallowing and voice as well as changes occurring secondary to pathology or to its treatment. These workers have focused on the oropharyngeal phase of swallowing. They pioneered the use of ultrasonic imaging to visualize tongue function during swallowing and clearly established the importance of oropharyngeal disturbances to the swallowing process. In addition, for the first time they have been able to show that alterations in salivary secretion, resulting from a number of pathologic or iatrogenic situations, lead to persistent disturbances of tongue movement during swallowing and an increased prevalence of clinical complaints among patients.

NIDR also funds a considerable extramural effort on salivary gland function and its effects on alimentary events. As noted, factors affecting saliva production directly affect the swallowing process. By using a noninvasive ultrasound imaging technique, scientists have compared tongue motion at rest and during speech production in normal older and younger adults. Although the older persons showed a significant diminution of tongue thickness during rest and changes in tongue movement during the production of certain phonemes, these changes do not appear to be of biologic significance. Healthy older persons are as capable of 'normal' speech production as are young persons.

SCIENTIFIC OPPORTUNITIES AND RESEARCH MANPOWER REQUIREMENTS

From data now available, it appears that the core problem with hearing in the aged lies more in the central than in the peripheral nervous system; it is a problem of speech intelligibility as well as of amplification. This requires new approaches to the design of prosthetic devices for hearing. There is a need for good epidemiologic data on impaired hearing and on the types of impaired hearing that develop during the aging process. There appears to be a total lack of such epidemiologic data for problems of voice and of swallowing in the elderly. While speech and swallowing changes associated with aging are not perceived as problems by the healthy elderly or their physicians, there is a need for good descriptive studies to establish the normal limits of oropharyngeal dynamics in the aged. In the absence of disease, there may be changes in oropharyngeal function that have impact on quality of life issues. These data are needed in order to estimate the magnitude of the effect of such disorders on this nation's public health as well as to link them as secondary to disease process or as manifestations of normal aging. There is the need for the continuance of basic studies in neuroscience in order to understand the control of sensory functions and cognitive processes and their underlying physiologic properties in the elderly so that normal aging can be better understood.

Critical to any expansion of this research endeavor is the recruitment of qualified investigators. There is a need for the appropriate professional clinical organizations to stimulate the development of a specialty of geriatric otolaryngology because there is a profound lack of such expertise at present. Mechanisms for training qualified clinicians to become researchers now exist, e.g., Physician Scientist Award and Clinical Investigator Award. The availability of these training opportunities needs to be made known to potential clinical researchers by their professional societies and by NIH.

The NIH will continue to encourage and to support fundamental and clinical research on the causes, the pathophysiology, and the treatment of dysfunction related to hearing, voice, and swallowing, three functions that frequently affect the elderly population. Research training in the neurosciences that focuses on otolaryngology, otopathology, audiology, and speech pathology should ensure continuing advances in these critical areas of investigation.

Chapter Five

SPEECH UNDERSTANDING AND AGING

JERRY V. TOBIAS, Ph.D., F.A.S.H.A., F.A.S.A.

Much of what I have to say here derives from the work of the National Academy of Sciences/National Research Council Working Group on Speech Understanding and Aging that was sponsored by the National Institute on Aging and that I chaired.[1] The report is long but worth reading, I think.

With the limited amount of space I have available, I will only be able to touch on a few of the Working Group's conclusions. Let me do that by selecting some of the kinds of problems that we thought were important and by working through some of the related issues that we felt were in need of new or expanded research. I am sure you will be struck, as we were, with the scientific community's current ignorance about a widely prevalent and highly important aspect of adult life.

Hearing problems increase with age; the person who invented the word "presbycusis" recognized that fact and people are getting older. This increase in age means that more and more people will have trouble with their hearing—especially with their hearing for speech.

Speech is the most important kind of sound that we listen to, and disruptions of the ability to understand speech can have tremendous consequences. We have all seen people whose hearing losses are far more handicapping than their audiometric findings might predict. These folks retire from work that they used to enjoy; they withdraw from social situations, especially ones that involve groups of people; they mistreat their friends and families; they separate themselves from the things that once pleased them; and they end up isolated, hostile, and lonely. The solitude that they have thrust upon them, or that they thrust upon themselves, is probably the most devastating result of their hearing loss.

Two of the things that led the National Institute on Aging to sponsor the Working Group's activities were (1) these serious consequences of hearing loss, especially for an aging population, and (2) the Institute's wish to sponsor research that will provide scientific explanations for the large number of questions about which we currently have mostly anecdotal answers. For so widespread a problem, we have a remarkably small number of controlled experiments and a concomitantly small amount of useful data.

In fact, we do not even have a standard vocabulary. Clinicians and researchers all recognize that comprehending what we hear is the important issue. But when we talk and write about comprehension, we use a number of not-quite-accurate terms; most commonly we call it "speech discrimination" or "speech intelligibility," but both of those expressions have special technical meanings that are different from the meanings we usually intend to convey. The first thing the Working Group did was to settle on a phrase that is hard to misinterpret: we called the process "speech understanding," and we hope that the usage will be widely adopted.

Now let me get to the specifics. As I discuss the background, it might seem as if the difficulties are insurmountable, but the truth is that, although the number of things that we do not know is large, most of the interesting questions are answerable. Still better, several recommended kinds of work are likely to lead to important and early payoffs. For example, whether we understand the link between hearing loss and age or not, it is still obvious that we can reduce the number of affected older individuals by improving hearing conversation among the younger population. So please do not feel totally pessimistic while I am summarizing knowledge gaps.

The topics that are most significant to speech understanding and aging can be organized into five major categories: (1) anatomy and physiology, (2) audiologic measurement, (3) noisy and degraded speech, (4) language and cognition, and (5) sensory aids. In each area, we know a good deal about the underlying science and about applications of that science to young normal listeners and to some listeners with auditory pathologies. But, when we look for a connection between those data and the aging population, the link is hard to find. As often as not, experiments that show a relation between age and hearing loss are countered by equally well-done experiments that show no relation. With that in mind, let me take the topics one at a time. I cannot cover them exhaustively here, so instead I will stress the parts that intrigue me the most.

ANATOMY AND PHYSIOLOGY

We do not know very much about the aging of physiological systems in general, and we know even less about the aging of auditory systems. If you decide to work in this area and try to correlate changes in the ear with general physiological age, you will discover—if you do not already know—that physiological age is poorly defined. To complicate your task even more, published studies of aging auditory systems are few and are limited in their applicability: only a few subjects, animal or human, have been examined, experimental techniques and designs have sometimes been flawed, auditory and neurological histories are commonly sketchy, and broad representative samples of ages and pathologies have not been included. It is uncomfortable to admit, but the fact is that the few things that we know—or believe that we know—are not well demonstrated.

If we want to improve our ability to differentiate the effects of trauma, of disease, of wear and tear, and of time-related or age-related degeneration, we need well-designed studies that use a wide spectrum of patients with a wide spectrum of diagnoses. If we want to estimate the physiological age of an auditory system, we need studies that include accurate evaluation of medical, genetic, social, and audiological factors, not at all an easy set of jobs to do successfully with the tools we have available today. For instance, we know that the handicap that results from poor speech understanding does not correlate highly with current tests of hearing for pure tones or of understanding of isolated words. Even when the results from pure-tone and word tests are combined, the correlation with handicap is poor. Therefore, audiological measurement cannot be limited to tone and word tests. However, suitable additions to the audiological armamentarium are only beginning to appear.

If we are to have a chance to expand the collection of facts on which we base our decisions about which anatomical and physiological changes are associated with aging and about whether and how much a particular set of changes is involved in a specific case, we need to expand the available data base. We need to develop and support colonies of animals selected to provide good models for the determination of auditory aging effects. We have to expand or build brain and temporal bone laboratories and give appropriately trained investigators enough support to keep them in those laboratories.

Similarly, the National Institute on Aging's Longitudinal Aging Program can contribute valuable information by routinely giving auditory tests to participants. We would gain even more important information if a significant proportion of those subjects permitted brain and temporal bone studies to be made after their deaths.

The Working Group concluded its discussion of anatomy and physiology with a list of answerable questions. Of course, some of them are easier to answer than others. Let me plagiarize those questions here:

1. How can we measure the physiological age of an auditory system?
2. How does the physiological age of the auditory system correlate with the physiological age of other organ systems?
3. Does neural damage increase with age?
4. How does audiological function correlate with neural structure?

Sometimes it is hard to remember, but we do not have adequate answers to any of these questions.

AUDIOLOGIC MEASUREMENT

Everyone who works with older people's hearing knows some of the methodological problems that interfere with getting clear answers to both clinical and laboratory questions. A major source of confusion has been the preponderance of studies that lump together heterogeneous groups of subjects for statistical analysis. This mixing of diagnoses, ages, and hearing losses disguises measurable features that may distinguish one pathology from another. A particularly useful early improvement in research methodology would be for scientists to look at pertinent subgroups of subjects separately—for example, people whose hearing losses are comparable or whose etiologies are similar. Pregrouping subjects would help to reveal the audiological characteristics that similar patients share.

Another typical methodological problem arises because data from tests of central auditory abilities are often contaminated by the patient's having problems that originate in the auditory periphery. Cochlear phenomena certainly affect test results, so if we want to make accurate tests of central auditory abilities, we need enough information about peripheral abilities to let us separate out the noncentral components. We have to conduct large scale studies of the influence of such factors as audiometric configuration, critical bandwidth, degree of hearing loss, and etiology of the loss. Once again, it is clear that audiometric tests of pure-tone sensitivity and word recognition are inadequate to measure hearing handicap, but a completely effective test battery has yet to be devised.

Here are some specific questions that the Working Group raised about measurement. Again, you will notice that they covered much more territory than I have been able to here. Please do read their full report.

1. How do subjects with related pathologies differ audiologically from other subjects?
2. What conductive hearing problems (such as canal collapse) affect the aged and to what degree?
3. How do medication and diet contribute to the decrement in auditory sensitivity seen in older patients?
4. Does the disparity between predicted and obtained speech understanding scores for the aging listener result simply from the statistical problem of predicting percentages of words understood from decibels of hearing loss or does it really represent a complex speech understanding problem?
5. How do identification and comprehension of speech signals vary with age and peripheral hearing loss?

NOISY AND DEGRADED SPEECH

Hearing-impaired subjects' auditory performance is below normal in the quiet listening conditions in which we normally measure hearing. It is reasonable to suppose that their hearing is even worse when the signal is partially masked and noise seems to make a bigger difference to old listeners than to young ones. Although young and old subjects show no measurable differences in the criteria on which they base their responses, younger listeners nevertheless judge their ability to understand noisy speech more accurately. Age-related changes in auditory processing, cognition, and attitude must account for the distinction, but so far the causes are obscure.

A particularly interesting aspect of speech degradation is only beginning to be recognized: the kind of sound we have always thought of as noise is just one of a variety of signal imperfections whose presence leads to deterioration in speech understanding. Reverberation, for example, is a common source of problems, but most masking research has been on noisy, not reverberating speech.

An even more fascinating set of problems originates in modern technology. We see new degradations to speech signals every day. Synthetic speech is becoming common. Television programs are being speeded up to meet time constraints. Speech signal redundancy is being reduced in a number of ways, which results in speech understanding getting harder for people who have a hard time anyway.

More and more frequently, we find speech that is being degraded in several ways simultaneously. We have a lot to learn about the relations among noise, temporal resolution, reverberation, and speech understanding.

Here are some specific research questions that the Working Group raised about degraded speech.

1. How does age affect the understanding of words heard in noise?
2. What proportion of the performance decrement that occurs when older listeners listen to noisy speech is attributable to masking and what proportion is attributable to other factors?
3. Are listeners with sensorineural losses affected by noise differently than are listeners with normal hearing?
4. How does reverberation affect speech understanding?
5. How do high frequency hearing loss and aging affect speeded-speech understanding?
6. What perceptual and cognitive problems do elderly individuals experience in trying to understand synthetic speech?
7. When several kinds of speech degradation arise at once, are the performance decrements additive?

LANGUAGE AND COGNITION

If you fail persistently to understand what is being said around you, you feel frustrated and discouraged. Those feelings in turn can lead to less aggressive listening and to a sense of resignation that can be truly handicapping. Such changes in listening strategy certainly do not represent aspects of auditory pathology in the usual sense, but they affect speech understanding just as surely as inner ear damage does.

The recent literature is filled with speculation about age-related slowing in mental activity and age-related deterioration in attention span. But we do not know whether or how much those sorts of cognitive changes influence speech understanding in quiet listening conditions. However, if you think about your own comprehension problems when you try to listen to a foreign speaker in noisy surroundings, you will recognize that slower mental activity, from whatever cause, can affect responses to speech under difficult listening conditions. Again, though, we have only limited research data to help to quantify the effects.

One positive sign is that people do not have to understand every word they hear except in clinical tests. In the real world, getting the gist of a message is enough to lead to an appropriate response. As the cognitive psychologists would say, we need analytic studies of language understanding that build not on word comprehension but on discourse comprehension.

Here are some specific research questions that the Working Group raised about language and cognition.

1. How does reduced working-memory capacity or mental slowing affect speech understanding as one grows older?
2. How do relative contributions of cognitive and sensory processes vary with age, hearing loss, and listening conditions?
3. Why does the ability to draw inferences that require the integration of new facts decline in old age when generic knowledge from semantic memory does not?
4. Does a listener's attitude regarding his or her hearing impairment affect communication success?

SENSORY AIDS

The invention of smart filters that adapt their characteristics to the noisiness of the signals that pass through them is leading to an exciting growth in digital hearing aid technology. We do not know yet whether adaptive filters actually improve speech understanding or only improve the perceived quality of the sound. However, if they only make listeners less negative about the sound that comes through their hearing aids, the filters are valuable.

New approaches to compression amplification can also increase the use of aids and may improve the understandability of the speech that comes through them.

Hearing aids are not the only technological means available today for assisting a depleted sensory system and increasing communication. Some obvious examples include cochlear implants, vibrotactile stimulators, teletypes, computer networks, closed-caption television, and the infrared transmitters that people can use in theaters and, in home versions, with television sets. All are being used to apparent advantage by sizable groups of people, but hardly any have received the kinds of comparative-value studies that would help an older person to make prudent decisions about which to select for himself or herself.

This topic, like the others, merits extended discussion, but my space is limited, so here are the specific research questions that the Working Group raised about sensory aids.

1. How are implants better than vibrators and how are vibrators better than implants?
2. How should compression amplification be used in hearing aids?
3. What kinds of computer networks would be most helpful and advantageous for the aging population?
4. Do digital hearing aids offer real improvement in speech understanding, do they improve the perceived quality of speech and thus increase the user's motivation to listen closely, or do they have no measurable effect at all?

CONCLUSION

I have only touched the edges of a few of the issues that the National Institute on Aging wants us all to learn more about. Your interest in the communication problems of the elderly should lead you to read the Working Group's full report and, for those with research training, time, and inclination, to help solve some of the mysteries.

Reference

1. Tobias JV, Bilger RC, Brody H, Gates GA, Haskell GB, Howard DV, Marshall LA, Nerbonne MA, Pickett JM. Speech understanding and aging. J Acoust Soc Am 1988; 83:859–895.

Chapter Six

MEDICAL/SURGICAL CARE: SHOULD AGE BE A VARIABLE?

RUE MOORE, A.B., M.Div.

Change is so common in the lives of a goodly number of people that it goes unnoticed. The usual exception, however, is that of the passing of time, called aging. In the early years of a person's life, there is much made of every little change, real or thought to be real, that is observed by those who have a vested interest in that which is called progress or the lack thereof. As time goes on and change continues at the normal or expected rate, less is made of the obvious.

Nevertheless, there does come a time when a person acknowledges that he is aged; the health care deliverers refer to him as a "geriatric patient." There is no universal accord as to when a person becomes aged and, therefore, a geriatric patient, nor is there agreement as to when it is proper to use either term. Both are labels, either self- or superimposed. There is agreement, though, that there is such a thing as aging, being old, and being cared for as such.

Present company excluded, if one is capable of seeing, hearing, or understanding, it is impossible to avoid the subject, irrespective of the source. Aging has become a topic of daily concern just shy of obsession in almost all forms of medium. This does not mean that the subject is a nonissue. It is a phenomenon that will not go away, and it requires the attention of the best thoughts and efforts that our society can produce to achieve a solution that is compassionate, equitable, and just.

At any given time in the life of a person, there are a number of choices and options that the individual can exercise. These are limited not only because the person is finite, but they vary with age, sex, geopolitical situation, and physical and mental condition.

The province of medicine is the care and cure of persons who are sick. As such, it is the business of intervening in the lives of those who seek relief from the sufferings and discomforts they experience. It is a work that is contranature. The interventions are made to correct or modify the "natural," which has been deemed undesirable by the person in whom such a process is occurring, and to maintain as many of the options or choices that one expects the person to have, given the age and the malady.

In the Western tradition of medicine, derived for the most part from the school of Hippocrates, the focus is on maintaining the health and well-being of the individual. The classic expression is, of course, "at least do no harm." A more recent expression derives from the Utilitarian philosophers' dictum to maximize the good and minimize the bad. Put in a different way: "In an ideal world we are morally required to choose the best of the goods. In the real world of clinical medicine we are morally required to choose the least of the evils." In the language of medicine this is the "risk-benefit calculus." Or to rephrase: "What are the short- and long-range consequences of the action proposed to be done to the patient?"

The work of medicine and/or surgery begins when a person presents himself or herself to a physician and is accepted as a patient. You are altogether familiar with what follows. Of prime concern is that which occurs after the diagnosis has been made—the information given to the patient and the patient's response.

Where the event occurs matters little. It is a given that the patient is stressed and very much interested to learn what the doctor has to say. The manner and the content of the telling, neither of which should be underestimated, determine the reactions of the patient. The manner is assumed to be always calm, compassionate, and empathic. The content can and does cover the range. It can be "good," in between, or "grim." In similar fashion, the reaction of the patient correlates with the prognosis and ranges from relief to despair.

There have been many well-conducted studies published in both lay and professional literature on the subject of what patients remember that their physicians said. The process is called 'selective perception'. It means that one hears what one wants to hear of what is said. Another process occurs that I call 'selective deception'. This has not been studied, but has been observed. Selective deception means that others hear what we want them to hear. Techniques employed in selective deception include some or all of the following: evading the subject, withholding information, obscuring the issue, using jargon, and misusing terms and names of objects.

Both selective perception and selective deception are used at times by some patients and some physicians. This should not be taken to mean that either party employs selection out of malice. Probably, given the setting, it is a function of the time spent during the communication. Further, there are no formal tests given that would determine whether or not the information given is understood, even though there usually is an opportunity given for the asking of questions. Parenthetically, one of the most frequent questions is, "What are my chances?" The usual answer is, "Well, 70 percent of the patients with your problem do well!" The real question was, "Will I live or die?" It was not answered, nor could it be. The percentage was for the universe and not for the individual. The patient wanted to know what was going to happen to *him*.

Germane to this discussion is the notion of autonomy. Autonomy is considered to be a cardinal right by most ethicists. It is a right that is not to be compromised, all things being equal, without grave reasons. In short, a person may determine his own fate insofar as he does not affect another's autonomy. However, a person may ask another to act for or upon him, given that the action is in the best interest of the one making the request and does not adversely affect the autonomy of the other. Two additional and related notions to autonomy are as follows. First is that which is called either "heroic" or "extraordinary" measures, from the patient's perspective. The second is that which is referred to as "the quality of life."

By definition, heroic or extraordinary is that which is done to a process deemed undesirable by the person in whom it is occurring and/or by the health care provider and that does not arrest, reverse, remove, or retard the aforesaid process. It is not morally or ethically necessary to continue such activity. The phrase "quality of life" means those qualities of life that the individual values. When the individual declares that sufficient diminutions have occurred so that continuation of life is no longer acceptable, the person is saying that there is not quality of life left. In other words, "My life no longer has any meaning. At best I'm only existing."

There are some other everyday usages that need to be changed because they lead to popular and professional confusion. As an example, "treatment and/or therapy" means anything that is done that has utility and/or benefit. If there is no utility or benefit, the activity is not treatment or therapy—the use of the term "respirator" for the machine that is a ventilator; saying that one is giving a patient a blood thinner when one is actually giving a medication that is an anticoagulant; the maintenance of life by artificial or mechanical means. There is no difference in kind between an aspirin and a contact lens, neither of which is produced by the human body. In that sense, both are artificial and/or mechanical. The actual difference is that the aspirin is more frequently and familiarly used. The list could go on because many more confusing terms are used. The point that is being made is that careful and proper use of the language and the means of medicine is to be worked at in order that the doers and receivers of medical and surgical care understand themselves and each other.

All that has been said so far is applicable to a person of any age. The crucial word is *person*! At the risk of being repetitious, "medical and surgical care" is the work of dealing with persons who are in some sense "sick." (Physicians are not professionally concerned with nonpersons.) The term used for that work is called "clinical judgement." This is the direct equivalent of the legal expression "reasonable." From the stance of ethics, the use of clinical judgement is what is expected of physicians. It is ordinary and usual. It is dealing with the reality of the situation, which has been determined by the use of any tools that are called for to discover the state of the person/patient, and, in concert with the person/patient, determining what can and will be done. That this is a discrete art and science should be declared not to be so in an open and honest admission. In so doing, the manner used should be all that is perceived to be human.

In those sad and painful times when the prognosis is the opposite of good, the physician's task is extremely difficult. It requires the mustering of all the resources the deliverer of the news can utilize. That is the privilege of being a physician: the doing of good when possible, the avoidance of further harm when possible, the living with the unavoidable at all times.

This has not been an exercise in scolding. Rather, this effort, such as it is, has been made to commend all of you for all of the difficult and painful efforts that you have and will make in your dealings with the human condition. Further, it has been made to encourage you to continue in your work of focussing on the best interest of the person using the skills of your craft, without age being considered a valid variable.

# PRESBYASTASIS: THE DYSEQUILIBRIUM OF AGING

Chapter Seven

PATHOLOGY OF PRESBYCUSIS

HAROLD F. SCHUKNECHT, M.D.

The durability of the auditory system, like other organ systems, is determined in great part by genetic factors and by the physical stress to which it is subjected during a lifetime. Moscicki et al,[1] utilizing a population from the Framingham Heart Study Cohort, found that women had significantly better hearing than men at 2 kHz and above. A multivariate model showed that age, sex, illness, family history of hearing loss, Meniere's disease, and noise exposure were significant risk factors, with age being by far the most critical risk factor.

The cells of the auditory sense organ and the neural pathways are "nonmitotics." They are among the most highly differentiated cells in the body. After specialized function has been established for them, they cannot reproduce and therefore can pursue only the course of aging and dying.

We can currently identify three definite types of presbycusis based on the selective atrophy of different morphologic structures in the cochlea, and suggest a fourth hypothetical type that needs further elucidation (Table 7–1). These types may occur singly or in combination. When they occur in isolated form, each is manifested by a characteristic pattern of functional disturbance, which can be identified by medical history, otologic examination, and auditory testing. The hearing losses are symmetrical in the two ears and slowly progressive.

SENSORY PRESBYCUSIS

The sensory type of presbycusis is recognized clinically as a bilateral symmetrical high-tone hearing loss characterized by an abruptly sloping threshold pattern. The involved basal end of the cochlea shows loss of both hair cells and sustentacular cells. On a pathologic basis, however, the sensory lesions caused by this genetically modulated aging effect cannot be clearly differentiated from those changes that result from a lifetime of use and abuse of the cochlea. The cytohistograms of aged subjects with abrupt high-tone hearing losses suggest that acoustic trauma is an important etiologic component of this type of hearing loss (Fig. 7–1).[2] The capability for word discrimination is inversely related to the range of frequencies involved in the hearing loss.

NEURAL PRESBYCUSIS

Neural presbycusis may begin at any age, but there is little hearing disability until late in life when the population of neural units falls below that required for effective processing of acoustic information. In a previous study,[3] we counted the neurons in the cochleas of 100 hearing ears of subjects whose

TABLE 7–1 Types of Presbycusis

Type	Location in Cochlea	Audiometric Profile	
		Pure Tones	Discrimination
Sensory	Basal end	High-tone abrupt slope	Related to frequency range
Neural	All turns	All frequencies	Severe loss
Strial	Apical region	All frequencies	Minimal loss
Cochlear Conductive	All turns basal > apical	High-tone gradual slope	Related to steepness of slope

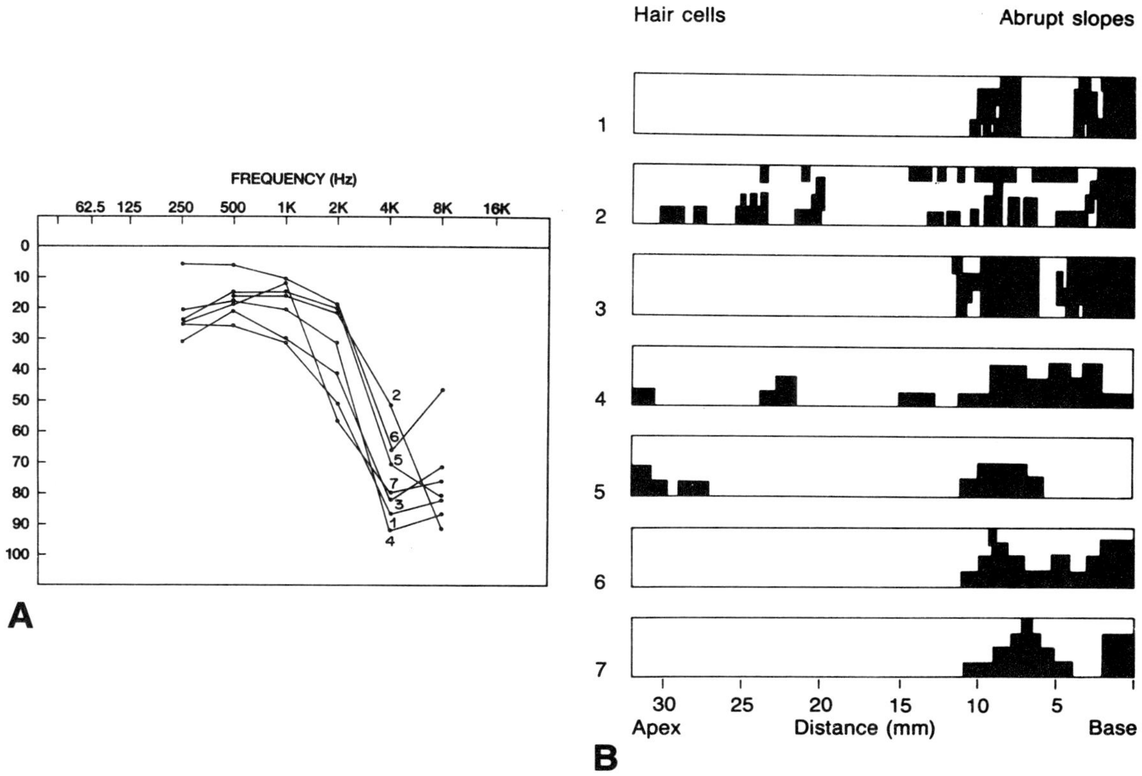

Figure 7-1 *A*, Audiograms of seven ears from six subjects showing abrupt sloping high-tone hearing losses. *B*, Cytohistograms of the seven ears show two principal areas of hair cell loss; one is located in the 7- to 10-mm regions (the locus for 4 kHz) and the other at the extreme basal ends of the cochleas. The first is probably caused by the wear and tear of a lifetime of use and the second by a genetically controlled effect of aging. From the functional standpoint, the first is more debilitating than the second because it invades the speech frequencies. The 4- and 5-mm regions have more hair cells present, which possibly accounts for the uptilts of the audiograms at 8 kHz.

ages spanned 9 decades and in whom there was no evidence of disease affecting the neurons. The neuronal populations ranged from 36,913 for those in the first decade of life to 18,626 for those in the ninth decade, thus showing a progressive loss of about 2,000 neurons per decade (Fig. 7-2). We have shown that the extent of loss of cochlear neurons in the 15- to 22-mm region, where the speech frequencies reside, correlates directly with the magnitude of the loss of word discrimination.[4] While neuronal losses may be limited to the basal end of the cochlea, thereby causing a high-tone loss,[5] a more typical pathologic finding is a diffuse loss in all three turns (Fig. 7-3).

The neuronal losses in the auditory system that occur with aging are not limited to the periphery. Arnesen[6] calculated the total number of neurons in the ventral and dorsal cochlear nuclei from serial sections in six subjects aged 76 to 89 years. There

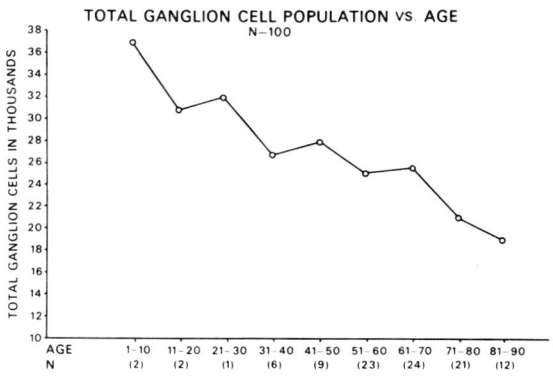

Figure 7-2 For ears with no known otologic disorders affecting the neurons there is a progressive loss of cochlear neurons as a function of aging. (From Otte J, Schuknecht HF, Kerr AG. Ganglion cell populations in normal and pathological human cochleae. Implications for cochlear implantation. Laryngoscope 1978; 88:1234.)

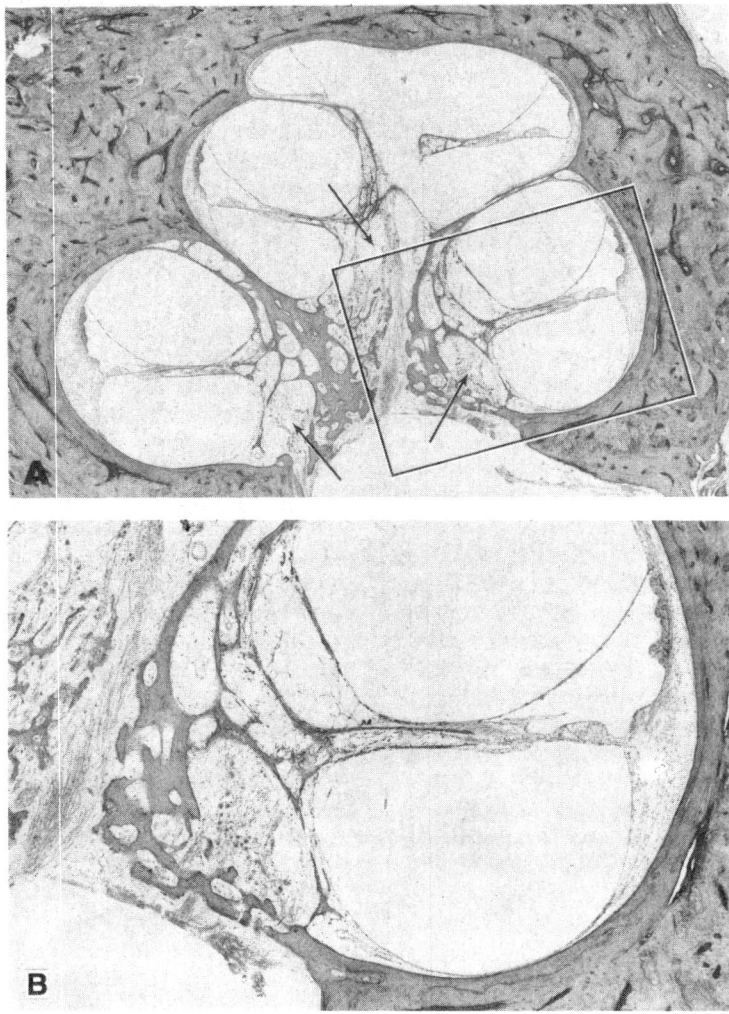

Figure 7–3 *A*, Midmodiolar section of the cochlea of a 91-year-old woman showing severe loss of cochlear neurons in all three turns. *B*, The organ of Corti, including the hair cell population and the stria vascularis, is normal.

was about a 50 percent loss of neurons when these numbers were compared to the numbers calculated for young subjects by other investigators.

STRIAL PRESBYCUSIS

Atrophy of the stria vascularis is a common pathologic entity that often affects several members of a family. The clinical feature that distinguishes this condition from other types of presbycusis is the flat pure-tone threshold audiometric pattern with preservation of the capability for word discrimination. We have shown that the magnitude of strial atrophy correlates positively with the extent of elevation of pure-tone thresholds (Fig. 7–4).[7]

Typically, there is patchy atrophy of the stria vascularis in the middle and apical turns of the cochlea.[8] The stria vascularis may contain cystic structures and basophilic deposits, but more commonly, there is simply a loss of strial tissue (Fig. 7–5). Apparently the loss of strial tissue affects some quality of endolymph, which in turn degrades the physical and chemical processes by which energy is made available to the sense organ.[9]

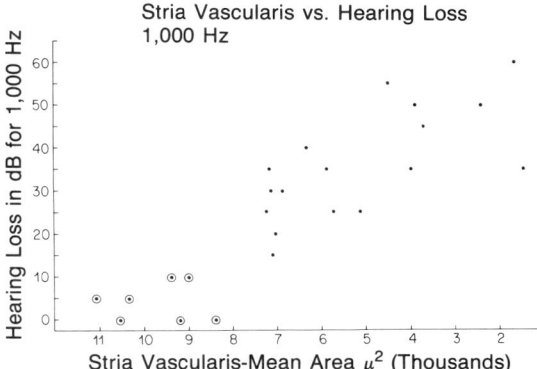

Figure 7-4 The quantity of strial tissue for 24 cochleas is plotted as a function of hearing threshold for 1,000 Hz. The circled points represent cochleas with normal pure-tone thresholds. The average age for the cases with strial atrophy is 70.6 years, and average for the normal cases is 53.4 years. (From Pauler M, Schuknecht HF, White JA. Atrophy of the stria vascularis as a cause of sensorineural hearing loss. Laryngoscope, in press.)

COCHLEAR CONDUCTIVE PRESBYCUSIS

Cochlear conductive presbycusis is a diagnosis derived by histologic exclusion of any consistent pathologic change. It usually first becomes evident in middle age and is characterized by the gradual sloping high-tone hearing loss. There are almost equal increments of loss for each octave from low to high frequencies. Word discrimination scores are inversely related to the steepness of the threshold gradient. In contradistinction to cochleas with abrupt high-tone hearing losses where sensory lesions were present, we[2] have been unable to demonstrate a consistent pathologic correlate in cochleas exhibiting gradual sloping high-tone losses (Fig. 7-6).

We speculate that such linear decrements of function are related to the physical-anatomic gradients that determine the resonance characteristics of the cochlear duct, for example, the width and thickness of the basilar membrane. The greatest threshold loss is for high frequencies, which have their locus of action in the basal end of the cochlea where the basilar membrane is thicker and narrower; the least loss is for low frequencies, which act mainly on the apical region of the cochlea where this membrane is thinner and wider. Support for the concept of an inner ear conductive hearing loss is found in the light and electron microscopic study of a single cochlea by Nadol.[5] This concerns an 81-year-old man who, by history, had a progressive bilateral hearing loss. In addition to severe atrophic changes in the organ of Corti, there was marked thickening of the basilar membrane due to an increase in the number of fibrillar layers.

SUMMARY

The types of presbycusis may be characterized as follows. 1. Sensory presbycusis is caused by degeneration of the organ of Corti and is manifested clinically by abrupt high-tone hearing loss with word discrimination inversely related to the frequency range involved. 2. Neural presbycusis is caused by a loss of cochlear neurons and is characterized by a severe loss of word discrimination. 3. Strial presbycusis results from a loss of stria vascularis and is manifested by a flat threshold pattern with excel-

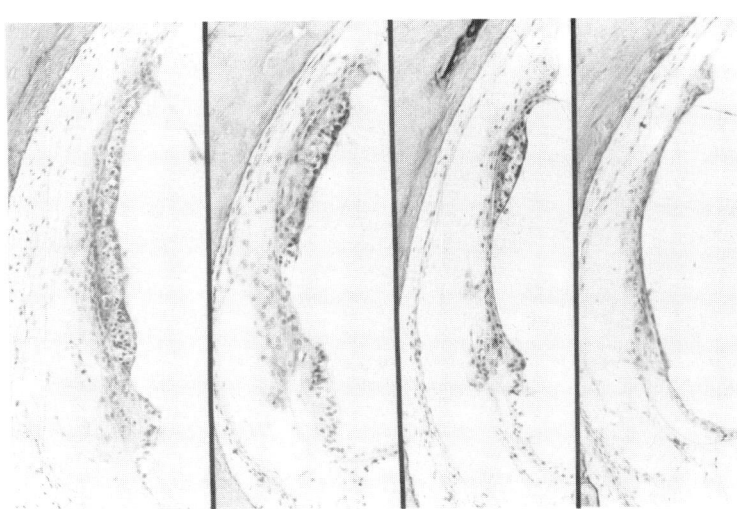

Figure 7-5 Views of the stria vascularis at selected locations show from left to right: normal stria, 40 percent loss, 75 percent loss, and total loss. Measurements were made with an image analysis computer system. (From Pauler M, Schuknecht HF, White JA. Atrophy of the stria vascularis as a cause of sensorineural hearing loss. Laryngoscope, in press.)

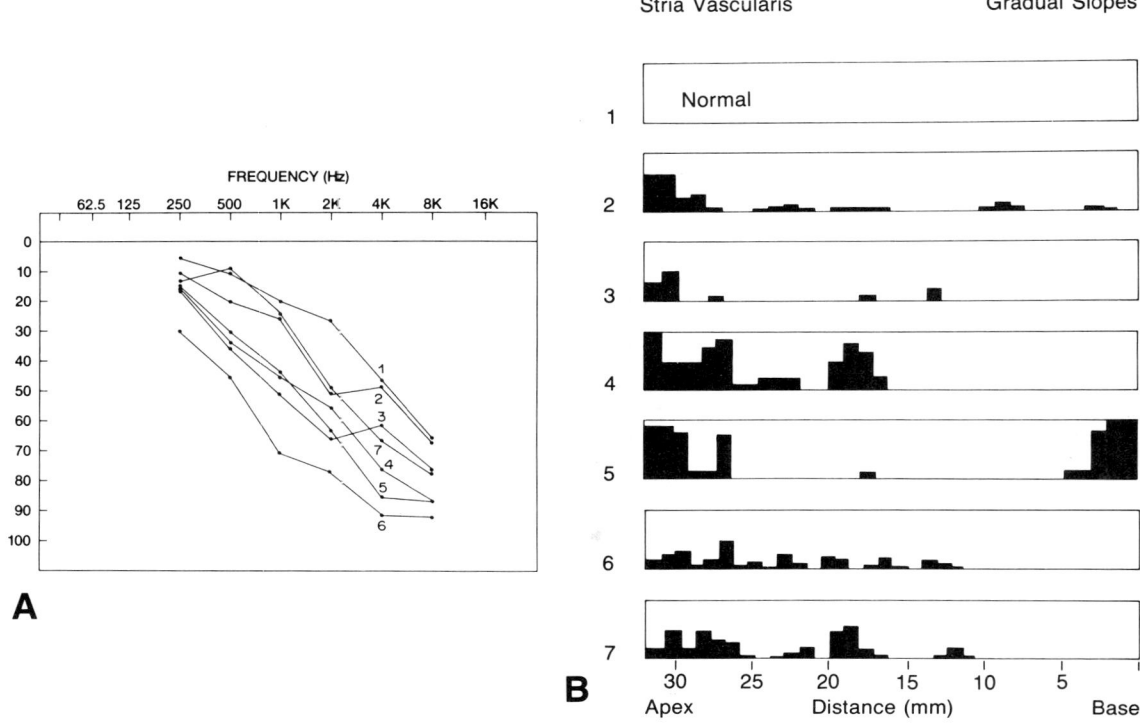

Figure 7-6 *A*, Audiograms of seven ears from six subjects with gradual sloping high-tone hearing losses. *B*, Cytohistograms show small patches of hair cell losses that are greater at the basal ends of the cochleas, but that do not correlate spatially with the audiometric thresholds. Also, there are no corresponding losses of cochlear neurons or stria vascularis.

lent preservation of word discrimination. 4. Inner ear conductive presbycusis is manifested by gradually sloping high-tone hearing losses and word discrimination that is inversely related to the steepness of the slope.

Combinations of the four principal types of presbycusis produce complex patterns of hearing loss. In the clinical management of patients with deafness of aging, it is important to understand the variable clinical expressions of the disorder. Presbycusis is not a single pathologic change with the only variable being the extent of involvement. There are at least four types of presbycusis, and when occurring in pure form, each responds predictably to the effectiveness of amplification devices.

This work was supported by Grant 5 R01 NS05881 from the National Institute of Neurological and Communicative Disorders and Stroke.

References

1. Moscicki EK, Elkins EF, Baum HM, McNamara PM. Hearing loss in the elderly: an epidemiologic study of the Framingham Heart Study Cohort. Ear Hear 1985; 6:184-190.
2. Ramadan H, Schuknecht HF. Is there a conductive type of presbycusis? Otolaryngol Head Neck Surg, in press.
3. Otte J, Schuknecht HF, Kerr AG. Ganglion cell populations in normal and pathological human cochleae. Implications for cochlear implantation. Laryngoscope 1978; 88:1231-1246.
4. Pauler M, Schuknecht HF, Thornton AR. Correlative studies of cochlear neuronal loss with speech discrimination and pure-tone thresholds. Arch Otorhinolaryngol 1986; 243:200-206.
5. Nadol JB Jr. Electron microscopic findings in presbycusic degeneration of the basal turn of the human cochlea. Otolaryngol Head Neck Surg 1979; 87:818-836.
6. Arnesen AR. Presbyacusis—loss of neurons in the human cochlear nuclei. J Larngol Otol 1982; 96:503-511.
7. Pauler M, Schuknecht HF, White JA. Atrophy of the stria vascularis as a cause of sensorineural hearing loss. Laryngoscope, in press.
8. Johnsson LG, Hawkins JE Jr. Symposium on basic ear research. II. Strial atrophy in clinical and experimental deafness. Laryngoscope 1972; 82:1105-1125.
9. Vosteen KH. Neue Aspekte zur Biologie und Pathologie des Innenohres. Arch Ohr Nas Kehlkheilk 1961; 178:1-104.

Chapter Eight

TINNITUS, DEPRESSION, AND AGING

ROBERT A. DOBIE, M.D.
WAYNE J. KATON, M.D.
MARK SULLIVAN, M.D., Ph.D.
CONNIE S. SAKAI, M.S.P.A.

George Reed[1] was probably first to quantify what all otologists had known for a long time: tinnitus is more common in older persons than in the young. In a group of 200 patients attending a tinnitus clinic, he found 64.5 percent were older than age 50. Reed believed that tinnitus prevalence decreased after age 70, but he had in fact only shown that the number of tinnitus patients decreased above that age. (The true prevalence among a particular age group would be the number of afflicted individuals divided by the total population of that age group.)

Others,[2,3] have also shown tinnitus prevalence to increase with age. However, the best data that addresses this question comes from Axellson and Ringdahl[4] in Gothenburg, Sweden. They mailed 3,600 questionnaires to 300 men and 300 women in each of 6 decade age groups, ranging from 20 to 29 to 70 to 79, and achieved a remarkable 66 percent response rate. Their data on tinnitus prevalence and age are summarized in Table 8-1. Prevalence was nearly constant from age 20 to 49, after which it more than doubled, and then again remained roughly constant from age 50 to 79. These data suggest that tinnitus is not a special problem of the elderly, but is considerably more common in the middle-aged and elderly than in the young. Severe tinnitus was defined in their questionnaire as tinnitus that "plagues me all day long." This category appeared to increase gradually up to age 49, then increased four-fold. Respondents in their 50s, 60s, and 70s had very similar prevalences; about 4 percent of each group complained of severe tinnitus.

Several authors have commented on psychological aspects of tinnitus. Reed[1] administered the Minnesota Multiphasic Personality Inventory (MMPI) to 100 tinnitus patients and reported simply that 34 percent were "neurotic." House[5] reported MMPI results on 132 patients; curiously, all were abnormal, with 48 cases in the "depressive range," 54 cases showing "neurotic conversion," and 30 cases demonstrating "borderline personality." A similar British study[6] showed elevated average scores for anxiety and depression in patients complaining of tinnitus.

The Tinnitus Research Clinic at the University of Washington has had a special interest in the psychiatric aspects of tinnitus for the past few years. While we have never focused on aging per se, our patients are, like Reed's, on the average older than the general population. We will present some of the data we have collected, then discuss these data in the context of what is known about interactions between aging and depression. We suspect that our findings regarding the prevalence and management of depression in tinnitus patients are generalizable to older tinnitus patients. However, special studies are clearly required to address these issues directly.

METHODS

We intensively studied 40 consecutive patients seen in our Tinnitus Research Clinic, each of whom had been referred after adequate otologic and audiologic evaluation had excluded treatable disease. The requirement for recent otologic evaluation and referral also ensured that this was a select group of patients for whom reassurance was not enough. In fact, many patients had already tried hearing aids, maskers, biofeedback, and/or drugs for their tinnitus, without success. Seventy-eight percent were male, and the average age was 49.4 years (standard deviation = 15.3 years). Most tinnitus matches were between 6 and 10 kHz, at a mean intensity of 10.3 dB sensation level (these are fairly typical of other series). A control group of 14 general otology patients was also enrolled and matched to the tinnitus

TABLE 8-1 Subjects Experiencing Tinnitus "Often" or "Always"

Age	Total Prevalence	Percent	Severe Cases	Percent
20–29	24/320	7.5%	1	0.3%
30–39	23/395	5.8%	2	0.5%
40–49	35/395	8.9%	4	1.0%
50–59	76/408	18.6%	17	4.2%
60–69	88/433	20.3%	16	3.7%
70–79	91/427	21.3%	18	4.2%
Total	337/2378	14.2%	58	2.4%

group for age, sex, and social class. The control patients had, on the average, more hearing loss than the tinnitus patients (49.6 dB versus 22.4 dB for the 0.5, 1, 2, 3 kHz pure-tone average), but none had tinnitus as a *presenting* complaint (some admitted to tinnitus that they considered mild).

Psychiatric assessment included a structured diagnostic interview (the National Institute of Mental Health Diagnostic Interview Schedule) that lasted about 1 hour, as well as the Hopkins Symptom Check List[7] (SCL-90), the Chronic Illness Problem Inventory[8], and other questionnaire instruments, which will not be discussed here. For greater detail regarding these tests, as well as detailed audiometric data, see Harrop-Griffiths et al[9] and Sullivan et al.[10] Psychiatric diagnoses used the criteria of the Diagnostic and Statistical Manual, 3rd edition (DSM-III) of the American Psychiatric Association.[11] A diagnosis of major depression required a predominant and persistent dysphoric mood plus a more than 2 week history of four of the eight following symptoms:

1. Appetite or weight change
2. Sleep changes
3. Psychomotor retardation or agitation
4. Decreased pleasure in usual activities
5. Decreased energy or increased fatigue
6. Feelings of worthlessness or inappropriate guilt
7. Decreased concentration
8. Recurrent thoughts of death, wishes to be dead, or suicide attempt.

In addition to our studies of the prevalence of psychiatric disorder in tinnitus, we have begun therapeutic trials of nortriptyline, a tricyclic drug, in depressed patients with tinnitus. Our initial trials have employed a single-blind nonrandomized placebo-controlled design. Patients first receive placebo for 2 weeks, although they believe they may receive the placebo at any time in the trial. They are then switched to nortriptyline, beginning at a low dose of 25 mg at bedtime. The dose is gradually increased to the point of tolerance or to the beginning of symptom relief. Serum drug levels are monitored to ensure therapeutic levels and patient compliance. After this dose adjustment period, treatment is continued for 6 weeks with daily diary and biweekly questionnaire assessment of tinnitus loudness, severity (each on a 0 to 7 scale), and duration (0 to 24 hours per day), and of depression (using the Hamilton Depression Scale). This study design was chosen as an efficient way to obtain a preliminary estimate of the magnitude of active and placebo effects in the hope of determining whether a more formal (and expensive) randomized controlled trial would be appropriate and how large a sample would be required.

At this writing, 10 patients have completed the therapeutic trial and data analysis; their results will be presented briefly.

RESULTS

A current major depression was found in 24 of 40 (60 percent) tinnitus patients, compared to 1 in 14 (7 percent) of controls ($p < 0.01$). Thirty-two of 40 (80 percent) had either a current or past major depression, compared to 3 in 14 (21 percent) of controls ($p < 0.02$). Other DSM-III diagnoses (alcoholism, panic disorder, phobic anxiety) were made with statistically indistinguishable frequency in both groups.

Tinnitus patients had higher average scores than controls ($p < 0.05$ in each case) on the SCL-90 scales for somatization, hostility, depression, obsessive-compulsive tendency, and phobia. When depressed tinnitus patients were analyzed separately from nondepressed patients, the latter group was not significantly different from controls on any subtest.

A similar pattern was seen for the Chronic Illness Problem Inventory: tinnitus patients had increased problems ($p < 0.05$) with sleep, cognition, sexual function, social activities, medical interactions, marital life, and illness focusing. Again, the depressed tinnitus patients accounted for all the differences in comparison with the control group.

Table 8-2 summarizes the preliminary results of the nortriptyline trial. Neither depression nor tinnitus responded frequently to placebo, while the majority of patients showed decreases in tinnitus loudness and severity and in depression after nortriptyline treatment. As expected, the Hamilton Depression Scale scores declined sharply (63 percent average decrease), with a more modest average decrease in tinnitus severity. Although 6 of 10 patients reported their tinnitus was less loud (by 16.7

TABLE 8-2 Patients Showing 25 Percent or Greater Improvement

Variable	Placebo	Nortriptyline	(Mean % Decrease)*
Depression+	2/10	8/10	(63.2%)
Tinnitus loudness	1/10	6/10	(16.7%)
Tinnitus severity	2/10	7/10	(32.7%)

* Mean percent decrease for entire group of 10
+ Hamilton Depression Scale

percent on average), this was not reflected in tinnitus matching retests.

Figure 8–1 shows a typical time course for one subject whose tinnitus severity dropped by 60 percent during treatment. No response was seen during the first 2 weeks (placebo), and a gradual response occurred thereafter, which did not plateau until 8 weeks into the study (6 weeks on nortriptyline, 4 weeks on full dosage).

DISCUSSION

The primary finding in our prevalence study was the strong association between severe tinnitus (severe enough to result in referral to a special clinic) and a diagnosis of active major depression. It must be stressed that this applies only to this highly selected group; most patients with tinnitus do not complain, and most who do complain require only reassurance. Still, the probability is high that a patient who is really distressed by tinnitus also is suffering from a major depressive episode. Further, depressed tinnitus patients had multiple significantly elevated scores for both psychiatric symptoms (SCL-90) and personal and social malfunctioning (Chronic Illness Problem Inventory), while nondepressed tinnitus patients were similar to controls in both tests. It would appear that depression accounts for, or is associated with, most of the severe distress and disability seen in tinnitus patients.

Hearing loss has been found to be associated with depression in the aged by Gilhome Herbst and Humphrey.[12] In a group of 217 patients over 70 years old, depression was seen in 41 percent of those with hearing loss ($\geq$ 35 dB in the better ear) and in 23 percent of those without hearing loss ($p < 0.01$). Our control group had worse hearing than our tinnitus patients, so we feel the high rate of depression seen in our study cannot simply be ascribed to hearing loss. The 7 percent prevalence of depression seen in our controls is close to the rate (6 percent) seen in unselected outpatients.[13] It seems likely that hearing loss and tinnitus, although arising from the same cochlear disorder, can independently increase the probability of major depression.

We cannot infer a simple causality of the form: "tinnitus causes depression." While many of our patients believed that to be the case, many also had had episodes of major depression prior to the onset of their tinnitus. In 32 patients with tinnitus and a current or past major depression, tinnitus preceded depression in 14, depression preceded tinnitus in 15, and the two began simultaneously (within a month or within the patients' limits of memory) in three.

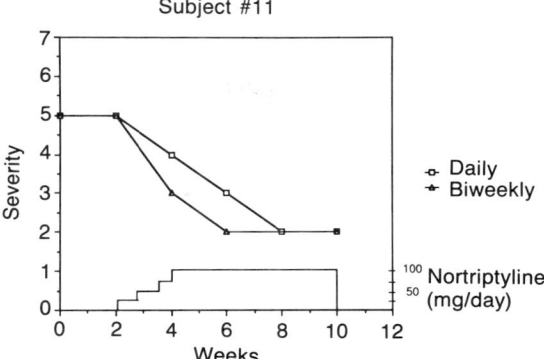

Figure 8–1 Tinnitus severity (0 to 7) as a function of time. Both the biweekly questionnaire data (triangles) and the means of daily diary entries (squares) are shown. Nortriptyline dose is also shown against the right-hand axis; it was increased from 25 mg to 100 mg nightly during weeks 2 and 4.

Mathew et al,[14] in discussing the physical symptoms of depressed patients, reported that 49 percent of 51 depressed patients complained of tinnitus compared to 12 percent of 51 controls. Does this suggest that depression causes tinnitus? This seems unlikely to us, but it is certainly plausible that depression could prevent or destroy the coping process that develops for most patients with tinnitus, thus changing an easily ignored symptom into an unbearable one. Depression has been demonstrated to cause amplification of disability associated with chronic medical illness.[15] In the irritable bowel syndrome, as with tinnitus, not all afflicted persons seek medical advice; those who do seek advice differ from those who don't (after controlling for severity of gastrointestinal symptoms) by having increased anxiety and depression.[16]

Our preliminary treatment results are encouraging. Nortriptyline, a tricyclic antidepressant given for a prolonged period after careful dose adjustment, appears to improve several symptoms in depressed tinnitus patients. Not surprisingly, the largest treatment effect appears to be a reduction in depressive symptoms. We expected patients' estimates of tinnitus severity ("How much does it bother you?") to decline as depression improved, but were surprised that many patients also reported decreases in tinnitus loudness. As stressed earlier, this study must be seen as providing preliminary information only. Patients were on placebo only 2 weeks, compared to 6 to 10 weeks on nortriptyline. During the entire study, they had frequent contact with a sympathetic physician. While no formal psychotherapy was carried out, we cannot unequivocally attribute our outcomes to drug alone. A formal double-blind randomized controlled trial will be necessary to determine whether nortriptyline is truly beneficial for depressed tinnitus patients.

There are many similarities between tinnitus and chronic pain. Each is often seen in a setting of peripheral denervation and represents a subjective complaint that can sometimes be ameliorated by masking (acoustic for tinnitus, vibratory for pain) or by electrical stimulation. Both respond poorly to nerve section and frequently coexist with depression. Tricyclic drugs have an analgesic action that is independent of their antidepressant action. Relief of chronic pain is often seen more quickly and at lower doses than required for antidepressive action. We have seen no indication so far of tinnitus relief prior to (or as great as) depression relief; most of our patients felt the major therapeutic benefit was in mood and coping ability, with little change in tinnitus per se. Nevertheless, the possibility of a specific effect on tinnitus cannot yet be ruled out.

More research is needed to focus specifically on tinnitus in the elderly. It seems likely that hearing loss and tinnitus could interact in a complex way to undermine the psychosocial well-being of older patients. The ameliorative effects of interventions such as counseling, hearing aid fitting, and antidepressive drugs should be assessed.

Rowe and Kahn[17] have stressed the need to intensively study individuals who are aging *successfully*, so that their adaptations can be applied to others. Factors like exercise, interesting activities, social support, and a sense of autonomy are important and modifiable extrinsic factors that can probably reduce the impact of tinnitus and other medical problems on the lives of older people. Even for younger people, it would be nice to know more about those who are well-adjusted to their tinnitus: how do they do it? Intrinsic factors such as personality and coping mechanisms must play a role, but there may be valuable lessons to be learned from such studies.

Most (nearly all?) tinnitus in the elderly comes from cochlear damage caused by excessive noise exposure and by age-related degeneration (presbycusis). Noise-induced hearing loss is preventable, and we should tell our younger noise-exposed patients about tinnitus to help motivate them to protect their ears. Despite the present enthusiasm about vascular inner ear disorders, presbycusis is probably not preventable, and tinnitus will continue to be a frequent companion of old age (and middle age). Most old people adjust successfully, and a few need help of the sort cursorily described herein.

References

1. Reed GF. An audiometric study of two hundred cases of subjective tinnitus. Arch Otolaryngol 1960; 71:94-104.
2. Hinchcliffe R. Prevalence of the commoner ear, nose, and throat conditions in the adult rural population of Great Britain. Br J Prev Soc Med 1961; 15:128-140.
3. Institute of Hearing Research. Epidemiology of tinnitus. In: CIBA Foundation Symposium 85. Tinnitus. London: Pitman, 1981:16.
4. Axelsson A, Ringdahl A. The prevalence of tinnitus. Acta Otolaryngol (in press).
5. House PR. Personality of the tinnitus patient. In: CIBA Foundation Symposium 85. Tinnitus. London: Pitman, 1981:193.
6. Stephens SD, Hallam RS. The Crown-Crisp experiential index in patients complaining of tinnitus. Br J Audiol 1985; 19:151-158.
7. Derogatis LR. SCL-90 Manual. Baltimore: Clinical Psychometric Research, 1977.
8. Kames LD, Naliboff BD, Henrich RL, et al. The chronic illness problem inventory: problem oriented psychosocial assessment of patients with chronic illness. Int J Psychiatry Med 1984; 14(1):65-74.
9. Harrop-Griffiths J, Katon W, Dobie R, Sakai C, Russo J. Chronic tinnitus: association with psychiatric diagnoses. Gen J Psychosomatic Res 1987; 31:613-622.
10. Sullivan MD, Katon W, Dobie R, Sakai C, Russo J, Harrop-Griffiths J. Disabling tinnitus: association with affective disorder. Gen Hosp Psychiatry (in press).
11. American Psychiatric Association, Committee on Nomenclature and Statistics. Diagnostic and Statistical Manual. 3rd ed. Washington, D.C.: American Psychiatric Association, 1980.
12. Gilhome Herbst KR, Humphrey CM. Hearing impairment and mental state in the elderly living at home. Br Med J 1980; 281:903-905.
13. Nielsen AC III, Williams TA. Depression in ambulatory medical patients: prevalence by self-report questionnaire and recognition by non-psychiatric physicians. Arch Gen Psychiatry 1980; 37:999-1004.
14. Mathew RJ, Weinman ML, Mirabi M. Physical symptoms of depression. Br J Psychiatry 1981; 139:293-296.
15. Wells KB, et al. Profiles of health and functioning for depressed and non-depressed adult outpatients of mental health and medical clinicians. Presented at American Psychiatric Association Meeting, Chicago, IL, 1987.
16. Drossman D, McKee D, Sandler RS, et al. Psychosocial factors in irritable bowel syndrome: a multivariate study of patients and nonpatients with IBS. Presented at Mental Disorders in General Health Care Settings: A Research Conference. Seattle, WA, June, 1987.
17. Rowe JW, Kahn RL. Human aging: usual and successful. Science 1987; 237:143-149.

Chapter Nine

COMMUNICATION ASSISTIVE DEVICES

DERALD E. BRACKMANN, M.D.

Hearing loss interferes with day to day communication on many occasions. Usually a hearing aid can help, but some situations may still present a problem. Listening might be difficult in a noisy restaurant or in a business meeting where the speaker is at a distance from the listener. Perhaps the television is not clear until it is so loud it drives friends and family out of the room. In addition, many people have difficulty hearing the telephone or the doorbell ring or safety alarms sound. In these difficult situations, a communication assistive device can enhance listening ability. This paper describes some communication devices for the hearing impaired. Details in regard to obtaining these devices may be obtained in a booklet available from the House Ear Institute, 256 S. Lake St., Los Angeles, California, 90057.

TELEPHONE AMPLIFIERS

Telephone amplifiers to increase the loudness of the telephone signal may be portable or nonportable. Several models have an adjustable volume control that enables adjustment of the signal to a comfortable level. Portable amplifiers are inexpensive and lightweight and may be carried in a pocket or purse. They fit directly over the ear piece of the telephone and are battery powered. They are ideal for travelers. The volume may be adjusted to a comfortable level. Nonportable amplifiers are of several types. One type is built into the handset of the telephone. There are two basic models: one with an adjustable volume control dial and one with a touchbar switch. The touchbar automatically returns the volume to its regular level when you hang up the phone and is ideal for a phone used by many people. Handset amplifiers are generally available from the telephone company.

TELEPHONE DEVICES FOR THE DEAF

The original telephone devices (TTYs) were teletypewriters like those used by news stations to transmit information over the telephone. The current telecommunication devices for the deaf, TDDs, allow a severely or profoundly hearing impaired person to directly call another person who has similar equipment. Telephone devices for the deaf are available in various styles and sizes: portable, semiportable, or desk models. Messages are displayed on the visual screen, and some TDDs have a paper printout for a permanent record of the conversation. In some states, telephone companies may provide (or rent) a TDD on request.

A unique type of TDD allows the deaf person to communicate through a code system with other parties who do not have a TDD. When the non-hearing impaired person presses a touch tone code, letters or words appear on the hearing impaired caller's device display. The hearing impaired person who has speech ability can use his or her own voice to reply.

Many standard answering machines are not able to record a TDD message. A machine with this capability is available for use with a TDD.

TELEVISION, RADIO, AND STEREO AMPLIFIERS

Listening to the television or radio in the presence of background noise is often frustrating for the hearing impaired person. In addition, the loud volume of the television set may be bothersome to normal hearing members of the family. With the use of an assistive listening device, the hearing impaired person may listen to the television, radio, or stereo at a comfortable loudness and without the interference of background noise.

Devices include those that connect to a hearing aid with direct audio input; head phones that connect to the listening jack of the television; listening loops for use with the telecoil on a hearing aid; or wireless infrared devices that send the television signal directly to the listener via a receiver. Many television sets are equipped with a private listening jack, which provides inexpensive help for hearing impaired patients. Several types of devices may be connected to the private listening jack, including standard headsets, induction coils, and pillow speakers. For television sets without a listening jack, devices are available that attach a microphone to the television speaker, amplify the sound, and present it to the patient through a pillow speaker. Complete induction loop kits are also available.

Infrared Systems

High-fidelity infrared systems convert audio signals into infrared waves (invisible light beams). The infrared transmitter is plugged into the wall socket, and the microphone is fastened with velcro to the front of the television speaker. The headset is lightweight and comfortable and has a volume control. The headset, powered by a rechargeable battery, converts the infrared energy back into amplified sound.

Television Caption Units

More than 40 hours a week of television programs have now been closed-captioned so hearing impaired viewers can read what they cannot hear. In addition, the National Captioning Institute has closed-captioned over 35 video cassettes of popular movies. Closed captions can be seen only on a television set with a decoding device, which can be purchased from several manufacturers for a moderate price.

SIGNALING DEVICES

An abundant number of signaling devices can visually alert the hearing impaired person to auditory signals that may not be heard. Most of these devices automatically flash a light to alert the person to the sound source. Others activate a vibrator to awaken a sleeping person. Signaling devices may be purchased individually, such as a telephone ring indicator, or in a complete alert system, which monitors phone, door, fire alarm, and even a crying baby. The most unique of the signaling devices is the hearing dog. Dogs are trained to listen and then alert their master when the appropriate sounds are heard.

PERSONAL AMPLIFICATION FOR LISTENING IN GROUPS AND PUBLIC PLACES

Many hearing impaired people have difficulty hearing and understanding in the presence of background noise. Listening in groups, meetings, or theaters can be affected by noise interference, room reverberation, and the distance between the listener and the talker. In these situations, it is important to have the speaker as close as possible to the listener.

Devices for One-on-One and Small Group Communication

These devices consist of a portable amplifying system. Signals from a hand-held microphone are amplified by a lightweight amplifier and then directed to the hearing impaired listener through ear phones. A variety of such devices are available.

Large Group and Theater Listening

Hearing impaired persons often have difficulty listening in the classroom, church, theater, or out-of-doors. Several systems are available to direct the amplified sound directly to the listener's ears.

Loop Induction System

A loop of wire encircles the room, thereby creating an electrical field that activates the hearing impaired person's hearing aid when the telecoil switch of the hearing aid is activated. The loop induction systems are relatively inexpensive to install.

Radio Frequency AM/FM Systems

These systems broadcast the auditory signal to special receivers, much like radio broadcasting. Frequency modulation systems (FM) are especially popular because they allow for more mobility, can be used outdoors, have a low operating cost, and are energy efficient.

Infrared Systems

Infrared systems for large theaters work on the same principle as described for television systems. Many theaters are now installing these devices. Because they are subject to interference from natural or artificial lighting, they may only be used indoors.

DEVICES FOR THE PROFESSIONAL

Many hearing impaired individuals do not use hearing aids, but still require amplification in some situations. The physician, for example, with a mild hearing loss may benefit from an electronic stethoscope. A nurse in a convalescent home may find a portable speaking tube useful to establish communication with hearing impaired patients.

CONCLUSION

A brief overview of the different types of assistive listening devices has been presented. These devices may be of great benefit for persons with all degrees of hearing impairment. Resource centers for further information are listed in the appendix.

From the Otologic Medical Group, Inc., Los Angeles; sponsored by a grant from the House Ear Institute, an affiliate of the University of Southern California School of Medicine, Los Angeles, California.

APPENDIX

Alexander Graham Bell
Association for the Deaf
3417 Volta Place, N.W.
Washington, D.C. 20007

American Academy of Otolaryngology–
Head & Neck Surgery
1101 Vermont N.W., Suite 302
Washington, D.C. 20005
(202) 289-4607

American Humane Association
9725 E. Hampden Avenue
Denver, Colorado 80231

AT & T Phone Company
National Special Needs Center
(800) 233-1222
(800) 833-3232
Directory TTY (800) 855-1155

Chicago Hearing Society
Charles A. Silberman Center
10 West Jackson Blvd., 4th Floor
Chicago, Illinois 60604

Consumer Organization of Hearing Impaired
P.O. Box 2538
Laurel, Maryland 20811

Fellendorf Associates, Inc.
P.O. Box 32227
Washington, D.C. 20007
(301) 593-1637

General Telephone
Handicap Assistance Center
(800) 352-7437
(800) 821-2858
(Repairs and first time TDDs)

Greater Los Angeles Council on Deafness, Inc.
(G.L.A.D.)
616 S. Westmoreland Avenue
Los Angeles, CA 90005
(213) 383-2220

National Association for Hearing and Speech
Action (NAHSA)
10801 Rockville Pike
Rockville, Maryland 20852
Helpline (800) 638-8255

National Captioning Institute (NCI)
5203 Leesburg Pike
Falls Church, VA 22041
(703) 998-2416

The National Information Center on Deafness
Gallaudet College
800 Florida Avenue, N.E.
Washington, D.C. 20002

National Technical Institute for the Deaf (NTID)
One Lomb Memorial Drive
P.O. Box 9887
Rochester, New York 14623
(716) 475-6824

Organization for Use of the Telephone, Inc. (O.U.T.)
P.O. Box 175
Owings Mills, Maryland 21117-0175
(301) 655-1827

Pacific Telephone
(800) 772-3140 (TDD)

Self Help for Hard of Hearing People, Inc. (SHHH)
4848 Battery Lane, Suite 100
Bethesda, Maryland 20814

Suzanne Pathy Speak-up Institute, Inc.
525 Park Avenue
New York, New York 10021
(212) 832-8286

Telecommunications for the Deaf, Inc.
814 Thayer Avenue
Silver Springs, Maryland 20910
(301) 589-3006

PRESBYCUSIS: THE HEARING LOSS OF AGING

INTRODUCTION

ARAM GLORIG, M.D.

My interest in the balance mechanism dates back, primarily, to when streptomycin was first used to treat tuberculosis. The patients became dizzy after use of this drug for a short while. I performed studies on the balance mechanism while in Washington, D.C., in 1946. We did caloric studies, and I did some refinements to Cawthorne Hallpike tests to try to control the temperature more accurately so that the stimulus was the same during the flow of the different temperatures of water. I also performed some table studies; we had a flat platform on which the patient was asked to rest on his hands and knees while we tilted the table back and forth to test the responses of the balance mechanism to the changes in position. I discovered that, after the use of streptomycin, there was a loss of control of the proprioceptor stimuli. I learned this by finding that, when a patient was asked to walk on a soft surface, he had difficulty maintaining an upright posture. This appeared to be due to the fact that he did not have a firm platform on which to walk and confirmed the complaints of many of these patients, i.e., inability to walk on an uneven surface, such as a thickly padded lawn surface. This also fitted in with the complaints that they had a great deal of difficulty maintaining an upright posture in the dark.

These findings confirmed the fact that there are three main mechanisms that seem to be related to maintaining an upright stature: (1) the proprioceptive senses from the muscles; (2) the visual system; and (3) the balance mechanism in the inner ear, the semicircular canals.

After considerable study, I concluded that the main problem with streptomycin toxicity was the fact that the semicircular canals were not responding properly: the cells of the semicircular canals did not allow the balance mechanism in the ears to provide the proper signals. The patient needed both the proprioceptor senses and the visual system in order to maintain any degree of steady uprightness.

After refining the caloric test, it appeared to be only a gross measure of the vestibular system as far as signal processing was concerned. To this day I feel that the caloric test is not a very refined test, but only provides gross information regarding the performance of the vestibular system; we need a much more refined method of testing the balance mechanism. It also became clear that the highly complex process of maintaining an upright position was one of the most difficult signal processing procedures with which we were provided, and that a fine balance between the proprioceptor system, the visual system, and the vestibular system was needed to accomplish this task.

I concluded that the refinement of this trisignal source was probably maintained in the cerebellum and was a tuning process of these three signal sources. The cerebellum was called on to compensate for changes occurring in any one of these three systems.

This became even clearer when the balance problems that accompany aging became evident. It became apparent that maintaining an upright position depended on the proper timing of the necessary signal processing, and that the aging process produced changes in this signal processing procedure. Therefore, compensatory processing became necessary in order to offset for these changes in this highly complex mechanism.

In my practice of the past 10 years, I have been called on to see numerous aged individuals who complain of problems in balance that do not show up well in any of the test procedures that we have for testing the balance mechanism. I have always believed that the aging changes produce a diminished rapidity of response so that, when one begins to experience a difference in balance, the various signal sources do not respond quickly enough to compensate rapidly enough to maintain complete stability. This gave me the idea that we might call this *presbyastasis*, which, to me, means a problem of stability in balance related to aging.

I was pleased when Dr. Goldstein invited me to organize the panel that will present two phases of the aging balance problem at this meeting. I felt it was high time that changes in the neurologic system related to presbyastasis were discussed. I would like to express my appreciation to Dr. Hugh Barber and Dr. Fred Linthicum for taking on this task and hope that it will provoke further study on this extremely important problem.

Further, I wish to express my gratitude to the American Academy of Otolaryngology–Head and Neck Surgery and to the National Institute of Aging for making it possible to have this very important conference.

In regard to this section, the Working Group on Goals and Mechanisms for Training Otolaryngologists in the Area of Geriatric Medicine questions the use of the term "Presbyastasis: The Dysequilibrium of Aging," since presbyastasis is a static process, whereas dysequilibrium implies an active process

Chapter Ten

PRESBYASTASIS

FRED H. LINTHICUM Jr., M.D.

Presbyastasis is a term coined by Belal and Glorig to describe the dysequilibrium that occurs with aging.[1] Degenerative changes and loss of structures have been reported in the otoconia, the vestibular epithelium, the vestibular nerves, Scarpa's ganglion, and the cerebellum. Changes in the cerebellum appear to have the greatest effect on balance in the aged. These changes begin to accelerate during the fifth decade of life. There is a paucity of information on the vestibular nuclei in the aged.

Degenerative changes in the otoconia caused by aging have been described by many authors. A summary by Ross, Johnsson, Peacor, and Allard includes a scanning electron microscopy demonstration of progressive degenerative changes in the otoconia.[2] The first change is a pitting of the surfaces of the structures, then cavitation in the surface of the otoconia, demineralization, and finally fragmentation. The resulting loss of mass is believed to decrease the responsiveness of the utricle to gravity and to linear acceleration. Schuknecht has demonstrated degenerated otoconial debris on the ampulla of the posterior semicircular canal that gives rise to positional balance disturbances.[3] He calls the condition *cupulolithiasis*.

Rosenhall and Rubin, describing changes of the sensory epithelium in the maculae and ampullae, included changes in the hairs; accumulations of inclusion bodies, including lipofuscin; vacuoles; and disappearance of some cells and replacement with scar tissue (Fig. 10–1). The decrease in the number of cells is particularly apparent after age 70.[4]

A decrease in the number of ganglion cells in Scarpa's ganglion begins about age 60.[5] The amount of loss varies among individuals between ages 60 and 80. There is a similar loss of nerve fibers between the vestibule and Scarpa's ganglion. This loss increases rather rapidly in the fifth decade, which is slightly earlier than the loss of ganglion cells.[6]

Van der Laan and Oosterveld, using caloric and torsion swing tests, found that the small frequency and large amplitude of nystagmus in children and young adults changes to a higher frequency, but smaller amplitude, in older adults. This change, which amounts to a 30 percent loss of sensitivity of the horizontal canal system with aging, may indicate a generalized loss of all vestibular sensory perceptions of about the same amount.[7] Microscopic evaluation of all of the receptors and neurons of the vestibular system structures reveals an increase in the amount of lipofuscin that occurs with advancing age (Fig. 10–2). The relationship of lipofuscin accumulation to cellular function and cellular death has not been established. It has been suggested that this accumulation could possibly decrease protein synthesis and interfere with intracellular transport.

Little data are available on changes in the vestibular nuclei in the brain stem. We have noticed the same accumulation of lipofuscin in the elderly vestibular nuclei, but we have not morphologically evaluated cell pathology and loss in humans.

There are a number of studies by Hutton, Nagel, and Loewenson[8] that track eye performance in

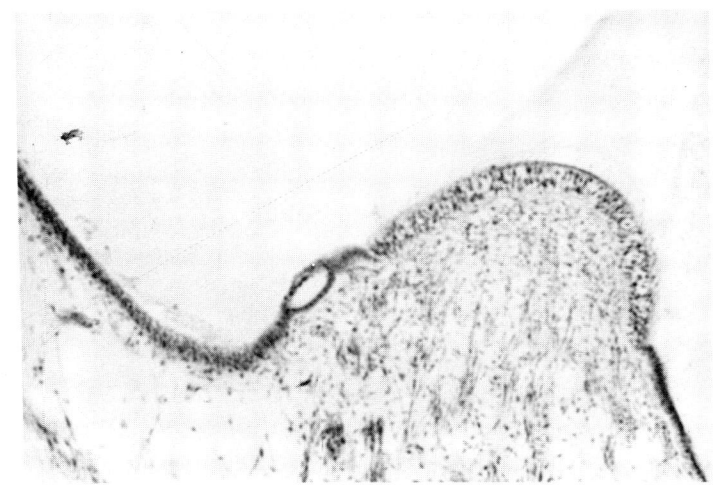

Figure 10–1 Semicircular canal ampulla demonstrating vacuoles in the sensory epithelium and cyst formation in the planum semilunatum; two changes found in aging individuals. (Hematoxylin and eosin [H & E] staining; magnification × 100).

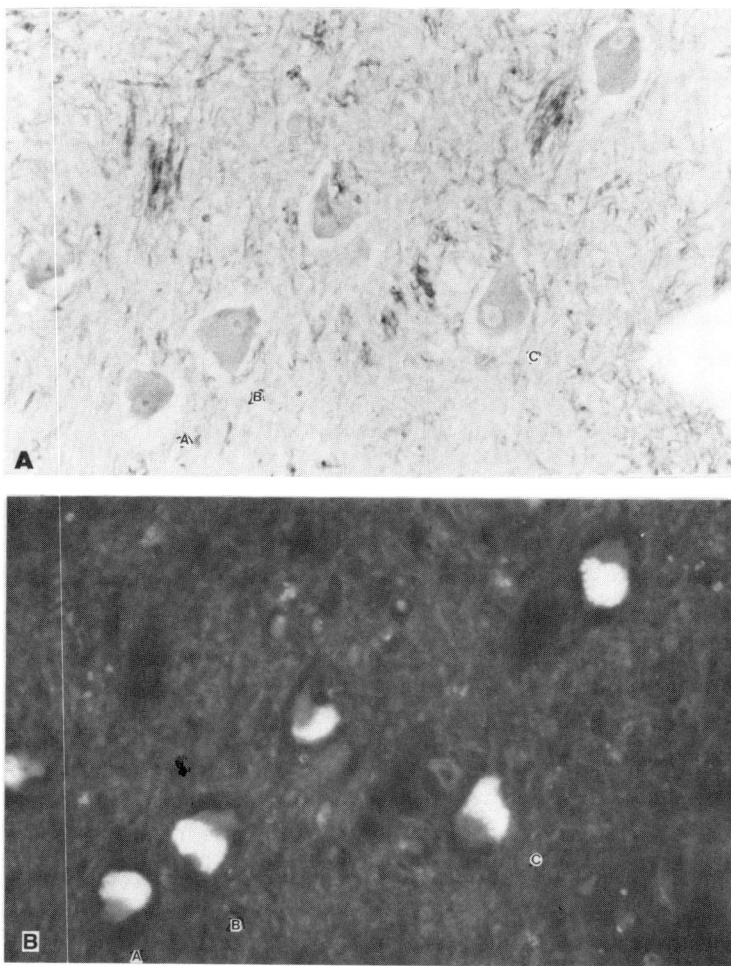

Figure 10–2 *A*, Nissl stain of neurons. Nissl substance appears as dark area adjacent to the nucleus. *B*, Fluorescent microphotograph of the same cells (A, B, C) showing large amount of lipofuscin (age pigment) occupying cell at the expense of the organelles. The reduction of organelles is felt by some to decrease the protein synthesis of the cells and to reduce their efficiency. (Magnification × 340)

elderly individuals. These studies showed a decrease in tracking ability with age. This substantiates our finding of abnormal tracking in 20 percent of individuals younger than 50 and in 80 percent of older individuals in their 60s and above (Fig. 10-3). This finding implicates the cerebellum as a major cause of eye tracking malfunction (Fig. 10-4).

The effect of cerebellar lesions on eye movements has been summarized by Morales-Garcia, Rios, Hoppe, and Fantuzzi.[9] They demonstrated that cerebellar damage adversely affects the ability to perform normal eye movements, which are mediated through the cerebellar ocular pathway. This system is independent of the vestibular system, which, however, can modify cerebellar ocular reflex by input into the cerebellum. The Purkinje's cells have an inhibitory influence on the input to the ocular muscles. Therefore, a reduction of this input results in abnormal muscular movements resulting in poor coordination of eye movements. A direct connection between the cerebellum and the vestibular nuclei has been demonstrated.[10] These projections involve primarily the Purkinje's cells.

Peterka, Black, Newell, and Schoenhoff found that 54 percent of people who fall on two or more posture test trials are 60 or older.[11] It therefore appears that the biggest effect of balance disturbances occurs in the cerebellar ocular system and the cere-

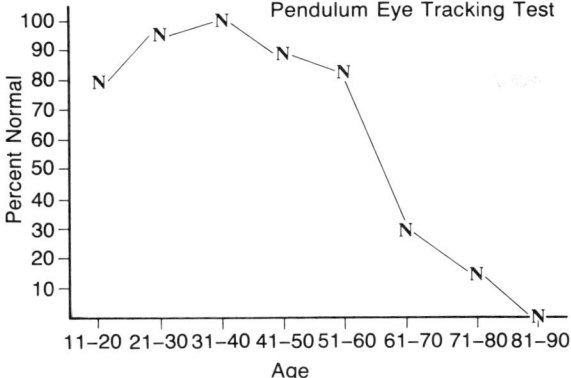

Figure 10-3 Graph demonstrating the percent (N) of 200 individuals without a history of balance or hearing problems and able to perform normal eye tracking tests. There is a marked decrease in tracking ability between ages 50 and 60.

bellar vestibular spinal system. Hall, Miller, and Corsellis, in their 1975 review of brain cell loss, note a concensus of opinions in the literature of a greater loss of Purkinje's cells in the cerebellum than in the rest of the brain.[12] They determined that there was a measurable diminishing in the number of cells beginning in the fifth decade. As with cells in Scarpa's ganglion, this number was variable. Some individuals in their ninth decade had a nearly normal number; others of the same age had a substantial reduction.

The balance mechanism, as tested by eye movement testing and postulography, showed more degeneration with age than the vestibular ocular reflexes, as determined by caloric and turning tests. This indicates that balance problems in the elderly are a result of loss of Purkinje's cells in the cerebellum. These cells have efferent control of the ocular motor system and the muscular system of the trunk, which depends on the cerebellum for coordination of muscular movements. Although the input from the vestibular system is reduced to about 30 percent in the elderly, this does not seem to explain the severe changes in the maintenance of posture. The cerebellar oculomotor and cerebellar spinal reflexes, on the other hand, seem to change rather rapidly at the end of the fifth decade. The role of the vestibular ganglia in the brain stem remains obscure because of the lack of morphologic data. The summary of the literature and our own data demonstrates some loss of sensory and neural structures from the end organ to the cerebellum and beyond in the central nervous system. Why particular types and groups of cells degenerate sooner than others needs more investigation.

References

1. Belal A Jr, Glorig A. Dysequilibrium of ageing (presbyastasis). J Laryngol Otol 1986; 100:1037-1041.
2. Ross MD, Johnsson L-G, Peacor D, Allard LF. Observations on normal and degenerating human otoconia. Ann Otol Rhinol Laryngol 1976; 85:310-326.
3. Schuknecht HF. Cupulolithiasis. Arch Otolaryngol 1969; 90:765-778.
4. Rosenhall U, Rubin W. Degenerative changes in the human vestibular sensory epithelia. Acta Otolaryngol 1975; 79:67-80.
5. Richter E. Quantitative study of human Scarpa's ganglion and vestibular sensory epithelia. Acta Otolaryngol 1980; 90:199-208.
6. Bergstrom B. Morphology of the vestibular nerve: II. The number of myelinated vestibular nerve fibers in man at various ages. Acta Otolaryngol 1973; 76:173-179.
7. Van der Laan FL, Oosterveld WJ. Age and vestibular function. Aerospace Med 1974; 45:540-547.
8. Hutton JT, Nagel JA, Loewenson RB. Variables affecting eye tracking performance. Electroencephalogr Clin Neurophysiol 1983; 56:414-419.
9. Morales-Garcia C, Rios E, Hoppe O, Fantuzzi H. Neurootological findings in cerebellar tumors. In: Graham MD, Kemink JL, eds. The vestibular system: neurophysiologic and clinical research. New York: Raven Press, 1987:421.
10. Gacek RR. The course and central termination of first order neurons supplying vestibular endorgans in the cat. Acta Otolaryngol [Suppl] 1969; (Suppl 254):1-66.
11. Peterka RJ, Black FO, Newell CD, Schoenhoff MB. Age-related changes in human vestibuloocular and vestibulospinal reflex function. (142A). In: Lim DJ, ed. Association for Research in Otolaryngology, 10th Midwinter Meeting, Clearwater Beach, FL, 1987: Abstracts. Columbus, OH: 1987: 112.
12. Hall TC, Miller AKH, Corsellis JAN. Variations in the human purkinje cell population according to age and sex. Neuropathol Appl Neurobiol 1975; 1:267-292.

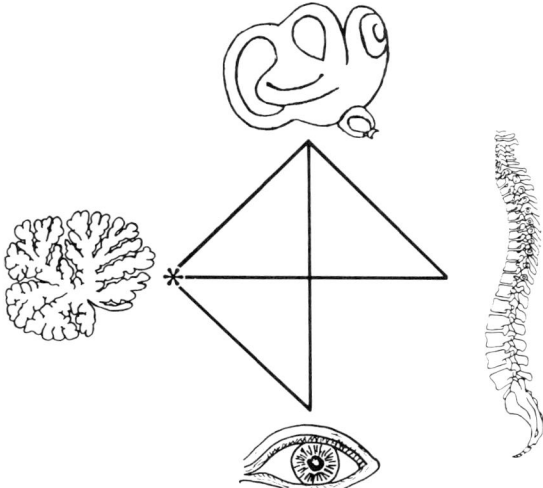

Figure 10-4 Diagram of the relationship of neural pathways controlling balance to the cerebellum. Impulses are afferent and efferent, the latter serving to control fine movement of the musculoskeletal system and eye movements, as well as to modify vestibular sensitivity.

Chapter Eleven

ATAXIA OF THE ELDERLY

HUGH O. BARBER, M.D., F.R.C.S.C.
BRIAN W. BLAKLEY, M.D., Ph.D., F.R.C.S.C.

FALLS AND IMBALANCE

Old people are afraid of falling, and with reason; the probability that a person will have a damaging fall by age 80 is about one in three[1] and women are affected more than men.[2] There is a huge health cost to society from femoral fracture alone, when considering the cumulative costs of acute care in hospital, possible complication, rehabilitation services, and, at times, prolonged care in a nursing home or similar institution. Wild et al[3] found that the inability to get up without help after falling altered prognosis; one-quarter of patients who lay on the floor for more than 1 hour died within 1 year, five times the rate expected for an age-matched group of control subjects.

Falls result from many causes, such as poor vision and tripping over objects, imbalance, drop spells in Meniere's disease,[4] syncope, postural hypotension, cardiac arrhythmia, Parkinsonism, and seizure disorders. Often the cause is not known.[1] Brocklehurst et al[5] reviewed the histories of 384 patients who had femur fracture from falls and estimated that perhaps 52 percent had some vestibular symptom preceding the attack. Loss of balance that was intermediate between a drop attack and an actual trip accounted for 32 percent.[5] Stelmach and Worringham[6] point out that, if a potential fall is imminent, sensory input must alert those centers responsible for response selection (to avoid the fall or to make a safe landing). Included in the alerting process are proprioception, vision, and vestibular senses. In aging, responses are slowed, especially "under conditions of time stress where there is limited opportunity for preparing the response in advance."[6]

Vision declines with age. Detection of passive movements of joints of the lower, but not upper, limbs declines in old age, and vibration sense in the lower limbs is also reduced.[6] Brocklehurst et al[7] found a high correlation between impaired vibration sense and body sway.

The vestibular system is subject to age changes. Rosenhall[8] studied the inner ears of 96 elderly individuals and found that the hair cell population decreased by 20 percent in the macular organs and by 40 percent in ampullary organs. Anniko[9] found that human Type I hair cells showed more age-related changes than Type II cells. Bergstrom[10] reported a 40 percent decline in human myelinated vestibular nerve fibers in old age. These morphologic changes do not transfer automatically to functional alteration, but there is evidence that vestibular function also changes with age. Bruner and Norris[11] found a decline of caloric reactivity after the seventh decade and cited other authors reporting a similar finding. In a more recent study, Karlsen et al[12] made similar observations. Studies in old people of the vestibulo-ocular response (VOR) to a wide range of frequencies of rotational stimuli appear to be lacking.

While falls result from a variety of causes, there seems to be good reason to suspect that vestibular and/or balance disorders may be a potent source.

ATAXIA OF THE ELDERLY

Patients with many kinds and causes of dizziness are seen in our Dizziness Unit.[13] Each patient receives a careful review from an experienced neurotologist and a series of standard laboratory tests of vestibular function, which, at present, does not include platform posturography. Recently we decided to group together under the category "Ataxia of the Elderly" all those patients over age 70 whose primary complaint was balance disturbance. Many of these patients had other head sensations, such as postural dizziness or lightheadedness, but in each case the first reason for attendance was imbalance, staggering, or fear of falling. All of these patients had the routine review referred to earlier, supplemented by appropriate radiologic and laboratory tests.

Ataxia of the elderly is much commoner in women than in men; in the age group 81 to 90, 89 percent of the patients were women. Figures 11–1 and 11–2 give diagnostic categories, established by

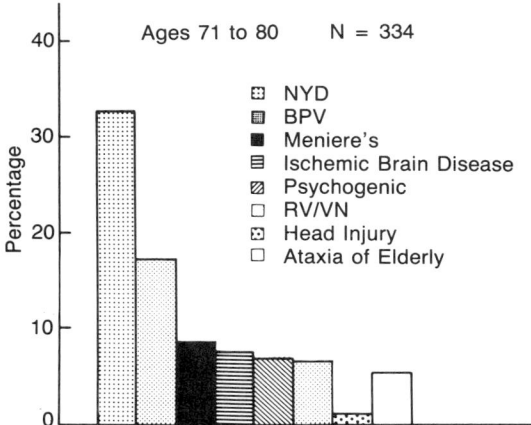

Figure 11-1 Diagnoses in eighth decade. NYD = undiagnosed, BPV = benign postural vertigo, RV/VN = recurrent vestibulopathy/vestibular neuronitis.

the Dizziness Unit, of patients in their eighth and ninth decades. The incidence of both ataxia of the elderly and ischemic brain disease (stroke, transient ischemic attack) doubles from one decade to the next.

Table 11-1 gives a list of most of the conditions considered responsible for ataxia of the elderly. While "undiagnosed" was the most common, a number of causes were identifiable.

CASE REPORTS

Case 1

A 72-year-old woman had the insidious onset of a sense of imbalance 2 years earlier. She would

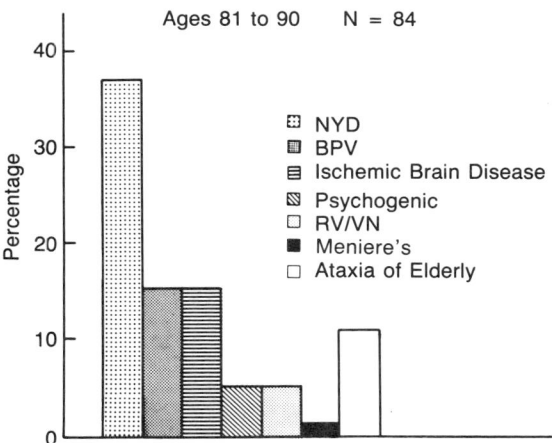

Figure 11-2 Diagnoses in ninth decade. Labeling as in Figure 11-1. Both ischemic brain disease and ataxia of the elderly are much more frequent than in the eighth decade (see Figure 11-1).

TABLE 11-1 Causes of Ataxia of the Elderly

Undiagnosed
Cerebellar degeneration
Bilateral vestibular loss
Unilateral vestibular loss—decompensation
Metabolic

start walking with good balance and then begin to waver to one side or to feel as if she was walking on a slant. Sometimes these feelings were accompanied by an abnormal head sensation, which she could not describe accurately. The symptoms had not progressed from onset. She had not fallen.

She was said to be borderline diabetic, had suffered a myocardial infarction 12 years earlier, and had a right carotid endarterectomy for an episode of slurred speech and left hemiparesis 7 years earlier.

On neurotologic examination, no clear physical abnormality was found. Electronystagmographic (ENG) recordings of ocular motor and vestibular function were normal. Hearing was normal for age, and auditory brain stem responses (ABR) were within normal limits. Computerized tomographic (CT) scanning was normal.

Comment: We considered this patient an example of ataxia of the elderly that was undiagnosed, a common circumstance. Many such patients have demonstrable gait ataxia, though she had none.

Case 2

A 78-year-old woman had relatively constant imbalance for about 5 years without a sense of spinning or lightheadedness. She had fallen several times. Auditory and focal neurologic symptoms were absent.

On examination, smooth ocular pursuit movements to the right were saccadic, and visual cancellation of a target moving with her as she moved her head at low frequency from left to right (VOR cancellation) was impaired.[14] Tandem gait was ataxic with eyes open and could not be performed with eyes closed. The audiogram, ENG, and CT were normal.

Comment: Here is a woman with ataxia and abnormal visual and vestibular function. The features point certainly to central nervous system (CNS) disease, but its nature is not known.

Case 3

A 71-year-old man was referred after several falls. In one fall, he had broken a rib, and in another he had fallen from a ladder. He thought that the falls were part of episodes of loss of balance, and he had no abnormal head sensations. His balance had been poor for the preceding 10 years, with episodes of staggering to either side. There were no auditory or focal neurologic symptoms.

On examination, finger-to-nose movements were somewhat dysmetric on each side. Tandem gait was very ataxic. Hearing and ENG examinations showed no significant abnormalities. CT (Fig. 11–3) showed cerebellar atrophy.

Comment: Probably the falls and ataxia in this patient have a common origin in the cerebellar atrophy.

Case 4

A lively 87-year-old woman had gradually increasing balance impairment for the preceding 2 or 3 years. The imbalance was much worse in the dark. Three or 4 years earlier, on several occasions she had visible circling of surroundings that lasted for "less than a minute", and she would have fallen had she not held on to something for support. She had had no falls. Auditory and focal neurologic symptoms were absent. Her general health was good.

On neurotologic examination, she lost three lines of the oscillopsia test.[14] Tandem gait was impossible for her. No other abnormalities were found.

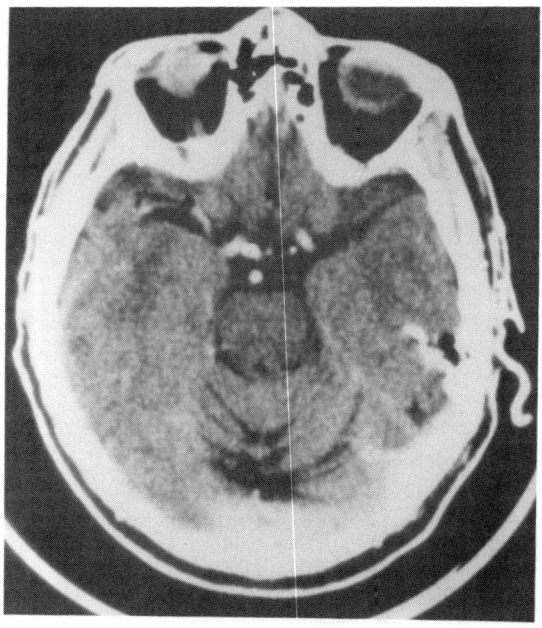

Figure 11–3 Case 3, CT scan. The cerebellar sulci are abnormally visible because of gyral atrophy.

Hearing was normal. ENG showed absent caloric responses bilaterally, and no eye movement response to sinusoidal rotational stimulation at 0.05 Hz (dark) was detected. CT was normal.

Comment: Bilateral vestibular loss of unknown cause explained this woman's ataxia. Clear evidence of CNS disease was lacking, and she had never received aminoglycosides. No cause has been identified in more than half of our cases of bilateral vestibular reduction or loss (unpublished data).

Case 5

An 84-year-old woman had increasing ataxia for several years that caused her to fall to one side quite often. Thirty years earlier she had had an episode of marked circling of surroundings, nausea, and severe imbalance, which gradually improved with a period of 10 to 14 days bed rest. Afterwards she had mild unsteadiness, especially with quick turns, but a considerable and progressive increase in her unsteadiness led to her referral. There were no auditory or focal neurologic symptoms. Her past health was good.

On neurotologic examination, the sole abnormality was a deviation to the right on tandem gait, with eyes closed only. Hearing was normal. ENG showed absent caloric response from the left side. CT was normal.

Comment: This woman had an episode of vestibular neuronitis 30 years earlier with a resulting permanent caloric loss on one side. She made a reasonably good compensatory response in the early months and years after this, but with advancing age and a declining neuron population in the brain, symptoms of decompensation appeared.

DISCUSSION

Balance disturbance, sometimes with falls, appears to be quite common in old age. Imbalance and fear of falls are certainly two reasons for elderly people's use of canes, though of course other reasons exist. With increasing interest in the afflictions of aging, we thought it reasonable to separate ataxia of the elderly from other conditions in order to focus attention on the condition and to gain skill in identification of its different causes. In most cases, using conventional methods of examination, no distinctive pathology has been identified, as in Case 1. The assumption that a natural decline in sense organ (eye, ear, proprioceptor) and brain function collaborate to cause ataxia in some people is not very appealing. We think it likely that further study will result in identification of specific abnormalities in these people.

Episodic and compensated unilateral, peripheral vestibular disorders do not usually produce persisting ataxia. Meniere's disease and recurrent vestibulopathy[15] are episodic, and the initial severe ataxia of vestibular neuronitis with persisting caloric loss is compensated for in a matter of weeks, though slight imbalance to a minor degree might persist indefinitely. However, recall that lasting ataxia results if animals with unilateral vestibular neurectomy are kept in the dark and restrained for only a few days after surgery.[16] We are confident that this experimental observation can be translated directly into clinical care of humans. *Early* movement and vision are essential for maximal compensatory recovery after such a lesion or its medical equivalent, severe vestibular neuronitis. Probably this requirement is even more critical in the older patient; the compensation process must require an effective neuronal pool, and it is reasonable to expect this pool's population and efficiency to diminish with advancing age.

Bilateral vestibular loss from any cause produces varying degrees of ataxia and, of course, may occur at any age. We have the clinical impression that, in this condition, staggering is usually more marked and disabling in older than younger people. Bilateral vestibular reduction is not a frequent cause of ataxia of the elderly in our material, but the probability that caloric activity diminishes after age 70 leads to the speculation that if the reduction is progressive, ataxia from this cause might be a relatively common occurrence in extremely old people.

The brain, especially the cerebellum, plays a key role in balance. Imbalance may result from primary cerebellar disease, mainly (in the elderly) from degeneration or ischemia, and this is a prominent candidate for the cause of our undiagnosed subgroup of ataxia of the elderly. A good cerebellum coordinates orientation signals from vestibular organs, vision, and position sensors, and has the capacity to repair the harmful effects (including ataxia) of defective visual and vestibular signals, at least. To a considerable extent, a good brain can cover up for the sins of defective orientation receptors. However, if that cover-up mechanism is getting old or anatomically or biochemically less effective, symptoms of a previously masked lesion may reappear, as in Case 5. Thus, the compensatory and/or adaptive capacity of the brain is probably a key player in imbalance of old people.

Table 11-2 gives an outline of our current investigation strategy in dealing with ataxia of the elderly. Review by a neurologist colleague is advisable in order to identify such conditions as Parkinsonism, posterior column disease, hypothyroidism, or diabetic neuropathy. All patients have brain imaging, which at our institution is CT scanning, although magnetic resonance imaging is preferred. We think it makes sense to attempt to obtain, by posturography, measured information on the vestibulospinal system and its relation to visual and vestibular function and expect to add this investigation to our study.

TABLE 11-2 Investigation of Ataxia of the Elderly

History, neurotologic examination
ENG
Neurologic consultation
Brain imaging
? Posturography

Better understanding of imbalance in the elderly will probably come from needed research in old people on such matters as vestibular function, motor responses to ordinary challenges, proprioceptive function, and visual-vestibular interaction. We need information on the brain's processing and transmitting systems, and on how these change in senescence. There is hope that effective means of altering some of the serious disabilities of aging can be found. Even now, the ataxia that may accompany severe hypothyroidism can be improved with thyroid replacement.

And the old can learn. Both young and old people perform slow tandem gait better with repetition. Stelmach and Worringham[6] note Begbies' finding in old people of a decrease in postural sway with practice. Who would have guessed, 15 or so years ago, that the incidence of stroke would decline in North America by about 5 percent yearly? Who can now predict the potentially great practical value of researches in neurochemistry? There is certainly a pressing need for advances in understanding and improving the health needs of the elderly, and surely good reason for optimism that these objectives can be achieved.

References

1. Issacs B. Are falls a manifestation of brain failure? Age Ageing 1978; 7(Suppl):97–105.
2. Gryfe CI, Amies A, Ashley MJ. A longitudinal study of falls in an elderly population: I. Incidence and morbidity. Age Ageing 1977; 6:201–210.
3. Wild D, Nayak USL, Isaacs B. How dangerous are falls in old people at home? Br Med J 1981; 282:266–286.

4. Tumarkin A. The otolithic catastrophe: a new syndrome. Br Med J 1936; 2:175–177.
5. Brocklehurst JC, Exton-Smith AN, Lempert Barber SM, et al. Fracture of the femur in old age: a two-centre study of associated clinical factors and the cause of the fall. Age Ageing 1978; 7:2–15.
6. Stelmach GE, Worringham CJ. Sensorimotor deficits related to postural stability. Implications for falling in the elderly. Clin Geriatric Med 1985; 1:679–694.
7. Brocklehurst JC, Robertson D, James-Groom P. Clinical correlates of sway in old age-sensory modalities. Age Ageing 1982; 11:1–10.
8. Rosenhall U. Degenerative patterns in the aging human vestibular neuro-epithelia. Acta Otolaryngol 1973; 76:208–220.
9. Anniko M. The aging vestibular hair cell. Am J Otolaryngol 1983; 4:151–160.
10. Bergstrom B. Morphology of the vestibular nerve. II. The number of myelinated nerve fibers in man at various ages. Acta Otolaryngol 1973; 76:173–179.
11. Bruner A, Norris TW. Age-related changes in caloric nystagmus. Acta Otolaryngol 1971; Suppl 282.
12. Karlsen EA, Hassanein RM, Goetzinger CP. The effects of age, sex, hearing loss and water temperature on caloric nystagmus. Laryngoscope 1981; 91:620–627.
13. Nedzelski JM, Barber HO, McIlmoyl L. J Otolaryngol 1986; 15:101–104.
14. Barber HO. Vestibular neurophysiology. Otolaryngol Head Neck Surg 1984; 92:55–58.
15. Leliever WC, Barber HO. Recurrent vestibulopathy. Laryngoscope 1981; 91:1–6.
16. Lacour M, Xerri C. Vestibular compensation: new perspectives. In: Flohr H, Precht W, eds. Lesion-induced neuronal plasticity in sensorimotor systems. New York: Springer-Verlag, 1981: 240.

THE AGING VOICE

Chapter Twelve

EVALUATION AND MANAGEMENT OF VOICE DISORDERS IN THE ELDERLY

MURRAY D. MORRISON, M.D., F.R.C.S.C.
LINDA A. RAMMAGE, B.A., M.Sc., S–LP(C)
HAMISH NICHOL, M.B., F.R.C.P.C.

INTRODUCTION

While the elderly patient may develop a voice disorder from those causative factors that affect all age groups, such as upper respiratory tract infections, he or she is also susceptible to "things" that have to do with getting or being old (Table 12–1). Firstly, there are those changes that are simply a normal part of the aging process. These "old voices" should not generally be considered to be disordered, but it is important for the otolaryngologist and speech pathologist to know and understand these changes in order to be in a position to help out when problems develop. We are all aware that some old men have a thin reedy voice that is higher in pitch than it used to be, and we also know women whose voices deepen with age. How far do these changes have to go before they cease to be normal? And who decides? When the older woman's voice gets too low in pitch, she is likely to unconsciously make muscular adjustments designed to raise the pitch. This works to a point, but soon the dysphonic voice is more a result of the muscular misuses brought on by the attempted compensations than of the original changes in the glottis. In a similar way, the old man with an easily tiring "glottal fry" voice and bowed-looking vocal cords is suffering as much from his subconscious attempt to drive the vocal pitch down to a more male-sounding level as he is from the muscle atrophy, fragmented collagen, and weakened elastin of his larynx. And how should these two hypothetical patients be treated? Should we coax them into accepting their "old voice" fate

TABLE 12–1 Voice Disorders in the Elderly

Changes due to normal aging
Unsuccessful compensatory voice use
Psychogenic dysphonia
Voice problems in neurologic disease
Miscellaneous causes: organic disease, reflux, iatrogenic causes

and help them out of their compensatory muscle misuse, or should we offer treatment designed to combat the aging changes, such as dissection or suction removal of submucosal tissue of Reinke's edema or early polypoidal degeneration?

Vocal folds are made up largely of voluntary muscle, and voluntary muscles move them about. This finely tuned neuromuscular system is prone to being knocked out of alignment by either psychologic or neurologic disease processes. Some forms of neurologic degenerative disorders, such as Parkinson's disease, affect the voice, and some psychopathologies cause dysphonia via the final common pathway of muscle misuse. Some of these psychological problems occur with prevalence in the elderly.

Finally, we must realize that older people are more prone to cancers, and this diagnosis must be ruled out in every case. Other systemic ailments that can play a part in dysphonia include lower respiratory problems and gastroesophageal reflux disease.

The clinical features of each of these disorder groups will be considered in detail after we review the steps that the clinician must take to establish a diagnosis.

HISTORY

Taking a history from anyone with a voice disorder is unique in that the most important physical features, other than those seen by laryngoscopy, can be observed or heard simultaneously with the collection of historical data. As the patient relates the ways in which the voice problem affects their activities or lifestyle, one can observe how the topic of conversation changes or does not change the voice. One listens for the expected sounds associated with aging and/or possible compensatory misuses, such as a breathy vocal fry in the old man or a hypertense dissonance in a woman. Nonverbal cues help elucidate the patient's mood or mental state. Agitation or depression may be evident, and it is important during the discussion to explore family, psychosocial, or occupational factors that may be associated in time or other ways with the voice disorder. There is not always a strong correlation between the severity of the dysphonia and the level of the patient's concern about it. When the mildly dysphonic voice complains bitterly, one must wonder why.

The history taking should enquire about general health and past medical history, since there may be relationships such as thyroid disease that may not be obvious to the patient. One should also enquire about symptoms that suggest gastroesophageal reflux, such as globus, postnasal drip, habitual throat-clearing, nighttime choking spells, sour acid taste, and heartburn, particularly if they are worse in the morning. Clean normal phonation requires relatively relaxed vocal fold approximation. Even if not the primary cause of the dysphonia, any active reflux disease impacts negatively on the voice because it tends to produce increased muscular tightness in the larynx and throat area generally. Smoking is almost always a factor in the more severe cases of polypoidal degeneration, particularly in older women, and of course may cause dysplastic and malignant change.

The patient's hearing ability and that of his or her spouse is a frequent factor in the management of a voice disorder.

PHYSICAL EXAMINATION

A full head and neck examination is required, and while one tends to focus on examination of the larynx, it is important to pay attention to other factors important in communication, including hearing, general alertness and mental status, any apparent tremors or movement disorders, any nonvocal speech problems such as dysarthria or abnormal resonance, and any voice related postural or musculoskeletal abnormalities.

Laryngoscopic features of various voice disorders are described in the succeeding section. Indirect mirror examination of the larynx is generally adequate and is often all that is available to the clinician. However, the flexible fiberoptic laryngoscope or rigid rod lens telescope, particularly when interfaced with a video camera, adds extra magnification and detail, which increases diagnostic precision. With these tools it is no longer necessary to submit the elderly patient to a general anesthetic in those instances when mirror visualization is not possible.

Stroboscopic laryngoscopy is another useful adjunct. In the elderly patient it can help to differentiate between functional and structural bowing or can demonstrate the reason for persistent dysphonia after laryngeal microsurgery by showing loss of a normal mucosal wave.

OTHER DOCUMENTATION

When possible, the patient's voice should be recorded as a clinical record as well as an aid to future therapy. During this recording session, the speech pathologist may begin to evaluate ways in which the voice patterns can be altered.

Most other objective measures of vocal function are still finding their way from research laboratories to everyday use in the clinic, but instruments can be purchased that perform an automated acoustic analysis (e.g., jitter, shimmer, harmonics-to-noise ratio). Other studies of glottic waveform such as electroglottography, photoglottography, and phonatory airflow studies can be performed. The full range of clinical usefulness of these measures is still to be established.

CLINICAL FEATURES OF VOICE DISORDERS IN THE ELDERLY

Normal Effects of Aging on the Larynx

Studies of the cartilaginous, mucosal, muscular, and connective tissue components of the larynx have yielded a general consensus about expected changes of normal aging (Table 12-2). Ossification of the cartilage begins near 25 years of age and is complete by age 65.[1] Islands of cartilage remain in the thyroid cartilage in the male, and preservation of cartilage exists in the upper portion of the female larynx. The cricoid may be nearly completely ossified.[1,2] The arytenoid undergoes ossification of the body and muscular process, with the apex remaining cartilaginous. In general, the onset of ossification is later and less extensive in women, and the entire process is variable between individuals. The ossification represents creation of true haversian systems with lamellae, osteocytes, and fat marrow. There is nothing to suggest that this ossification process is directly related to laryngeal dysfunction except where changes occur in the cricoarytenoid joints. Kahn and Kahane[3] have shown that older articular surfaces undergo fibrillation and other changes in collagen fiber arrangement, as well as ossification that may limit the range of arytenoid excursion. When this leads to an inadequate posterior

TABLE 12-2 Voice Effects of Aging

Atrophic changes
  Mostly in males
  Increased pitch
  Thin, reedy voice

Edema and polypoid change
  Females
  Lower pitched voice
  Pharyngeal formants also lower
  Smoking relationship

Vocal stability
  Wobbling and tremolo (S.D. fo and jitter)
  Physical conditioning versus age

---

glottic closure, there may be a degree of air leakage that alters voice quality and intensity.

The connective tissue changes are quite uniform, but again a sex difference exists. In the male, the elastin fibers are fewer, fragmented, and clumped in groups. The absolute number of collagen fibers is decreased after age 50, with the remaining fibers being thinner. They are also seen to separate from each other and become more wavy. In females, the dense packing and linear relationship is preserved. The muscles of the larynx show general thinning and decreased fiber density, as well as fragmentation of the intermuscular septae.[1,2] Sato and Tauchi[4] have shown a significant decrease in the number of both red and white muscle fibers with some increase in fiber volume after 50 years of age. After age 80 the changes are even more significant, but while the loss of red fibers is compensated to some degree by increased fiber volume, the white fibers simply are reduced in number. Finally, there is a decrease in the number of fibroblasts seen in the conus elasticus. These changes are more prevalent in male than in female larynges.[1,2]

The aforementioned changes tend to occur parallel to each other and in accompaniment with mucosal changes. The mucous membrane is thinned and atrophic. Mucous glands become atrophic and reduced in number. Metaplasia of the epithelium is seen. The underlying tissue may be subject to fatty infiltration, and the number of lymphatic channels is reduced.[2,5]

Laryngeal findings on physical examination are familiar to practising laryngologists. One study[6] found 39 percent of male and 47 percent of female larynges examined to have significant abnormalities. Honjo and Isshiki found that 67 percent of these males had a glottic gap, a similar portion had atrophy, and 56 percent had edema. Females had significant edema in 74 percent, a glottic gap in 58 percent, and only 26 percent had atrophy. About one in 10 in each sex had vocal cord sulci.

Mysak[7] compared middle-aged sons to their elderly fathers and discovered an increasing fundamental frequency of speech with advancing years from middle age onwards. Hollien and Shipp[8] studied males from age 20 to 80 and, in addition to confirming this trend, established that the curve was saucer-shaped when younger subjects were included. They theorized that the vocal cords were thickest in the 40s and 50s with the increasing fundamental frequency being secondary to thinning and stiffening of the vocal cords.

Several studies have shown that the vocal fundamental frequency becomes lower in aging females.[9,10] This is generally felt to be related to Reinke's edema and polypoidal changes. However, Linville and Fisher[10,11] have shown that the first formant frequency is also reduced for both phonated and whispered voice, thus suggesting that both phonatory and resonance features play a role in defining age characteristics of women's voices.

There is less agreement among studies of pitch range. McGlone and Hollien[12] determined that pitch range was largely preserved in elderly women, whereas Ptacek[13] found a loss of the high-tone production in both sexes, and Luchsinger's study supported this.[5] Aronsen's[14] larger series supported the preservation of pitch range in both sexes. Methodology differences in each series may be responsible for the apparently conflicting results.

Ramig[15,16] has shown that fundamental frequency changes and quality differences, manifest by actual jitter and shimmer scores as well as by phonation time and range, may be caused as much or more by general physical condition as by actual chronological age. Other age-related voice changes include a wobbling of the voice, attributed to irregular respirations, and the tremulous voice or "senile tremolo." Some of these changes can be demonstrated as increased fundamental frequency standard deviation and altered jitter scores.[17]

In summary, it seems that there are two altered states in the larynx that develop with aging. One state is a thickened, chronically edematous larynx, with phonation in the lower part of the voice range and a husky or muffled timbre. Atrophic changes predominate in the other state. These patients develop a squeaky voice from using the upper end of their range, and the vocal timbre is thin and reedy.

Pitch changes with aging are noted in the preceding literature review and occur more noticeably in males than in females. In the male, the voice is deepest in the fourth and fifth decades and rises later in life apparently because of the decreased bulk and elasticity of the vocal cords. Terms used to describe vocal quality changes resulting from this rise include "thin," "reedy," and "breathy." Pitch change is not noted so significantly among females. Even if a rise in vocal pitch among females in later life were present, it would not be perceived as a problem since the higher pitch would be considered sociably acceptable and therefore not likely to result in a functional misuse because of a failed attempt at compensation.

Some degree of polypoidal degeneration of the vocal cords with Reinke's space edema has been described as developing in older persons. Distinct from the atrophic changes already described, these polypoidal thickenings are more noticeable in females since they result in a drop of the vocal pitch and lead to a harsh and/or breathy voice. This more masculine sounding voice, which occurs mainly in older women who have smoked for many years, is socially unacceptable to the patient. Consequently, the woman with early polypoidal changes and a deepening pitch is at risk for developing ventricular band functional misuse related to inappropriate approach to compensation. Any early polypoidal change in the male vocal cord causes a deepening of the pitch, which results in the maintenance of a younger and more masculine sound. Consequently, this is not perceived as a problem and no attempt at compensation would occur.

Disorders Due to Attempts to Compensate for Normal Aging Process

As already described, the aging process in the male larynx involves muscle atrophy and loss of elasticity. The normal voice effect is increased pitch and thinning of the vocal tone. Attempts to compensate for this result in a gravelly and vocal fry type of phonation with easy fatiguing of the voice and consequent increased vocal effort (Table 12-3). The audible breathiness and fry correlates with apparent shortening and bowing of the true vocal cords on indirect laryngoscopy. Less bowing may be noted if vocal cord lengthening can be achieved by higher-pitched phonation, and the voice may become considerably less dysphonic when the patient is encouraged to speak in a higher range.

In females with developing polypoidal degeneration of the vocal folds, the most common compensatory misuse is a squeezing of the larynx in an attempt to increase vocal pitch (see Table 12-3). This may be quite dramatic and marked to the stage of

TABLE 12-3 Unsuccessful Compensatory Voice Use

Male
    Attempts to drop pitch
    Gravelly, breathy, glottal fry
    Easy fatigue
    Apparently bowed vocal cords

Female
    Attempts to raise pitch
    Squeezed, strained
    Effortful voice
    Variable ventricular band adduction

ventricular band dysphonia, or may be associated only with a mild false cord adduction and an apparent increased tension in the true vocal cords with increased vocal effort. Phonation becomes easier and clearer when the patient is encouraged to allow the vocal tone to drop to a more physiologic level consistent with the polypoid change.

Psychogenic Dysphonia in the Elderly

Psychogenic voice disorders may be produced by various psychopathologic processes, including tensional, hypochondriacal, depressive equivalent, and symbolic processes (Table 12-4). Tensional symptoms arise from the overactivity of the autonomic and voluntary nervous systems in individuals who are unduly aroused and anxious. Since speech is a significant part of our social interaction, any voice difficulty can well lead to anxiety about human relationships, and this anxiety, once aroused, tends to perpetuate itself. Depressive equivalent symptoms may arise in those individuals who are not complaining overtly of depression, but who may be suppressing the impulse to cry or to express anger verbally. In older patients, loneliness or separation from family frequently may lead to depressions that result in a vocal muscular misuse. Symbolic symptoms occur in those who convert a psychologic conflict into a somatic symptom; this is generally termed a conversion hysteria and, while more often related to a hypoadduction of the true cords with whisper phonation, it can also be seen in patients with ventricular band adduction.

There is, logically, considerable overlap between those patients who have dysphonia as a result of attempting to compensate for age-related changes and those patients who have purely psychogenic functional dysphonias. Consequently, when evalu-

TABLE 12-4 Psychogenic Dysphonia in the Elderly

Process	Includes
Tensional	Overactive neural activity with anxiety
Depressive	Suppressed cry or anger; loneliness
Symbolic	Conversion to a somatic symptom
Hypochondriacal	Self-fulfilling anticipation of poor voice

ating an elderly female patient with adducting false cords and with either tightly adducted true cords, giving a high pitched squeaky voice, or low tension glottic bowing, yielding a lower pitched breathy voice, it may be difficult for the clinician to determine just how much is purely psychogenic and how much is compensatory misuse. The relative ease with which changes can be enticed during a voice therapy program may help sort this out.

Voice Disorders Associated with Neurologic Degenerative Processes

Neurologic diseases tend to occur more commonly in elderly persons, and as would be expected, voice difficulties associated with these present from time to time. There are a number of general neurologic diseases in which the voice may be abnormal, but these seldom present a diagnostic problem for the otolaryngologist since they are rarely the presenting symptom. Examples include stroke, amyotrophic lateral sclerosis, pseudobulbar palsy, and so on. However, dysphonia on occasion may be the presenting symptom of a neurologic disorder (Table 12-5). Essential tremor, although usually presenting in the dominant hand, may present as a vocal tremor that is a more or less regular fluctuation of pitch and/or loudness during speech or singing at a rate of 4 to 12 cycles per second. It may be associated with essential tremor in the head and neck, face, mandible, or tongue, as well as in the upper limbs. Tremor of the voice is consistent throughout all phonatory efforts; it is usually most evident during sustained phonation of a single vowel in the middle to lower end of the pitch range and is often intensified with efforts to increase loudness. A vocal tremor results in a rhythmic quavering quality.

A flat monotone voice with loss of expression and rhythm may be a presenting symptom of Parkinson's disease. The voice often is low in volume and energy. The diagnosis is confirmed by resolution of the problem following treatment with anti-Parkinsonian drugs.

Focal dystonias in the head and neck can result in prolonged muscle spasms leading to blepharal spasm, oral mandibular dystonia, or laryngeal dystonia. As with the other focal dystonias of spasmodic torticollis or writer's cramp, these tend to be refractory to most forms of treatment.

Miscellaneous Causes of Dysphonia in the Elderly

Cancers of the larynx and other tumors in this area may, of course, produce voice changes, and while these disorders make up an important segment of the elderly dysphonic population, they will not be considered here.

Gastroesophageal reflux disease is a common accompaniment of other processes producing dysphonia and in many cases is the basic underlying etiologic factor (Table 12-6). When reflux is present, many patients develop an "acid laryngitis" that consists principally of erythema around the posterior glottis, sometimes with ulceration and contact granuloma formation. These findings are associated with symptoms of globus, habitual throat-clearing, postnasal drip, and voice changes that are often worse in the morning. Often, the larynx may look more normal, and the voice changes are related to increased laryngeal muscle tension. The hyperfunctional voice use is probably associated with a generalized increase in tonus, related to chronic esophageal irritation, and an upwardly referred sensation through the vagally-mediated pathway, thus leading to a reflex-induced muscular tension as well as to the pharyngolaryngeal symptom complex. In patients with functional voice misuse related to other causative factors, it is often apparent that the overall treatment is easier and more effective when the chronic gastric reflux is controlled.

Laryngeal trauma in this age group is more

TABLE 12-5 Neurologic Disease and Dysphonia

May be presenting symptom in
  Essential tremor
  Parkinson's disease
  Focal dystonias

Not usual presenting symptom in
  Stroke
  Amyotrophic lateral sclerosis
  Pseudobulbar palsy

TABLE 12-6 Miscellaneous Causes of Dsyphonia in the Elderly

Gastroesophageal reflux
   Direct: acid laryngitis
   Indirect: reflex hypertonicity

Laryngeal trauma
   Usually iatrogenic, following surgery
      for polypoidal degeneration

Tumors

---

often than not iatrogenic. A too common example is the elderly female patient with mild or moderate polypoidal degeneration or Reinke's edema who undergoes removal of the polypoid tissue only to develop much more severe dysphonia because of scarring of the surface of the vocal cord and subsequent tethering of the overlying mucosa. The resultant loss of the mucosal wave is clearly visible with stroboscopy. Once established, this condition may produce longstanding dysphonia for which most treatments are ineffective.

TREATMENT OF VOICE DISORDERS IN THE ELDERLY

Counseling

Often the elderly patient needs only to be reassured that the changes they are detecting in their voice do not represent any life-threatening illness. Helping them to understand why things are changing as they are, in some cases is all the treatment needed.

Voice Therapy

Voice therapy for voice disorders in the elderly is frequently focused on reduction of muscular misuses that accompany attempts by the patient to compensate for the changes that have occurred. The therapy program may be directed towards encouraging the upward adjustment of vocal pitch in the elderly male with thinning vocal cords, coupled with any necessary alterations of respiratory support and resonance. In the female, it may consist of encouraging her to accept a deeper vocal pitch and to develop an easier more relaxed style of laryngeal muscle use.

Psychological Management

Counseling by the laryngologist and the speech pathologist, as well as the actual voice therapy program, makes up a major portion of the management of the psychological component of the dysphonia. The reassurance and attentive care that patients receive during this process cannot help but have positive therapeutic effects. However, in some cases where associated anxiety and/or depression is a major causative factor in the dysphonia, management may be more difficult without assistance from a psychologist or psychiatrist.

The indications for psychiatric referral (Table 12-7) in these situations include a strong coincidental psychological event that occurred with the onset of the dysphonia, or the clinician's intuition as to how important psychological factors may or may *not* be. The word "not" has been highlighted in this case because, when explaining to a patient why you feel it is necessary that a psychologist or psychiatrist become involved in the evaluation process, it is often useful to indicate that the major psychological factors may not be relevant, but that you do not have the background training or expertise to be able to answer that particular question. During a voice therapy program, a patient may appear to become less motivated to achieve changes or may respond inappropriately to improvement in the voice that can be demonstrated with the help of the speech pathologist, and these factors may suggest that psychiatric help may be beneficial. Similarly, when the dysphonia recurs after a period of recovery and the reason for the recurrence is obscure, then further search into psychological processes may be appropriate. Finally, the patient may recognize the strong relationship between the dysphonia and psychological factors and may express an interest in seeing the Voice Clinic psychiatric consultant, either at the time of the

TABLE 12-7 Reasons for a Psychiatry Referral

At initial assessment
   Coincident psychological event with onset of dysphonia
   Cause and effect relationship unclear

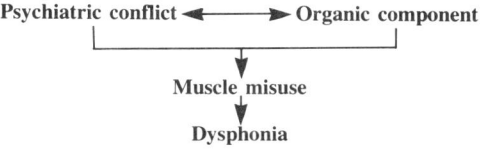

   Patient requests psychiatry referral

During voice therapy program
   Reduced motivation
   Inappropriate response to demonstrated improvement
   Recurrence of dysphonia after recovery
   Patient requests psychiatry referral

initial assessment or during the voice therapy program.

Sometimes voice disorders in elderly people are part of their general social situations. They may find themselves living alone in an apartment with little opportunity to use their voices except on the telephone. Encouragement to alter their social situation to permit more free direct voice use might be helpful.

Medical Management

Direct medical management of dysphonia depends on the cause. Since this often involves management of neurologic disorders, this subject will not be covered here. The point has already been made about managing problems of chronic gastroesophageal reflux when associated with a dysphonia, and this is often a most useful medical adjunct to treatment.

Surgical Management

Conservatism in surgery should be the general rule when managing patients with voice disorders, particularly when treating a patient with polypoidal degeneration. If this is of sufficient size to warrant surgical treatment, and if altering the voice use through a therapy program has not been sufficiently successful, then reduction in the amount of polypoidal degeneration may occasionally be warranted. This should entail removal of the Reinke's space edema tissue only, if at all possible, with maintenance of the epithelial cover. This can be accomplished by making an incision laterally along the superior aspect of the vocal cord and reflecting the mucosal flap medially toward the free margin. Cup forceps, alligator forceps, or suction can then be used to ease the gelatinous polypoidal tissue away from the underlying vocalis muscle. Following this, the mucosa can be draped back over the vocal cord. Fibrin glues such as Tisseel can be helpful in keeping the mucosa in place.

The management of dysphonia associated with scarring and mucosal tethering following vocal cord stripping can be extremely difficult and good results are hard to obtain. These dysphonias are often unresponsive to voice therapy, and injection of the cords with substances such as Teflon is generally not helpful. The use of collagen to inject the vocal cords submucosally is still being evaluated, but may hold some promise.

References

1. Pressman JJ, Keleman G. Physiology of the larynx. Physiol Rev 1955; 35:513-515.
2. Kahane JC. A survey of age-related changes in the connective tissues of the human adult larynx. In: Bless DM, Abbs JH, eds. Vocal cord physiology. San Diego: College-Hill Press, 1983:44.
3. Kahn AR, Kahane JC. India ink pinprick assessment of age-related changes in the cricoarytenoid joint (CAJ) articular surfaces. J Speech Hear Res 1986; 4:536-543.
4. Sato T, Tauchi H: Age changes in human vocal muscle. Mech Ageing Dev 1982 Jan: 18(1):67-74.
5. Luchsinger R, Arnold G. Vocal involution or seniscence of the voice. In: Voice-speech-language. Belmont, CA: Wadsworth Publishing Co, 1965:135.
6. Honjo I, Isshiki N. Laryngoscopic and vocal characteristics of aged persons. Osaka, Japan: Kansai Medical University, 1979.
7. Mysak ED. Pitch and duration characteristics of older males. J Speech Hear Res 1959; 2:46-54.
8. Hollien H, Shipp T. Speaking fundamental frequency and chronologic age in males. J Speech Hear Res 1972; 15:155-159.
9. Morgan EE, Rastatter M. Variability of voice fundamental frequency in elderly female speakers. Percept Mot Skills 1986; 1:215-218.
10. Linville SE, Fisher HB. Acoustic characteristics of perceived versus actual vocal age in controlled phonation by adult females. J Acoust Soc Am 1985; 78(1 Pt 1):40-48.
11. Linville SE, Fisher HB. Acoustic characteristics of women's voices with advancing age. J Gerontol 1985; 3:324-330.
12. McGlone R, Hollien H. Vocal pitch characteristics of aged women. J Speech Hear Res 1963; 6:164-170.
13. Ptacek P, Sander EK, Malone WH, Jackson CCR. Phonatory and related changes with advanced age. J Speech Hear Res 1966; 9:353-360.
14. Aronsen AE. Clinical voice disorders: an interdisciplinary approach. New York: Thieme-Stratton, 1980:51.
15. Ramig LA, Ringel RL. Effects of physiological aging on selected acoustic characteristics of voice. J Speech Hear Res 1983; 1:22-30.
16. Ramig LA. Effects of physiological aging on vowel spectral noise. J Gerontol 1983; 2:223-225.
17. Linville SE, Korabic EW. Fundamental frequency stability characteristics of elderly women's voices. J Acoust Soc Am 1987; 4:1196-1199.

Chapter Thirteen

DIAGNOSIS OF NEUROMUSCULAR VOICE IMPAIRMENT

DAVID G. HANSON, M.D., F.A.C.S.
PAUL H. WARD, M.D., F.A.C.S.
BRUCE R. GERRATT, Ph.D.
GEORGE BERCI, M.D.
GERALD S. BERKE, M.D.

Voice dysfunction in the elderly patient may be associated with neuromuscular impairment of laryngeal control, which is difficult to diagnose with standard indirect mirror evaluation of the laryngeal structures. This paper, presented before the conference on Geriatric Otorhinolaryngology, March 25, 1988, reviews some of the techniques that aid in the diagnosis of voice impairment by providing documented objective data. Case reports provide several illustrative examples of geriatric voice disorders of neurologic origin. The paper was presented with a video tape, *Physiologic Assessment of Vocal Fold Movement*.

The diagnosis of the cause of voice impairment for most patients is usually evident on completion of a history and a careful physical examination. A majority of phonatory disorders seen in children and young and middle-aged adults are associated with abnormalities of vocal fold structure or glottal configuration. Usually these anatomic abnormalities are readily apparent to the experienced examiner. The diagnosis of voice impairment when the laryngeal structures evidence no anatomic abnormality may be a much greater challenge. As the patient population lives longer, voice pathology involving the control of laryngeal structures will be encountered more commonly. Neuromuscular problems affecting the larynx and pharynx may be particularly difficult to detect and to define using standard indirect mirror laryngoscopy.

In recent years, major advances have been made in our ability to document the appearance of the larynx. Telescopic and fiberoptic laryngoscopes have improved the ability to examine the movements of the laryngeal structures as well as the hypopharynx and tongue. The wide angle view necessary to see movements of these structures in relation to each other is not possible with most indirect mirror examinations. Most importantly, telescopes have allowed practical documentation of the examination by cine and video photography. Commercially available systems provide immediate "hard copy" in the clinic for demonstrating the findings to the patient and the referring physician, as well as for documentation in the medical record.

Repeated review of cine or video documented examination with slow speed or with stop frame analysis has enhanced our ability to define neuromuscular dysfunction that results in visible movement or position disturbance. Video recording has now essentially replaced more expensive and cumbersome cine photography. Laryngostroboscopy, used for many years in laboratories for study of normal laryngeal function, is now being applied to patients in conjunction with video docmentation of the stroboscopic image.[1]

There have also been considerable advances in our ability to assess objectively the characteristics of phonatory function at both the level of vocal fold vibration and of the resulting acoustic signal. Digital recording and computer-assisted signal processing techniques have greatly changed the feasibility of documenting and analyzing such high speed events as vocal fold vibration and acoustic voice signals. This technology has had an important impact on voice-related research.[2] Voice and glottographic signal analysis techniques are also being adapted for the evaluation of patient populations.[3] Thus, more objective assessments of voice impairment are becoming practical.

Development and assessment of objective measurement techniques for clinical use are tasks that require a broad multidisciplinary approach to phonatory physiology and pathophysiology. In a clinical setting, the contemporary voice pathology laboratory provides investigators with the capacity to document telescopic and stroboscopic laryngeal examinations, glottographic measures of vibration, air flow and pressure measures, and high quality reproductions of the acoustic voice signal. Available computing facilities allow simultaneous digital recording of multiple signals for subsequent automated or interactive analysis of the data.

The vibratory movements of the vocal folds that

actually produce voice occur faster than the eye can follow. Therefore, objective measures of these vibratory movements offer advantages over purely visual examination techniques. Measures that reflect the vibratory movements of the vocal folds are termed "glottographic." Techniques such as electroglottography (EGG)[4] and photoglottography (PGG)[5] have shown promise as objective measures of vocal fold vibratory function. In a recent study of well-defined surgical lesions of the peripheral nerve supply of the larynx, measurements from photoglottography significantly distinguished between different types of nerve injury. The measure speed quotient[6] differentiated among data from patients with recurrent paralysis, superior laryngeal paralysis, idiopathic paralysis, and vagal paralysis, and normal speakers.[7] We are currently investigating the hypothesis that the morphology of particular glottographic signal patterns may be characteristic and perhaps diagnostic of different pathologic conditions, such as strain, paralysis, rigidity, spasticity, asymmetry of muscular tone, and tremor.[8-10]

The vibratory physiology of voice production is complex; however, multiple simultaneous measures such as glottography and stroboscopy provide complementary perspectives on the three-dimensional relationships of glottal configuration during vibration. The combination of glottographic signals with documented stroboscopy offers additional validation of these techniques.[11] Stroboscopic images help to interpret the physiologic significance of glottographic patterns. Figure 13-1A demonstrates a single frame photograph with an exposure time of 80 millionths of a second during the unzipping of the upper edges of the vocal folds. The photograph was made with a 24-kilolux flash (B & K stroboscope model 4914) using 35-mm film processed at 4,000 ISO. The relationship of the photographic image to a simultaneously recorded photoglottography signal is shown in Figure 13-1B. The photograph was taken just at the point, during the opening of the glottis, at which the last strands of mucus had separated across the glottis. Note that after this point, the impedance represented in the electroglottography (EGG) signal levels off, representing the complete separation of the vocal folds. Animal model work seems to confirm the potential utility of glottographic measures for description of specific abnormalities of vocal fold vibration.[12-14]

The following cases illustrate how currently available objective documentation techniques may be applied to the evaluation of difficult voice impairment diagnoses.

CASE 1

A 67-year-old male professional voice user had consulted six different otolaryngologists regarding his troublesome voice abnormality. He described progressive fatigue and deterioration of his voice with use. Typically his voice was weak and breathy by the end of the day. He had been told that mirror

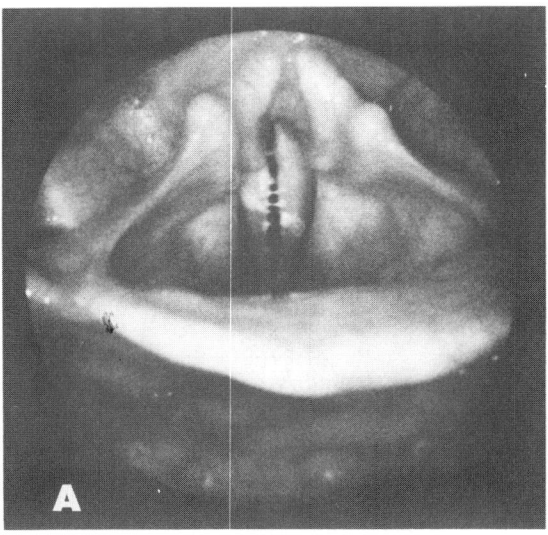
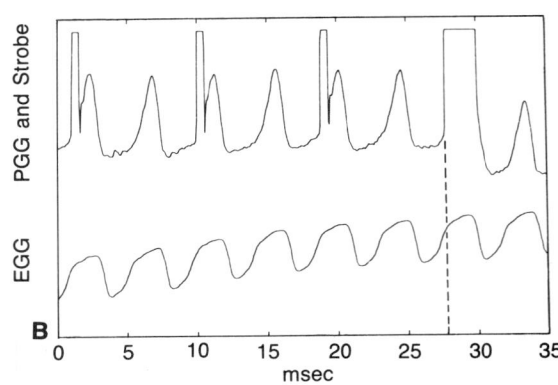

Figure 13-1 *A*, The photograph was taken via a 90-degree telescope (K. Storz) with an Olympus OM2 SLR camera with 1,000 ISO film, processed at 4,000 ISO. The duration of the exposure was determined by an 80-μsec flash of a B & K stroboscope. The relationship of this glottal configuration to the glottal cycle as recorded by glottography is shown in *B*. The clipped spikes represent 5-μsec flashes of the strobe superimposed on a PGG signal obtained with a separate constant light source. The photo was taken at the first part of the large clipped peak. This peak in the PGG signal was longer than the 80 μsec of the actual flash because of the recovery time of the photosensor after the extremely bright 24-kilolux strobe.

examination of his larynx was normal and had been referred for speech therapy, which appeared to have had little beneficial effect. Video documented laryngoscopy showed a normal range of laryngeal movement. However, on close examination during phonation, it was apparent that, although the vocal processes were firmly approximated, the vocal folds appeared rigid and bowed. Figure 13-2A shows a Polaroid reproduction of the video picture of this man's larynx. This configuration of the folds is, in our experience, characteristic of the effects of Parkinson's disease on the larynx.[15] The quality of this type of documentation is not as crisp as that obtained with a single lens reflex camera (see Fig. 13-1A). However, it is much simpler to capture the desired view from previously recorded video tape. Figure 13-2B demonstrates, for further comparison of reso-

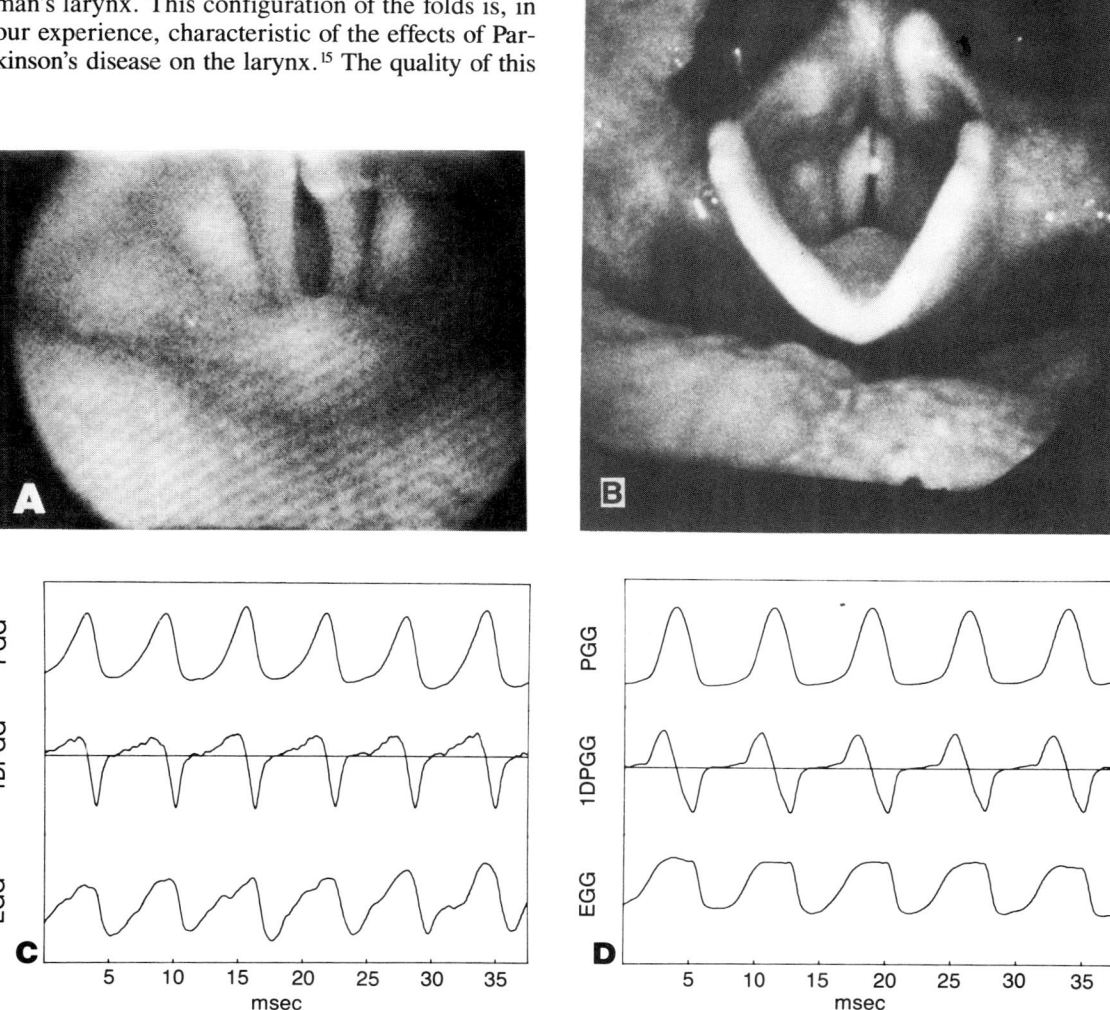

Figure 13-2 *A*, The configuration of the vocal folds during phonation showed bowing even though the vocal processes were firmly approximated. This picture is typical of the laryngeal configuration often seen in association with Parkinson's disease. The photograph is a Polaroid generated from a video signal. *B*, For comparison with *A*, a single frame is reproduced from 16-mm film. This photo shows the larynx of a patient with Parkinson's disease. With the vocal processes firmly approximated, the glottic aperture remains open anteriorly. These patients often have mucous stringing across the glottis at the vocal processes. The resolution obtained with 16-mm film is superior to that from a video signal image. However, cine documentation is more expensive and is not available for immediate reviewing in the clinic. *C*, PGG, first derivative (lDPGG) or velocity of the PGG, and EGG signals show a pattern that is characteristic for laryngeal dysfunction associated with Parkinson's disease. *D*, Glottographic signals typical for normal phonation in modal register for a male voice. For comparison with the patient data, note the relative symmetry of opening and closing phases. The plateau in impedance of the EGG, which is associated with full separation of the vocal folds, occurs well before peak glottal aperture as measured by PGG.

lution, a photograph of another larynx affected by Parkinson's disease reproduced from a single frame of 16-mm cine film.

Photoglottography and electroglottography were also recorded for this patient and these signals are demonstrated in Figure 13-2C. These can be compared to typical glottographic signals for a normal modal male voice seen in Figure 13-2D. The PGG signal, reflecting cross-sectional glottal area, indicated that there was not a well-defined baseline of a closed period. There was also asymmetry of opening and closing phases in the open period, which are reflected in the opening and closing velocity (IDPGG). The EGG signal, reflecting vocal fold contact area, was noisy (often associated with poor vocal fold approximation during the "closed" phase) and showed maximal impedance (associated with maximum separation of vocal folds) that occurred quite late in relation to the peak glottic area seen in the PGG. These characteristics of the glottographic signals are typical of patterns seen in patients who have involvement of the laryngeal muscles with Parkinson's disease.[6,8]

Comment

On the basis of this evaluation, it was recommended that the patient have a neurologic consultation. At the time, we were able to tell the patient that his voice dysfunction was the result of a neuromuscular control problem. Vocal rehabilitation oriented toward the observed pathology was more effective in helping the patient to cope with his laryngeal dysfunction than prior therapy had been. Two years later, on the basis of subsequent development of other symptoms and signs, the diagnosis of Parkinson's disease was confirmed.

CASE 2

Figure 13-3A demonstrates glottographic signals from a 70-year-old gentleman who also complained of a weak breathy voice. On documented laryngoscope his vocal folds did not approximate firmly during phonation and appeared myasthenic. In attempting to obtain closure during phonation, the patient "squeezed" the supraglottic masculature (see Fig. 13-3B). This may have represented a form of compensation for the apparent laxity of the folds. There were several elements in the waveforms of this patient's glottographic recordings that differentiated them from recordings of patients with Parkinson's disease who also exhibited bowing of the folds. The opening movements of the upper edges of the folds, seen after a distinct change in slope at the point marked with an arrowhead, correspond well with flattening of impedance seen in the EGG signal. This flattening of the EGG impedance indicates that the folds lose contact with each other at this point. The maximal impedance (least contact) occurred before the peak glottal aperture indicated in the PGG signal. This contrasts with the data recorded in our laboratory for many patients with Parkinson's disease. As observed in Figure 13-2C, the peak impedance of the EGG in the Parkinsonian patient occurred well after the peak glottal aperture at a point close to greatest closing of the glottal aperture. The simultaneously recorded glottographic sig-

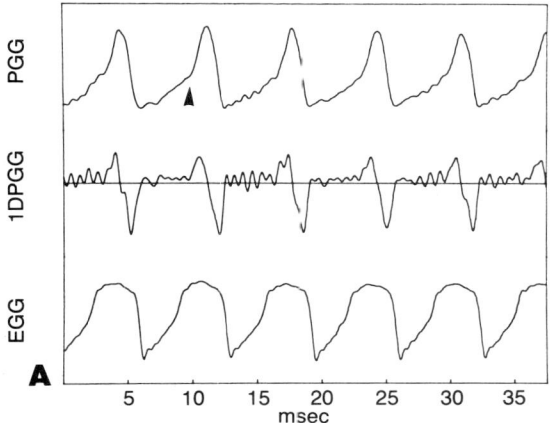 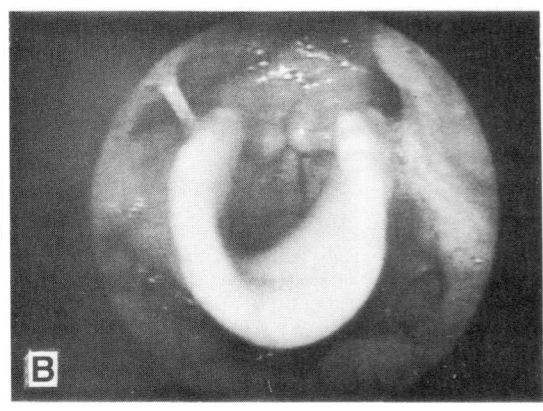

Figure 13-3 *A*, Glottographic signals from a patient with myasthenia laryngis. *B*, During phonation the supraglottic structures were often constricted, perhaps as a compensatory response to the bowed, inefficient closure associated with the myasthenic pattern.

nals show physiologic patterns of vibration that contrast between the patient with Parkinson's disease and the patient with myasthenia laryngis, even though the phonatory posture of their laryngeal structures was not dissimilar.

Comment

This man's voice has remained relatively unchanged for over 5 years. He has developed no sign of neurologic abnormalities, and on examination, his vocal folds continue to approximate in the configuration that has been termed myasthenia laryngis.

CASE 3

A 68-year-old previously healthy male complained of gradual onset of hoarseness without other symptoms. On documented video laryngoscopy he had a right vocal cord paresis. Examination, endoscopy, and a computed tomography (CT) scan failed to show a cause for the paresis. Glottographic signals for this patient are demonstrated in Figure 13-4A. The configuration of the PGG signals indicates notably greater velocity of opening phase in comparison to closing phase. Peak impedance of the EGG signal occurred prior to the peak glottic aperture indicated in the PGG. When these PGG signals are compared to representative signals recorded from paralysis patients and reported by Hanson, Gerratt, Karin, and Berke[7] (see Fig. 13-4B), it appears that the signals are most similar to patterns seen for peripheral recurrent laryngeal nerve injury.

Comment

In our experience, laryngeal nerve paralysis that, after follow-up, is truly idiopathic, has almost always involved both recurrent laryngeal and superior laryngeal nerves.[16] Therefore, a progressive isolated recurrent nerve paresis suggested a neoplastic process in spite of the negative CT scan. A subsequent magnetic resonance imaging (MRI) scan showed the poorly differentiated thyroid carcinoma that was responsible for the paresis.

CASE 4

A 62-year-old woman presented for consideration of botulinum toxin injection for treatment of spastic dysphonia. The patient had seen over 20 physicians and had spent thousands of dollars on speech and psychiatric therapy without apparent benefit. Other than her voice dysfunction, she had no complaints. Documented telescopic and fiberoptic laryngoscopy clearly showed tremor of the intrinsic laryngeal muscles. The movements occurred at about 4.5 to 10 cycles per second and were present constantly, during respiration as well as phonation. When the patient attempted to superimpose phonation on these movements, the resulting voice was strained with irregular pitch and loudness variation and frequent voice interruptions. Simultaneously recorded data from photoglottography, electroglottography, and acoustic signals are shown in Figure 13-5 and demonstrate the effect of the tumor on at-

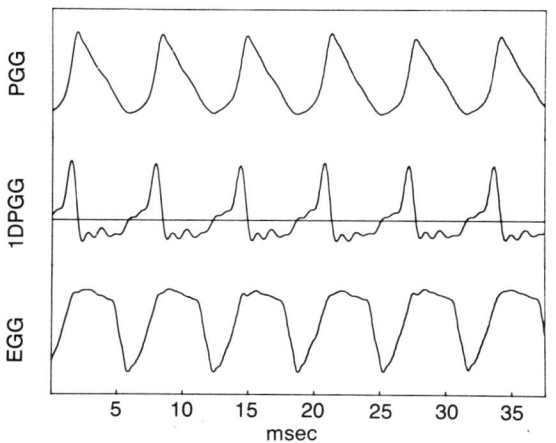
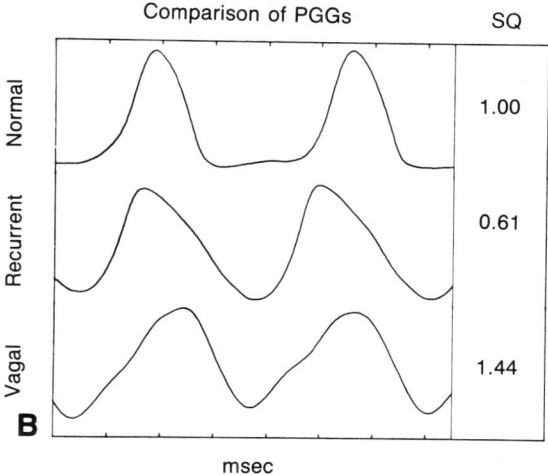

Figure 13-4 *A*, Glottographic signals that are typical for flaccid recurrent laryngeal nerve paralysis. *B*, Comparison of photoglottographic signals recorded from patients with recurrent laryngeal nerve paralysis and vagal nerve paralysis in comparison to normal signals. The ratio of the opening phase to the closing phase is the speed quotient (SQ).

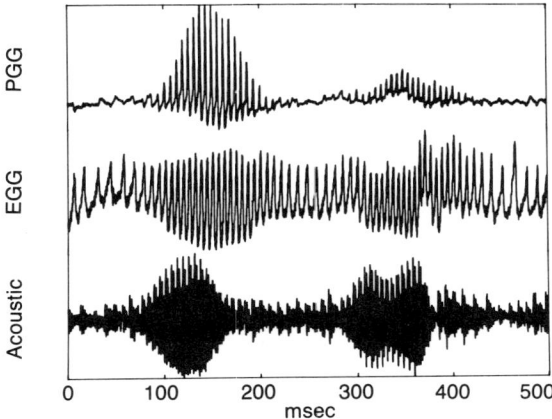

Figure 13–5 Glottographic signals recorded over a half second demonstrate the time varying effects of tremor on the vibratory cycles. Simultaneously recorded signals from PGG, EGG, and the acoustic voice signal are shown.

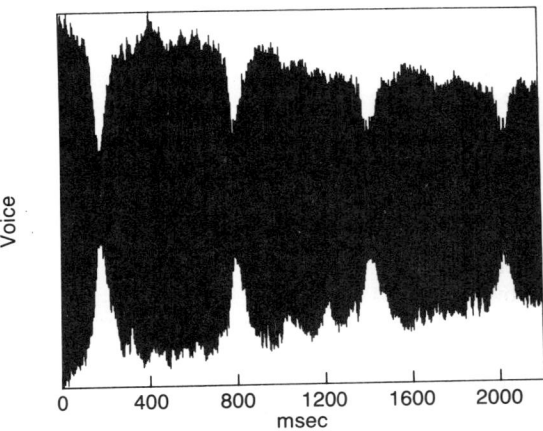

Figure 13–6 The two seconds of acoustic voice signal demonstrate the effects of myoclonus of the laryngeal and pharyngeal muscles.

tempts to maintain a steady vowel production. The cause of this isolated laryngeal tremor was not discovered.

Comment

Although this woman had been examined by several competent otolaryngologists, it appeared that prolonged examination of the respiratory movements of the larynx had not been accomplished. Unfortunately, this woman wasted years in frustration and considerable sums of money being treated ineffectively for the wrong diagnosis.

CASE 5

A 64-year-old woman was referred for evaluation of spastic dysphonia. The patient, a trained professional singer, had noted gradual onset of extreme difficulty in speaking or singing. Her voice was described as effortful, with rhythmic variations in intensity and pitch. Examination with a mirror and with the 90-degree telescope was difficult, but showed hyperadduction of the vocal folds in phonation. The experienced examiner was not successful in observing respiratory movements clearly. A flexible fiberoptic telescope was therefore introduced. Monitoring of the patient's hypopharynx showed a regular rhythmic jerking of the larynx at about 2 Hz. Figure 13–6 demonstrates the patient's voice signal for a period of 2 seconds during attempted prolonged phonation of the vowel /a/. The jerking movement, also present during quiet respiration, was assymmetrical, primarily to the left side. (A videotape of this movement was presented with the paper.) The magnitude of the myoclonic movement appeared to change with the respiratory cycle and was more prominent at the end of inspiration. During phonation, the attempt to superimpose voicing on the myoclonic movements of the larynx resulted in the observed voice pathology.

Comment

Myoclonus of muscles supplied by the vagal nerve is thought to result from a supranuclear brain stem lesion. Subsequent neurologic evaluation, including a good quality MRI, failed to localize a specific lesion in this patient. In our experience, a specific lesion is usually not identified in patients who demonstrate palatolaryngopharyngeal myoclonis.

CASE 6

A 62-year-old professional actor was hospitalized with acute vertigo, complete loss of the ability to swallow, and hoarseness. He also had minor weakness of his left arm. Within 3 days he regained his voice and most swallowing function. Within 3 weeks he was relatively asymptomatic. The patient presented 2 months later because of recurring harshness in his voice. He complained that his voice fatigued rapidly with use. Laryngoscopy revealed small midcord hemorrhages and early polypoid degeneration. Laryngeal movements appeared to be grossly normal. After voice rest, the appearance of the larynx returned to normal. Figure 13–7A shows the configuration of the cords as they separated just after phonation. There was a subtle difference in the appearance of the two vocal folds. However, after voice rest there were no anatomic lesions of the epithelium. Slow motion review of video-documented laryngoscopy showed a slight lag in the movements of the left vocal fold in relation to the right side. In addition, there was slight bowing of the left fold. There appeared to be full abduction and adduction of the vocal folds with no other apparent abnormal movements. However, in contrast to 30 previous years of successful voice use as a professional, the patient complained of significant deterioration in his vocal control and strength. On several occasions he was observed to have laryngeal findings that are usually considered signs of vocal abuse. Reinke's edema, focal hemorrhages, and small nodules readily responded to voice rest. Glottographic signals, seen in Figure 13–7B, were recorded 2 months after what was diagnosed on CT scan as a small left lateral medullary infarct. At the time of recording, the patient's larynx appeared as seen in Figure 13–7A. PGG signals showed a prolonged opening phase compared to the closing phase (see Fig. 13–7B). The ratio of the duration of these phases resulted in a speed quotient of 2.1, which was several standard deviations above the range of normal values. The configuration of the PGG and EGG signals showed a delay of the peak impedance of the EGG signal in relation to the peak glottic aperture indicated in the PGG signal. The pattern was most similar to the patterns that are characteristic of vagal or idiopathic vagal paralysis.[7] On multiple glottographic recordings, elevation of speed quotient has persisted for over a year since his vascular accident.

Comment

Modified video barium swallows of this patient continued to show spasticity of the cricopharyngeus muscle, which was associated with mild symptomatic dysphagia. Long after gross movements of the laryngeal muscles had returned to normal by visual examination, objective measures continued to show the effects of vagal paresis after an extremely discrete upper motoneuron lesion.

DISCUSSION

These cases represent a few examples of voice disorders that may not be adequately discerned by traditional diagnostic evaluations. In our experience, voice dysfunction caused by neurologic disease is not uncommon, particularly in the geriatric population. Voice disorders resulting from neuromuscular dysfunction can have devastating effects on the social interactions and economic security of patients who previously took their voice quality for granted. Yet laryngologic, neurologic, and speech pathology

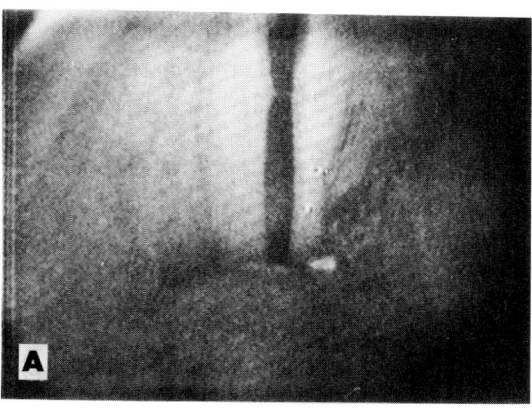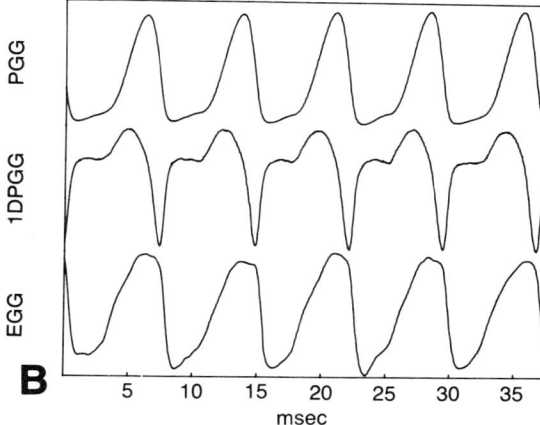

Figure 13–7 *A*, Visible epithelial abnormality of the vocal folds in Case 6 was not evident after a period of voice rest. Subtle differences in the configuration of the two vocal folds are apparent on single frame analysis. *B*, Glottographic signals from Case 6, recorded after recovery of gross laryngeal movements 2 months after a small left lateral medullary infarct. Measured SQ was elevated and remained at pathologic values on continued subsequent follow-up.

textbooks and literature offer relatively little information about these disorders and their treatments.

Effective remedies and rehabilitation of these problems will necessarily lag behind the capability to provide an accurate diagnosis and to objectively evaluate the efficacy of treatment. However, increasingly accessible technology for objective documentation of phonatory physiology appears to offer encouraging opportunities for a more sophisticated understanding and treatment of these disorders of phonation.

References

1. Kitzing P. Stroboscopy—a pertinent laryngological examination. J Otolaryngol 1985; 14:151–157.
2. Daniloff R. Laryngeal function in phonation and respiration. (Book Review). ASHA 1988; 30:60–61.
3. Kitzing P. Glottography, the electrophysical investigation of phonatory biomechanics. Acta Otorhinolaryngol Bel 1986; 40:863–878.
4. Fabre P. Un procédé électrique percutane d'inscription de l'accolement glottique au cours de phonation: glottographque de haute frequence. Bull Acad Natl Med 1957; 121:66–69.
5. Sonesson B. A method for studying the vibratory movements of the vocal cords. J Laryngol Otol 1959; 73:732–737.
6. Timcke R, von Leden H, Moore P. Laryngeal vibrations: measurements of the glottic wave. Part 1. The normal vibratory cycle. Arch Otolaryngol 1958; 68:1–9.
7. Hanson DG, Gerratt BR, Karin RR, Berke GS. Glottographic measures of vocal fold vibration: an examination of laryngeal paralysis. Laryngoscope 1988; 98(5):541–549.
8. Gerratt BR, Hanson DG, Berke GS. Glottographic measures of laryngeal function in individuals with abnormal motor control. In: Harris K, Sasaki C, Baer T, eds. Vocal fold physiology: laryngeal function in phonation and respiration. San Diego: College Hill, 1987:521.
9. Kitzing P. Clinical application of combined electro- and photo- glottography. IALP Conference Proceedings. Copenhagen: IALP 1977; 1:528–539.
10. Hanson DG, Gerratt BR, Ward PH. Glottographic measures of vocal dysfunction: a preliminary report. Ann Otol Rhinol Laryngol 1983; 92:413–420.
11. Hanson DG, Gerratt BR, Berke G. Simultaneous photoglottography and stroboscopy. Proceedings of the International Conference on Voice, XXth Congress of IALP. Kerume: University of Kerume, 1986:33.
12. Berke GS, Hantke DR, Hanson DG. An experimental model to test the effect of change in tension and mass on laryngeal vibration in-vivo. Proceedings of the International Conference on Voice, XXth Congress of IALP. Vol II. Kerume: University of Kerume, 1986:1.
13. Berke GS, Moore DM, Hantke D, Hanson DG, Gerratt BR. Laryngeal modeling: theoretical, in-vitro, in-vivo. Laryngoscope 1987; 7:871–881.
14. Moore DM, Berke GS, Hanson DG, Ward PH. Videostroboscopy of the canine larynx: the effects of asymmetrical laryngeal tension. Laryngoscope 1987; 7:543–553.
15. Hanson DG, Gerratt BR, Ward PH. Cinegraphic observations of laryngeal function in Parkinson's disease. Laryngoscope 1984; 94:348–353.
16. Ward PH, Berci G. Observations on so-called idiopathic vocal cord paralysis. Ann Otol Rhinol Laryngol 1982; 91:558–563.

Chapter Fourteen

OBJECTIVE EVALUATION OF VOICE DYSFUNCTION IN THE ELDERLY

RAYMOND H. COLTON, Ph.D.

INTRODUCTION

The voice has been said to be a mirror on the self. In the case of disease, the voice reflects any anomalies that affect the vibratory characteristics of the vocal folds. One of the early signs of cancer of the throat is a change in the quality of voice, specifically the development of hoarseness.

The voice also reflects the growth of an individual. The young infant can only cry to reflect his inner state, but, after he has learned the symbol code for his language, can communicate much more effectively. The voice is part of this symbol code and reflects the physical growth of the individual through changes of pitch and quality of the voice. During the tempestuous adolescent years, there is rapid growth and rapid change in the voice. When adulthood is attained, these changes subside, but throughout the adult years subtle changes in the voice occur that reflect the growth of the individual intellectually, socially, or physically. It is also true that the voice may reflect the decline in these functions, especially those that occur in the later years of an individual's life.

The purpose of this paper is to review the information that exists on the objective evaluation of the voice characteristics of the elderly. The focus will be on those characteristics that differentiate the young from the old voice, and the attempt will be made to describe the normal elderly voice. The techniques to be discussed are objective and quantitative, even in those instances where the perceptual features of the voice are reviewed. Diseases, pathologies, or other problems with the voice affect these characteristics, although in different ways that depend on the nature of the disease, pathology, or other malfunction. The analysis of normal voice function can provide information about the characteristics of the normal elderly voice as well as the abnormal elderly voice. Clinicians working with the abnormal elderly voice must be able to distinguish it from the normal elderly voice.

PERCEPTUAL CHARACTERISTICS OF THE ELDERLY VOICE

There have been several studies in which the perceptual voice characteristics of the aged have been investigated. Two fundamental conclusions may be drawn from these studies. First, within limits, the age of a person can be reliably estimated from tape recorded samples of his or her voice. Second, there are distinct perceptual characteristics of the older versus younger voice. In fact, it appears that, between these two extremes of age, there are unique characteristics of voice that enable listeners to correctly estimate approximately the speaker's age.

Age Estimations from the Voice

Ptacek and Sander[1] asked listeners to place recordings of speakers sustaining the vowel /a/ or reading a passage into age groups of under 35 and over 65. As shown in Table 14–1, listeners placed the sustained vowels of the speakers into the correct age group 78 percent of the time, whereas the reading passage was correctly classified 99 percent of the time. Later, Shipp and Hollien[2] asked their listeners to judge the age decade of 175 male talkers. The correlation between perceived age and chronologic age in the direct estimation of age task was 0.88. It is apparent that listeners are capable of estimating the ages of subjects from their voices. Similar results have been reported for female talkers.[3,4]

Perceptual Features of the Elderly Voice

Given that listeners can correctly perceive age in the voice, what features are they using to accomplish this task? Information about the perceptual features of the elderly voice has been available from several studies. Ryan and Burk[5] asked 40 speakers

TABLE 14-1 Perceptual Characteristics of Aging

Perceived Versus Chronologic Age

Percent correct age group classification*

Vowels	Backward Speech	Forward Speech
78%	87%	99%

Judged age on a seven point scale† (2= 20-29 years, 3= 30-39 years, and so on)

Chronologic Age in Decades

20-29	30-39	40-49	50-59	60-69	70-79	80-89
2.8	3.6	4.2	4.8	5.1	5.9	6.6

Perceptual Features of Age Decades‡

Rank	20-30	30-40	40-50	50-60
1	High pitch	Low pitch	Low pitch	Hoarseness
2	Rapid rate	Precise articulation	Hoarseness	Low pitch
3	Precise articulation	Clear quality	Slow rate	Imprecise articulation
4	Clear quality	Moderate pitch	Imprecise articulation	Breathiness
5	Semantic content	Moderate rate	High pitch	Long pauses

* Data from Ptacek P, Sander E. Age recognition from voice. J Speech Hear Res 1966; 9:273-277.
† Data from Shipp T, Hollien H. Perception of the aging male voice. J Speech Hear Res 1969; 12:703-710.
‡ Data from Hartman D, Danhauer J. Perceptual features of speech for males in four perceived age decades. J Acoust Soc Am 1976; 59:713-715.

of varying ages to read the Rainbow passage. Five experienced speech pathologists identified as many perceptual features as possible from the 40 recordings. Eighteen experienced listeners rated the 40 speakers by using 10 of the most common features reported by the smaller observer group. Estimates of the age of the speakers were obtained, as well as five acoustic measures: mean dB sound pressure level (SPL), words per minute, words per minute per sentence, mean fundamental frequency, and standard deviation of fundamental frequency. Multiple regressions were obtained between the perceptual and acoustic variables with estimated age being the dependent variable. Five of the perceptual dimensions were highly correlated with estimated age. These were (1) air loss, (2) laryngeal tension, (3) voice tremor, (4) imprecise consonants, and (5) slow rate. Only one acoustic variable, mean fundamental frequency, had a high correlation with estimated age in the multiple regression analysis. Obviously, perceptual features were the most important in classifying the ages of these talkers. It is curious that none of the other acoustic variables correlated with estimated age or with the perceptual dimensions. One explanation is that the acoustic variables measured were not appropriate, although the two measures of reading rate should be related to the perceptual feature of slow rate.

In another study, Hartman and Danhauer[6] asked 46 subjects between the ages of 25 and 70 years to engage in spontaneous conversation, which was recorded. Small random samples of these conversations were presented to 20 listeners who were asked to write down the perceptual features they heard in the voice recordings. The features were arranged according to the age decade, 20 to 30, 30 to 40, 40 to 50, 50 to 60 (see Table 14-1). Features associated with the 20 to 30 decade included high pitch, rapid rate, precise articulation, clear quality, hypernasality, and semantic content. Features associated with the 50 to 60 age decade included hoarseness, low pitch, imprecise articulation, breathiness, slow rate, and long pauses. Similar results were reported by Hartman[7], probably because it appears to be the same study.

Ryan and Capadano[8] had 98 students, mostly male, rate the reading passages of speakers from various age groups. There were three tasks: (1) rate the speaker on six seven-interval bipolar adjective scales, (2) guess the age of the speaker, and (3) write down the salient voice characteristics. For female speakers, there was a significant correlation (0.93) between chronologic and perceived age. The features of importance to the listeners were pitch, tone, and volume. In general, the voices of older women were perceived as reserved, passive, out-of-it, and inflexible when compared to the voices of younger women. For the male speakers, there was a correlation of 0.81 between chronologic and estimated age. The perceptual features of importance to the listeners were pitch, volume, speed, clarity, and authority. The voices of older men sounded less flexible than younger men.

These data support the conclusion that age can be correctly estimated from the voices of speakers and that there are several perceptual features that listeners attend to when listening to voices. Some of these features (e.g., hoarseness, low pitch, precision of articulation, speaking rate) are associated with aging, with young speakers on one end of the continuum and older speakers on the other end.

Perceptual judgments, when properly obtained, can be reliable and valid. There is, in fact, considerable face validity to perceptual judgments of experienced listeners. The problem is usually to obtain the desired judgments and to obtain them consistently. Although one could argue to the contrary, perceptual judgments are often not thought to be objective. Fortunately, for many of the perceptual features of voice, there are acoustic correlates that can be measured objectively. Most often, it is convenient to obtain the acoustic data and then to relate them to the desired or hypothesized perceptual features. A brief review of some acoustic features of the elderly voice will be presented after a discussion of considerations in obtaining objective measurements.

OBJECTIVE MEASUREMENTS OF VOICE FUNCTION

There are many methods available to measure the characteristics of the voice. Some of these methods involve the measurement of the perceptual features of the voice, others focus on the acoustic characteristics of the voice, and still others focus on the physiology of voice function. Many of these methods are objective and yield quantitative information of the function of the voice.

Many of these methods are also noninvasive. That is, they do not involve the insertion of needles, catheters, or other foreign objects into the body. These methods are desirable for patient comfort and cooperation and should also minimally interfere with the normal physiology of the voice. Furthermore, most of these methods are simple to use and the data easy to obtain from the patient. In the study of the elderly, these advantages should be obvious.

There exists considerable commercial equipment that is well-suited to collect the desired data on the voice. In many cases, the experimenter need only decide on the kind of data to be collected and then search for the equipment item that best meets that need. In other cases, the equipment is not available commercially and must be obtained from other clinics or laboratories that have expertise in the procedure desired. In most cases, a computer is desirable, not only for data collection, but also for data analysis and storage.

In order to collect and analyze data on voice function, there must be tasks for the patient to do. Selection of these tasks should be made according to the desired function to be studied, but should also be chosen to sample the range of function to be studied, especially if the aim of the procedure is to examine the limits of function. One should also design the tasks to sample a function several times in order to estimate its consistency. In some cases, the specific speech samples may be limited by the instrumentation to be used. For example, if one plans to view the vocal folds with a laryngeal mirror, the patient must produce a vowel that will enable the experimenter to see the vocal folds. Other procedures may require certain vowels or syllables to be used in order to perform optimally.

Finally, one must design the procedure for data collection with the subject or patient in mind. After all, the subject must understand what he or she is to do before one can expect him or her to perform the task. Explanations should be clear and thorough. One should demonstrate, if possible, and should always be prepared to explain what is happening. Most patients also appreciate an explanation of what the information means to them, and if possible, such explanations should be forthcoming. One should be always aware of other limitations that may interfere with the collection of the data. For example, a subject may be hard of hearing and misunderstand your directions or not hear your speech sample if you present it orally. Many elderly patients need glasses to be able to read passages. It usually takes little effort to properly prepare the samples to be used and to prepare the subject for the experimental task to be performed.

ACOUSTIC CHARACTERISTICS OF THE ELDERLY VOICE

There are many acoustic features of voice that can be measured and may correlate with the perceptual features of the elderly voice. These acoustic features include fundamental frequency, variation of fundamental frequency (short- and long-term), fundamental frequency range, vocal intensity, variation of vocal intensity (short- and long-term), vocal intensity range, spectrum, reading rate, format frequencies, voice onset time, burst duration, pauses, and vowel duration. Many of these variables have been measured in the voices of the elderly and will be briefly reviewed.

Fundamental Frequency

There are several measures of fundamental frequency that should be considered when examining the acoustic characteristics of the elderly voice. Many of these same measures are used to describe the voice of persons with voice problems. It is important to be aware of the differences between normal voices and abnormal voices and between young and old voices on these measures if one is to correctly interpret the meaning of changes in these measurements.

Average Speaking Fundamental Frequency

Average speaking fundamental frequency refers to the average value of fundamental frequency measured during speaking or reading. It is an estimate of an individual typical pitch level for everyday speaking situations. The typical values for young adult males range between 100 to 125 Hz[9-11] and for females between 200 and 220 Hz.[9,12,13] As is shown in Table 14-2, as the male voice ages, there is a tendency for the fundamental frequency to increase, especially in the 6th and 7th decades of life.[10,14-17] For females, there is a tendency for fundamental frequency to decrease as a function of aging.[13,18] The magnitudes of the frequency changes as a result of aging are small in both males and females (less than 30 Hz in males, 10 Hz in females). Consequently, although there are some changes of speaking fundamental frequency as a result of aging, these changes are small and probably have little significance.

Variability of Fundamental Frequency

There are two ways to analyze the magnitude of fundamental frequency variation that occurs in the voice. The first, which is called short-term in this paper, refers to the rapid changes of frequency that may occur between adjacent cycles of vibration. This phenomena is often referred to as a frequency perturbation and often reported in percent. The second index of variability may be referred to as long-term variability and reflects the variation of fundamental frequency that occurs during normal speaking. Much of this variability occurs because of the linguistic characteristics of the message, the emotional mood of the situation, or the personal characteristics of the speaker. It reflects the degree of control the speaker has during speech. Both measures may reflect the same or different aspects of the physiologic system used to produce speech and voice.

TABLE 14-2 Speaking Fundamental Frequency as a Function of Age

From Hollien and Shipp, 1972* (males)

Age Decade	Mean Age	Fundamental Frequency
20–29	24.4	120
30–39	34.9	112
40–49	45.4	107
50–59	54.3	118
60–69	64.6	112
70–79	74.7	132
80–89	83.6	146

From Wilcox and Horii, 1980[†]
Young group: 124 Hz
Old group: 122.4 Hz

Female Subjects

Author(s)	Age	Fundamental Frequency
McGlone and Hollien[‡]	65–79	196.6
McGlone and Hollien[‡]	80–94	199.8
Benjamin[§]	68–94	180.2
Stoicheff[#]	60–69	199.7
Stoicheff[#]	>70	202.2

* Data from Hollien H, Shipp T. Speaking fundamental frequency and chronologic age in males. J Speech Hear Res 1972; 15:155–159.
† Data from Wilcox KA, Horii Y. Age and changes in vocal jitter. J Gerontol 1980; 35:194–198.
‡ Data from McGlone R, Hollien H. Vocal pitch characteristics of aged women. J Speech Hear Res 1963; 6:164–170.
§ Data from Benjamin B. Frequency variability in the aged voice. J Gerontol 1981; 36:722–726.
# Data from Stoicheff ML. Speaking fundamental characteristics of nonsmoking adults. J Speech Hear Res 1981; 24:437–441.

Frequency Perturbation. Frequency perturbation or jitter is the cycle-to-cycle change of frequency (or period) that occurs during speech. Since this measure supposedly reflects the stability of the vibrating vocal folds, it is usually measured on samples where the subject is intending to produce a stable and single frequency. Thus, most of our measurements of perturbation are made on sustained vowels. Perturbation increases when the fundamental frequency increases. Therefore, most investigators use a ratio measure (jitter ratio, jitter factor) to remove the effects of fundamental frequency from the measurement.

Several studies have investigated the frequency perturbation produced at different ages.[11,19-21] In general, frequency perturbation is increased in the elderly (Table 14-3). However, factors such as vowel used[11] and physical condition[20,21] affect the magnitude of perturbation measured. Ramig and Ringel[20] studied several acoustic characteristics of the voices of older subjects by dividing their subjects into those in good physical condition and those in poor physical condition. The groupings were made on the basis of the results of several physiologic tests, including resting heart rate, systolic blood pressure, diastolic blood pressure, percentage of body fat, forced vital capacity, and adjusted forced vital capacity. In each age group, the eight subjects who had the best performance on these measures comprised the good physical condition group and the eight subjects who had the worst performance on these measures comprised the poor physical condition group. In general, subjects in all age groups in good physical condition produced lower levels of perturbation than speakers in poor physical condition (see Table 14-3). Furthermore, young speakers in poor physical condition had jitter levels slightly higher than old speakers in good physical condition and were comparable to older speakers in poor physical condition. Thus, it is possible that an elderly patient in good physical condition will have perturbation measures comparable to a younger speaker. An older patient in poor physical condition could exhibit perturbation measures comparable to a patient with a vocal pathology. One must be aware of the physical characteristics of the subject before interpreting the results of studies on frequency perturbation.

TABLE 14-3 Frequency Perturbation in the Aged Voice

From Wilcox and Horii, 1980* (jitter)

Group	/i/	/a/	/u/
Young	0.61	0.53	0.51
Old	0.76	0.84	0.58

From Benjamin, 1981† (percent)

Group	Young	Old
Males	4.54	14.44
Females	0.79	6.09

From Ramig and Ringel, 1983‡ (percent)

Group	Age	/i/	/a/	/u/
Young				
Good condition	29.5	0.686	0.424	0.714
Poor condition	32.2	0.827	0.497	0.881
Middle age				
Good condition	53.0	0.691	0.501	0.650
Poor condition	52.6	0.955	0.700	0.678
Old age				
Good condition	67.5	0.759	0.596	0.738
Poor condition	69.1	0.817	0.646	0.815

From Ringel and Chodzko-Zajko, 1987§ (percent)

Group	Good Condition	Poor Condition
Young	0.40	0.51
Old	0.59	0.69

* Data from Wilcox KA, Horii Y. Age and changes in vocal jitter. J Gerontol 1980; 35:194-198.
† Data from Benjamin B. Frequency variability in the aged voice. J Gerontol 1981; 36:722-726.
‡ Data from Ramig L, Ringel R. Effects of physiological aging on selected acoustic characteristics of voice. J Speech Hear Res 1983; 26:22-30.
§ Data from Ringel RL, Chodzko-Zajko WJ. Vocal indices of biological age. J Voice 1987; 1:31-37.

In order to develop an index that might be used as a control for the effects of physical condition, Chodzko-Zajko and Ringel[22] performed a factor analysis on seven physiologic variables including lean body weight, systolic blood pressure, diastolic blood pressure, forced vital capacity, forced expiratory volume, serum triglyceride, and serum total cholesterol-high density lipoprotein ratio. Three factors were identified: pulmonary function, blood lipids and body weight, and blood pressure. A weighted combination of these three factors was used to produce an Index of Physiologic Status (IPS). Subjects in good physical condition were selected from those who had scored at least one-half a standard deviation above the mean for the entire group, whereas subjects in the poor physical condition group were chosen if they had scores at least one-half a standard deviation below the mean for the group. Various acoustic measures were analyzed in the voices of these subjects, including jitter. As shown in Table 14–3, the subjects in poor physical condition had greater jitter than those in good condition, but unlike the results from Ramig and Ringel[20], the older subjects in good physical condition had slightly greater jitter than the younger subjects in poor physical condition. Although not tested by these authors, one might expect that these differences would not be significant statistically.

Standard Deviation of Fundamental Frequency (Pitch Sigma). The longer-term index of variability, which may also reflect the degree of control of the voice, is often referred to as pitch sigma.[12] It is simply the standard deviation of the frequency measurement during a reading or a spontaneous conversation. Mysak[15] reported that his elderly subjects tended to exhibit greater variability than his middle-age subjects (Table 14–4). Stoicheff[13] and Linville and Fisher[3] report similar findings for female speakers. An interesting observation of Stoicheff[13] was that older women who had not entered or who were in menopause had less variability than women who had completed menopause. These results lend support to Segre's[23] report that, in senescence, the voice is more monotone. Stoicheff[13] also reports that the fundamental frequencies of the postmenopausal women were lower than those of premenopausal women or women in menopause. However, the magnitude of the change (about 20 Hz) is much smaller than the three or four tone drop claimed by Segre.

Fundamental Frequency Range

The range of fundamental frequencies an individual can produce is often referred to as phonational range and reflects the physiologic limits of the individual voice. Therefore, one would expect changes in phonational range as an individual ages because of the changes in the cartilages, connective tissue, and muscles that accompany aging.[24]

TABLE 14–4 Variability of Fundamental Frequency (Standard Deviation)

From Mysak, 1959* (males)		
Group	Oral	Impromptu
Middle age	2.9	2.9
Older group I	3.0	2.8
Older group II	3.3	3.4
From Stoicheff, 1981† (females, reading)		
Age Group	Mean Age	SD of FF
20–29	24.6	3.78
30–39	35.4	3.92
40–49	46.4	4.00
50–59	54.5	4.33
60–69	65.8	4.25
>70	75.4	4.70
From Linville and Fisher, 1985‡		
Group	Age Range	SD of FF
Young	25–35	1.47
Middle	45–55	1.68
Old	70–80	2.52

* Data from Mysak ED. Pitch and duration characteristics of older males. J Speech Hear Res 1959; 2:46–54.
† Data from Stoicheff ML. Speaking fundamental characteristics of nonsmoking adults. J Speech Hear Res 1981; 24:437–441.
‡ Data from Linville S, Fisher H. Acoustic characteristics of women's voices with advancing age. J Gerontol 1985; 40:324–330.

Ptacek, Sander, Maloney, and Jackson[25] reported much smaller phonational ranges for their group of older subjects (males: 76.8; females: 76.9 years) than for their group of younger subjects (males: 27.6; females: 23.5 years). The two groups of older female subjects in the McGlone and Hollien[18] study also had a smaller total phonational range. On the other hand, Benjamin[19] reported data showing that the older groups, both males and females, exhibited phonational ranges slightly larger than the younger subject group. Differences of procedure may possibly explain these disparate findings.

Linville[26] also reported on the effects of aging on the phonational ranges of elderly women. In general, elderly speakers produced lower high frequency limits and consequently had a smaller total phonational range than the younger speakers. Middle-aged women who had completed menopause produced significantly lower low frequency limits and higher high frequency limits than middle-aged women who had not completed menopause. As expected, the total phonational ranges of the postmenopausal women were significantly greater than the premenopausal group.

Vocal Intensity

Average Intensity During Speaking

Ryan[27] measured the average intensity produced by subjects in several age groups during a reading passage (see Table 14-4). Middle-aged speakers produced average intensities of 69.2 dB (oral reading) and 68.1 dB (impromptu speaking). Speakers aged 70 to 79 produced intensity levels of 71.3 dB (oral reading) and 70.7 (impromptu speaking). These data suggest that older speakers tend to speak a little louder, on the average, than younger speakers. Ryan pointed out that all of his subjects possessed hearing within normal limits. He argued that aging affects the sensory processes in the larynx and the respiratory system and therefore feedback from these systems is diminished. The result is that the person may tend to speak a little louder in order to overcome these slight deficiencies.

Short-Term Variability of Intensity: Shimmer

Ramig and Ringel[20] and Ringel and Chodzko-Zajko[21] analyzed the shimmer in the voices of their subjects of varying age and varying physical condition. As is shown in Table 14-5, Ramig and Ringel's[20] subjects in the two older age groups who were classified in good physical condition had lower shimmer values than those in all three age groups in poor physical condition. The young subjects, whether in good or poor physical condition, exhibited similar shimmer values. Older subjects in good physical condition had a higher shimmer value than the young subjects in poor physical condition. This result suggests that aging affects the vibratory characteristics of the vocal folds towards greater instability and may contribute to the perceptual impression that older subjects are hoarse or rough-sounding.

Later data from Ringel and Chodzko-Zajko[21] suggest that older subjects have greater shimmer, but that subjects in poor physical condition show greater shimmer than subjects in good physical condition no matter what their age (see Table 14-5). The difference between the two physical condition groups was greater for the older subjects.

Maximum Intensity Range

Maximum intensity range or maximum dynamic range refers to the range of vocal intensities an individual can produce. Most dynamic range measurements have been made without control of fundamental frequency, although there is some data to suggest that differences will be found if the fundamental frequency at which the range measurements are made is controlled.[28,29]

Ptacek et al[25] reported slightly lower maximum intensity ranges for their group of geriatric men and women. Morris and Brown[30] reported that their younger speakers had significantly lower minimum intensity levels and significantly greater maximum intensity levels than their older speakers. However, no significant differences of speaking intensity level were found between the two groups.

Acoustic Spectrum

Acoustic spectrum is usually considered to be the primary acoustic correlate of the perceptual feature of vocal quality. In view of the results of research concerned with the perceptual features of aging voice, it is curious that little data exist concerning the spectral characteristics of the aging voice.

Ramig[31] analyzed the spectral noise occurring in spectrograms of young and old subjects in good and poor physical condition. In general, older speakers in poor physical condition had greater spectral noise than older speakers in good physical conditions or than younger speakers regardless of physical condition.

Colton[29] analyzed sustained vowels and sentences produced by 35 males and 27 females between the ages of 40 and 70 years. The mean age of the male group was 56.17 years, whereas the mean age of the female group was 57.48 years. The spectrum in 23 one-third octave bands was analyzed and averaged over the time of the utterances. Principal components analysis of the 23 frequency bands was performed to reveal three spectral factors: the first correlated with the frequency bands, 6,400, 8,000, and 10,000 Hz; the second correlated with the frequency bands 800, 1,000, and 1,260 Hz; the third correlated with the frequency bands 100 and 125 Hz. Estimates of these spectral factors were computed for each subject and each speech sample. The results illustrate the spectral differences between the four speech samples (/a/, /i/, and two sentences) and between the males and females. The original intent of this study was to gather some baseline spectral data to which spectral analyses of patient voices could be compared. However, this technique may be used to compare the spectral variations associated with aging. Such a study of aging is currently in progress.

Rate of Speaking

As reported in several studies of the perceptual features of the aging voice (see Table 14-1), reading rate tended to be slower in the older speakers. One would expect that an analysis of reading rate from the acoustic recordings would reveal differences between older and younger speakers.

Mysak[15] reported lower reading rates of older subjects, but rates of speaking during spontaneous conversation were similar for the middle age and for

TABLE 14–5 Vocal Intensity in Aging (Summary from Previous Studies)

Average Speaking Intensity
From Ryan, 1972* (in dB)

Age Group	Oral	Impromptu
40–49	69.1	68.1
50–59	69.7	68.7
60–69	69.3	68.6
70–79	71.3	70.7

Short-Term Variability: Shimmer
From Ramig and Ringel, 1983† (in dB); comfortable duration

Group	Age	/i/	/a/	/u/
Young				
Good condition	29.5	0.276	0.275	0.305
Poor condition	32.2	0.224	0.274	0.303
Middle age				
Good condition	53.0	0.044	0.160	0.100
Poor condition	52.6	0.089	0.298	0.076
Old age				
Good condition	67.5	0.268	0.364	0.214
Poor condition	69.1	0.290	0.426	0.227

From Ringel and Chodzko-Zajko, 1987‡ (in dB)

		Condition	
Group	Age	Good	Poor
Young	29.5	0.20	0.29
Middle	53.0	0.28	0.34
Old	67.5	0.31	0.52

Maximum Intensity Levels
From Ptacek et al, 1966§ (in dB)

Group	Males	Females
Young	105.8	106.2
Old	100.5	98.6

* Data from Ryan WJ. Acoustic aspects of the aging voice. J Gerontol 1972; 27:265-268.
† Data from Ramig L, Ringel R. Effects of physiological aging on selected acoustic characteristics of voice. J Speech Hear Res 1983; 26:22-30.
‡ Data from Ringel RL, Chodzko-Zajko WJ. Vocal indices of biological age. J Voice 1987; 1:31-37.
§ Data from Ptacek PH, Sander E, Maloney W, Jackson CC. Phonatory and related changes with advanced age. J Speech Hear Res 1966; 9:353-360.

two older speaking groups. Ryan[27] also reported a tendency for oral reading rate to show a decrease as a function of age, but the differences of rate between the younger and older speaking groups during spontaneous conversation were small.

These small differences between old and young speakers in speaking or reading rate are puzzling when considering the reports of other investigators (e.g., Ryan and Burk[5]) who state that rate of articulation is an important perceptual feature of voice and one that distinguishes older from younger voices. However, this discrepancy may mean that rate of speaking, as measured in words per minute or words per minute per sentence, may not be the appropriate acoustic correlate of the perceptual feature of rate. Rather, it may be more important to look at the rate or duration of individual speech elements (e.g., vowels and consonants).

Oyer and Deal[32] analyzed pause times in a reading passage produced by 24 males and females equally distributed in the 5th, 6th, and 7th decades of life. The oldest group (7th decade) required a significantly longer time to read the passage than the younger group. Apparently, the oldest group did not produce longer pause times (i.e., period of silence), but tended to produce more instances of low level acoustic energy during the reading.

Morris and Brown[30] measured the consonant and vowel durations for their groups of young and old female speakers. They found that the older speakers produced significantly longer vowel and consonant durations than the younger speakers.

Another acoustic variable that may be related to the perception of slower speaking rate in the elderly is voice onset time (VOT). VOT is the time from the release of the burst in a stop consonant to the onset of voicing by the vocal folds. It is a significant acoustic clue for distinguishing between a voiced (e.g., /b/) and an unvoiced consonant (e.g., /p/). Several studies have analyzed the speech of older subjects for variations in voice onset time.

Sweeting and Baken[33] studied the VOTs of men and women in three age groups, 25 to 39, 65 to 74, and over 75 years of age. They reported no statistically significant differences between the various age groups. Neiman, Klich, and Shuey[34] also reported no statistically significant differences between their younger and older women subjects. Morris and Brown[30] also failed to find any statistically significant differences in VOT between their younger and older women subjects. These data suggest that, when older subjects speak slower, they do not do so by varying the length of voice onset time. They may increase vowel duration, or perhaps they increase the time of other acoustic features of consonants like burst duration, silent interval, or friction duration.

PHYSIOLOGIC CHARACTERISTICS

Few studies have been done on the physiologic characteristics of the aged voice. This state of affairs is curious, considering the multitude of data that exists on the acoustic characteristics. The little data that does exist concerns vital capacity, intraoral air pressure, and laryngoscopic features.

Vital Capacity

Ptacek et al[25] reported lower vital capacities in their older speaker group when compared to their younger speaker group. Others[35-37] have reported smaller vital capacities in older populations. However, it is difficult to evaluate the significance of the lower elderly vital capacities for speech purposes. Most speech production occurs between 40 and 60 percent of an individual's vital capacity range. Even in singing, individuals rarely phonate at vital capacities greater than 70 percent of their range.[38] Thus, it seems unlikely that the elderly need the full vital capacity range. What may be of more significance to speech production is the control of the egressive breath stream. Here, the elderly show less lung elasticity and compliance[39] than younger speakers. They may not, therefore, be able to control the steady air flow and pressure necessary for speech production, at least not to the degree that younger speakers can.

Intraoral Breath Pressure

Ptacek et al[25] also measured the magnitude of pressure created in the oral cavity when their subjects produced speech. Although this measure is most directly related to force of articulation, indirectly it may mirror the pressure available below the vocal folds. In some cases, intraoral pressure is a good estimate of lung pressure.[40,41] Ptacek et al[25] reported much lower intraoral pressures for their elderly group. On the other hand, Morris and Brown[30] reported no significant differences of intraoral breath pressure between their young and old subject groups. Thus, it is unclear about the capabilities of elderly speakers to vary air pressures within the oral cavity and the pressures required from the thorax.

Laryngoscopic Observations

Several investigations were done on the characteristics of the larynx and vocal folds as viewed from above. Most used living subjects, whereas one investigation based observations on autopsy material.

Segre[23] noted yellowish discoloration of the vocal folds, atrophy of the ventricular folds, loss of normal tension, and a fissure in the middle or anterior one-third of the glottis. However, he does not report the details of his experimental procedure.

Honjo and Isshiki[42] studied the larynges of 20 elderly men and 20 elderly women laryngoscopically. Their findings, reported in Table 14-6, show that older larynges tend to have yellowish cords, edema, atrophy, and an incomplete glottal closure. However, these authors did not make objective measurements of these features, nor did they compare their findings to those of a younger control group.

Mueller, Sweeney, and Baribeau[43] studied 25 old larynges (mean age 81 years) and 10 young larynges (mean age 44.7 years) postmortem (see Table 14-6). They noted bowing, atrophy, and a cordal sulcus in the older group. Seventy-five percent of the older larynges demonstrated an arrowhead configuration of the vocal folds, whereas none of the control group demonstrated this.

There have been many studies in which the anatomical and structural changes of aging have been reported. These involve the analysis of material after death, and although pertinent to the analysis of voice function in the elderly, they are beyond the scope of this paper. A good review of these findings may be found in a chapter by Kahane.[24]

SUMMARY AND CONCLUSIONS

The aging voice exhibits different perceptual characteristics. People can hear the aging voice. They are also able to place voices in approximate age groups based on hearing the voices. They may do so by listening for certain characteristics, such as higher than normal pitch, hoarseness, or breathiness, as well as longer production times for vowels and consonants or more low level acoustic energy.

The aging voice exhibits different acoustic characteristics than a younger voice. An aged voice has a slightly different fundamental frequency than a younger voice, although the direction of the difference depends on the sex of the speaker. Elderly speakers tend to be more variable in their fundamental frequency, both long-term and short-term. Elderly speakers may be louder or softer when they speak, depending on the extent of physiologic decline in their muscles and connective tissue. Older speakers tend to show greater noise in their voices, which may correlate with the greater hoarseness or breathiness that listeners perceive. It is possible that the overall spectral characteristics of the aged voice may

TABLE 14-6 Summary of Some of the Laryngoscopic Characteristics of Aging

From Segre, 1971*

Yellowish discoloration of vocal folds
Atrophy of the ventricular folds
Loss of normal tension
Fissure in mid or anterior 1/3 of glottis

From Behrendt and Strauch, 1965†

Keratosis of mucous membrane
Increased elastic and collagen fibers in submucous tissue
Fat degeneration of muscles

From Honjo and Isshiki, 1980‡

Feature	Men	Women
N subjects	20	20
Yellow or dark folds	39%	47%
Edema	56%	74%
Atrophy	67%	26%
Glottal opening	67%	58%
Sulcus	10%	10%

* Data from Segre R. Senescence of the voice. Eye Ear Nose Throat Monthly 1971; 50:223-233.
† Data from Behrendt W, Strauch G. Die Feinstruk des menschlichen Stimmbandes abhängig vom Lebensalter. Arch Ohr Nas Kehlkopfh 1965; 184:510-520.
‡ Data from Honjo I, Isshiki N. Laryngoscopic and voice characteristics of aged persons. Arch Otolaryngol 1980; 106:149-150.

also be different, although little data exist to support that conclusion. Finally, the aged voice tends to have a slower rate and longer vowels and consonants. There are little data available of the timing of speech production by the elderly.

Laryngoscopically, there appear to be several characteristics of aging, including tissue color change, edema, atrophy, and incomplete glottal closure. However, these data are based on a small number of subjects with inadequate comparative data for younger subjects.

Finally, there are little data on the vibratory characteristics, muscle activity, or aerodynamics of the elderly voice. The need for these data is apparent in view of the extensive acoustic changes and the extensive anatomical changes that occur as a result of aging.

References

1. Ptacek P, Sander E. Age recognition from voice. J Speech Hear Res 1966; 9:273–277.
2. Shipp T, Hollien H. Perception of the aging male voice. J Speech Hear Res 1969; 12:703–710.
3. Linville S, Fisher H. Acoustic characteristics of women's voices with advancing age. J Gerontol 1985; 40:324–330.
4. Linville S, Korabic E. Elderly listener's estimates of vocal age in adult females. J Acoust Soc Am 1986; 80:692–694.
5. Ryan WJ, Burk KW. Perceptual and acoustic correlates of aging in the speech of males. J Commun Disord 1974; 7:181–192.
6. Hartman D, Danhauer J. Perceptual features of speech for males in four perceived age decades. J Acoust Soc Am 1976; 59:713–715.
7. Hartman D. The perceptual identity and characteristics of aging in normal male adult speakers. J Commun Disord 1979; 12:53–61.
8. Ryan EB, Capadano HL. Age perceptions and evaluative reactions toward adult speakers. J Gerontol 1978; 33:98–102.
9. Fitch JL, Holbrook A. Modal vocal fundamental frequency of young adults. Arch Otolaryngol 1970; 92:379–382.
10. Hollien H, Shipp T. Speaking fundamental frequency and chronologic age in males. J Speech Hear Res 1972; 15:155–159.
11. Wilcox KA, Horii Y. Age and changes in vocal jitter. J Gerontol 1980; 35:194–198.
12. Linke CE. A study of pitch characteristics of female voices and their relationship to vocal effectiveness. Folia Phoniatr 1973; 25:173–185.
13. Stoicheff ML. Speaking fundamental characteristics of non-smoking adults. J Speech Hear Res 1981; 24:437–441.
14. Mysak E, Hanley TD. Aging processes in speech: pitch and duration characteristics. J Gerontol 1958; 13:309–313.
15. Mysak ED. Pitch and duration characteristics of older males. J Speech Hear Res 1959; 2:46–54.
16. Mysak E, Hanley T. Vocal aging. Geriatrics 1959; 14:652–656.
17. Kent R, Burkard R. Changes in the acoustic correlates of speech production. In: Beasley D, Davis G, eds. Aging communication processes and disorders. New York: Grune & Stratton, 1981:47.
18. McGlone R, Hollien H. Vocal pitch characteristics of aged women. J Speech Hear Res 1963; 6:164–170.
19. Benjamin B. Frequency variability in the aged voice. J Gerontol 1981; 36:722–726.
20. Ramig L, Ringel R. Effects of physiological aging on selected acoustic characteristics of voice. J Speech Hear Res 1983; 26:22–30.
21. Ringel RL, Chodzko-Zajko WJ. Vocal indices of biological age. J Voice 1987; 1:31–37.
22. Chodzko-Zajko WJ, Ringel RL. Physiological fitness measures and sensory and motor performance in aging. Experimental Gerontology 1987; 22:317–328.
23. Segre R. Senescence of the voice. Eye Ear Nose Throat Monthly 1971; 50:223–233.
24. Kahane J. Anatomic and physiologic changes in the aging peripheral speech mechanism. In: Beasley D, Davis G, eds. Aging communication processes and disorders. New York: Grune & Stratton, 1981:21.
25. Ptacek PH, Sander E, Maloney W, Jackson CC. Phonatory and related changes with advanced age. J Speech Hear Res 1966; 9:353–360.
26. Linville SE. Maximum phonational frequency range capabilities of women's voices with advancing age. Folia Phoniatr 1987; 39:297–301.
27. Ryan WJ. Acoustic aspects of the aging voice. J Gerontol 1972; 27:265–268.
28. Kent RD, Kent JF, Rosenbek JC. Maximum performance tests of speech production. J Speech Hear Disord 1987; 52:367–387.
29. Colton RH. Spectral characteristics of older speakers. 1987; unpublished manuscript.
30. Morris RJ, Brown WS. Age-related voice measures among adult women. J Voice 1987; 1:38–43.
31. Ramig L. Effects of physiological aging on vowel spectral noise. J Gerontol 1983; 38:223–225.
32. Oyer HJ, Deal LV. Temporal aspects of speech and the aging process. Folia Phoniatr 1985; 37:109–112.
33. Sweeting PM, Baken RJ. Voice onset time in a normal-aged population. J Speech Hear Res 1982; 25:129–134.
34. Neiman GS, Klich RJ, Shuey EM. Voice onset time in young and 70-year-old women. J Speech Hear Res 1983; 26:118–123.
35. Shock N. The physiology of aging. Sci Am 1962; 206:100–110.
36. Norris AH, Shock NW, Landowne M, Falzone J. Pulmonary function studies: age differences in lung volumes and bellows function. Gerontologica 1956; 11:379–387.
37. Hoit JD, Hixon T. Age and speech breathing. J Speech Hear Res 1987; 30:351–368.
38. Proctor DF. Breathing mechanics during phonation and singing. In: Wyke B, ed. Ventilatory and phonatory control mechanisms. London: Oxford University Press, 1974:39.
39. Turner JM, Mead J, Wohl ME. Elasticity of human lungs in relation to age. J Appl Physiol 1968; 25:664–671.
40. Rothenberg M. The breath stream dynamics of simple-released-plosive production. Bibliotheca Phon 1968; 6:1–117.
41. Smitheran J, Hixon T. A clinical method for estimating laryngeal airway resistance during vowel production. J Speech Hear Dis 1981; 46:138–146.
42. Honjo I, Isshiki N. Laryngoscopic and voice characteristics of aged persons. Arch Otolaryngol 1980; 106:149–150.
43. Mueller PB, Sweeney RJ, Baribeau LJ. Acoustic and morphologic study of the senescent voice. Ear Nose Throat J 1984; 63:71–75.

SMELL, TASTE, AND AGING

CLINICAL DISORDERS OF OLFACTION AND GUSTATION IN THE AGED

JAMES B. SNOW Jr., M.D.

INTRODUCTION

The senses of smell and taste determine the flavor and palatability of beverages and foods and serve, with the trigeminal system, as monitors of dangerous volatiles such as natural gas, air pollutants, and smoke. Disturbances of these important senses in the elderly cause considerable sensory and psychological consequences and are indicative of a number of serious diseases, including degenerative disorders of the central nervous system such as Korsakoff's psychosis, Parkinson's disease, and Alzheimer's disease, intracranial neoplasms, head trauma, viral infections, autoimmune disease, and neurotoxicity.

The qualitative sensations of smell are mediated by specialized receptors in the olfactory neuroepithelium, while a number of chemicals are capable of producing sensations of coolness, warmth, sharpness, and irritation through receptors in the nose, oral cavity, pharynx, and larynx subserved by the trigeminal, glossopharyngeal, and vagal nerves. Other chemicals stimulate receptors in taste buds subserved by the facial, glossopharyngeal, and vagal nerves. Therefore, it is appropriate to consider these sensations in the context of a chemosensory system that includes olfactory, trigeminal, and taste perception of most chemical substances. A few chemicals such as phenyl ethyl alcohol, a rose-like odorant, are almost pure olfactory stimulants, but most odorants have varying degrees of olfactory and trigeminal stimulation.

ANATOMY

The human olfactory neuroepithelium is located in the superior part of the nasal cavities and occupies the area of the cribriform plate and the superior portions of the lateral walls and nasal septum. The olfactory neuroepithelium differs from the respiratory epithelium by being thicker (average of 70 μm compared to 45 μm), by containing Bowman's glands, and by having cilia that lack dynein arms needed for intrinsic mobility. The olfactory neuroepithelium contains an orderly zonal distribution of bipolar olfactory receptor cells, microvillar cells, sustentacular cells, and basal cells.

The olfactory receptor cells number approximately 6 million and contain a unique protein, the olfactory marker protein, which appears to be correlated with their functional integrity. A bulb-shaped modification of the tips of the dendrite of each receptor cell, known as the olfactory knob or vesicle, projects into the mucus layer and has 10 to 30 cilia. It is generally believed that the receptor sites for odorant molecules are located on the cilia.

The microvillar cells, of which there are 600,000, are found adjacent to the receptor cells at the surface of the neuroepithelium. The sustentacular cells are distributed throughout the neuroepithelium. The basal cells are the progenitors of the other cell types in the olfactory neuroepithelium, including the bipolar receptor cells. The basal cells are adjacent to the lamina propria during their resting phase and undergo profound structural and functional changes as they differentiate. The receptor cells are regularly replenished from the basal cells, and this is the only known renewal of primary sensory neurons.[1]

The unmyelinated axonal processes of the olfactory receptor cells are grouped together as fila and pass through the cribriform plate and terminate in spherical masses of neuropile, called glomeruli, which are located in single and double layers at the margin of the olfactory bulb. These terminations consist of complex arborizations in which multiple synaptic contacts are made with the dendrites of mitral, tufted, and periglomerular cells. Since many more nerve fibers enter glomeruli than leave them, the glomeruli are a focus of a high degree of convergence of information.

The principal secondary neurons in the olfactory system are the mitral cells, the largest cells in the olfactory bulb. The primary dendrite of each mitral cell extends into a single glomerulus. The mitral cell axons project through the internal plexiform layer and proceed caudally within the granule cell layer. The tufted cells are located between the glomeruli and the mitral cell layer and have dendritic processes that often project to more than one glomerulus.

The axons of the mitral and tufted cells proceed to the higher centers in the limbic system, including the anterior olfactory nucleus, the prepyriform cortex, the periamygdaloid cortex, the olfactory tubercle, the nucleus of the lateral olfactory tract, and the corticomedial nucleus of the amygdala.

The taste receptor cells are in the taste buds, which are spherical groups of cells arranged like the segments of a citrus fruit. At the epithelial surface, the taste bud has a pore that leads into a space into which microvilli of the receptor cells project. The taste buds are located in the foliate papillae on the lateral margin of the tongue, the fungiform papillae on the dorsum of the tongue, the circumvallate papillae at the junction of the anterior two-thirds and the base of the tongue, the palate, and the epiglottis. The taste buds have a similar structure in each of these locations. Unlike the olfactory system, the receptor cells are not primary neurons. Gustatory afferent fibers contact the individual taste receptor cells.

The sensory branch of the chorda tympani nerve of the facial nerve subserves taste along the lateral margin of the tongue. The greater superficial petrosal branch of the facial nerve provides taste afferents from the palate. The lingual branch of the glossopharyngeal nerve subserves taste from the circumvallate papillae. The internal branch of the superior laryngeal nerve of the vagus nerve provides the taste afferents from the epiglottis.

The cell bodies of the taste afferents are unipolar, and the single process is T-shaped with central and peripheral branches. The cell bodies of the fibers of the chorda tympani and the greater superficial petrosal nerves are located in the geniculate ganglion of the facial nerve. The cell bodies of the taste afferents of the lingual branch of the glossopharyngeal nerve are in the superior and petrosal ganglia, and the cell bodies of the taste afferents of the vagus nerve are in the jugular and nodose ganglia.

The taste afferents terminate in the nucleus of the tractus solitarius in the brain stem. The afferent division of the nervus intermedius of the facial nerve carries the central branches of the cells in the geniculate ganglion to the cephalic portion of the nucleus, while the fasiculus solitarius carries the central branches in the ganglia of the glossopharyngeal and vagal nerves to the middle and caudal portions of the nucleus.

The central pathway from the nucleus of the tractus solitarius projects to the ipsilateral parabrachial nucleus of the pons. Two divergent pathways project from the parabrachial nuclei.[2] One pathway ascends to the gustatory relay in the dorsal thalamus, synapses, and continues to the insular cortex. The other pathway goes to the ventral forebrain, including the lateral hypothalamus, substantia innominata, central nucleus of the amygdala, and stria terminalis. There is also evidence for a direct pathway from the parabrachial nuclei to the cortex. Olfaction and gustation appear to be unique among sensory systems in that at least some fibers bypass the thalamus.

PHYSIOLOGY

Odorant molecules are absorbed in the mucus covering the olfactory neuroepithelium, diffuse to the cilia on the dendritic processes of the olfactory receptor cells, and reversibly bind to protein receptor sites. Binding causes conformational changes in the receptor proteins that induce intracellular biochemical events culminating in the development of action potentials in the primary receptor neurons. Perceived intensity appears to be coded by the relative number of activated afferent neurons. Unlike intensity coding, little is known about quality coding. Individual receptor cells are responsive to a wide range of odorants, which suggests that more than one type of receptor site is present on each cell. In most instances, the response spectra overlap extensively. Odor quality perception may be related to the spatial distribution of receptor cells within the olfactory neuroepithelium. For example, the anterior region of the salamander's olfactory neuroepithelium is more responsive to propanol than the posterior region, while the reverse is true for pinene. This phenomenon occurs at several concentrations of these stimuli.

Tastant molecules reach the receptor cells through the pore of the taste bud. Four qualities of taste are recognized: sweet, sour, salty, and bitter. Individual gustatory afferent fibers respond to a number of different chemicals. Response patterns of gustatory afferent fibers can be grouped into classes based on the stimulus chemicals that produce the greatest response. For example, for the sucrose-best response neurons, the second-best stimulus is nearly always sodium chloride. Since individual gustatory afferents respond to a large number of chemicals, the across-fiber-pattern theory of gustatory coding evolved, while the best-stimulus analysis led to the concept of labeled afferents. It appears that labeled afferents are important for establishing gross quality sensation; and the across-fiber-pattern within a best-stimulus category, and perhaps among categories, is important for discrimination of chemicals within qualities. Intensity appears to be coded by the quantity of neural activity.

PATHOLOGY

The olfactory neuroepithelium and its central connections are a phylogenetically-ancient system in which the first order neurons are in direct contact with the chemical environment. They are particularly vulnerable to repeated viral infections and chemical injuries over the course of a lifetime. Fortunately, the receptor cells are unique in their regenerative capacity. After injury, the receptor cells are replaced with new cells arising from the basal cells. The new cells are capable of reestablishing connections in the olfactory bulb. A similar phenomenon occurs when the olfactory fila are transected.[1]

Pathologic changes in the human olfactory system should be interpreted in the context of the usual findings in the neuroepithelium in individuals who did not have olfactory dysfunction during life. In the human fetus, the olfactory neuroepithelium covers the roof of the nasal cavities and extends for a considerable distance to the superior part of the lateral walls of the nasal cavities and the nasal septum in a continuous sheet. In adults, the olfactory neuroepithelium occupies a relatively much smaller area and has widespread degeneration.[3] The degeneration is evidenced by loss of the zonal distribution of receptor, sustentacular, and basal cells, loss of receptor cells, dilatation of Bowman's glands, and gland-like invagination of respiratory epithelium into the lamina propria. Much of the area thought to be occupied by olfactory neuroepithelium is replaced with respiratory epithelium. The intercalation of respiratory epithelium occurs throughout the majority of the area usually thought to be occupied by olfactory neuroepithelium. This process of degeneration and replacement of olfactory neuroepithelium increases with age.[4] However, it begins early in adult life and is clearly evident in the second and third decades of life. It may correlate with the known diminution in olfactory sensitivity that occurs with aging.[5] It is conceivable that repeated viral upper respiratory infections and exposure to environmental neurotoxic chemicals produce this damage to the olfactory neuroepithelium.

The olfactory pathway is a principal means of entry of viruses into the central nervous system. Histopathologic changes can be observed throughout the olfactory system in animals inoculated with viral agents, regardless of whether intranasal, intracorneal, or intraperitoneal routes are used. Necrosis of the olfactory bulbs and tracts and of the prepyriform cortex is commonly observed in rodents inoculated with viruses.

Likewise, volatile toxic chemicals such as chlorine, N-methyl-forminino-methylester, 1,2-dibromo-3-chloropropane, and 1,2-dibromoethane induce structural changes in the olfactory neuroepithelium.

Transection of the olfactory fila in their fixed positions at the cribriform plate results from acceleration and deceleration impacts in which the brain moves independently from the skull. Head injuries also result in intracranial hemorrhage, which, at least in laboratory animals, causes degeneration of the olfactory neuroepithelium without transection of the olfactory fila.[6]

Experimentally-induced ischemia in the gerbil, which has an incomplete circle of Willis, results in damage to the olfactory neuroepithelium and its central connections.[7] It is of interest that the olfactory bulb is particularly resistant to ischemia.

Agents that affect cell turnover, neurotoxic drugs, and radiation therapy to the head are well-recognized causes of damage to the olfactory neuroepithelium.

Taste buds have the ability to regenerate after various forms of injury. Inflammatory and degenerative diseases of the oral cavity, viral infections, endocrine disorders, heavy metal intoxication, drugs that affect cell turnover, radiation therapy to the oral cavity and pharynx, neoplasms, transection of taste afferent fibers, xerostomia, and bacterial colonization of the taste bud pore are known causes of gustatory loss. Taste buds degenerate when their gustatory afferents are transected, but remain intact when their somatosensory afferents are severed. Aging itself appears to be less of a determinant of gustatory sensitivity than it is for olfactory sensitivity.

CLINICAL EVALUATION

Diminution of smell and taste perception in the elderly is a frequently-encountered clinical problem. Chemosensory dysfunction seriously affects the quality of life of many elderly individuals. The clinical evaluation of the elderly does not substantially differ from the clinical evaluation of younger patients with smell and taste complaints. The natural history of the evolution of the patient's complaint is of fundamental importance in establishing an etiologic diagnosis. The physical findings, particularly in the nasal cavities, oral cavity, and pharynx, often provide important clues as to the mechanism and cause of the impairment. Computed tomography with enhancement and magnetic resonance imaging play an important part in demonstrating the cause of olfactory dysfunction and in excluding evidence of anterior cranial fossa neoplasms and fractures.

Quantification of the loss or distortion of the senses of smell and taste by psychophysical techniques provides objective evidence to corroborate the patient's complaint, to determine the severity of the impairment, to monitor the efficacy of therapy, and to establish the degree of permanent impairment.

PSYCHOPHYSICAL EVALUATION

Patients with a loss of the sense of smell often complain of a loss of the sense of taste, even though their perception of sweet, sour, salty, and bitter stimuli remains normal. This occurs because they cannot discriminate flavors of food and beverage, which is an olfactory function.

Patients with a complaint of a loss of the sense of smell, loss of the sense of taste, or both should have their senses of smell and taste measured.

The first step in our sensory evaluation is to determine the degree to which qualitative sensations are perceived. For this assessment, we use the University of Pennsylvania Smell Identification Test (UPSIT), a 40-item forced-choice odor test consisting of four booklets containing ten odorants each, one odorant per page.[8] The stimuli are embedded in microencapsulated crystals 10 to 50 μm in diameter located on strips at the bottom of each page. Above each odorized strip is a multiple-choice item with four possible responses. For example, one of the items reads, "This odor smells most like: (a) chocolate; (b) banana; (c) onion; or (d) fruit punch," and the subject is required to choose one of the alternatives, even if no odor is perceived. The forced-choice aspect of the test encourages the subject to sample each odorant and provides a basis for detecting malingering.

The UPSIT is highly reliable with a short-term, test-retest reliability of $r=0.95$. There are normative data that allow direct comparison of a patient's score with controls of the same gender and age so that the result can be expressed as a percentile of the norm.[9] It is sensitive to gender and age differences. There is a decrement in sensitivity with age, which becomes abrupt at 65 years of age.

The second step in our olfactory testing is to determine the detection threshold for the rose-like odorant phenyl ethyl alcohol. Sensitivity for each side of the nose is determined with a detection threshold for phenyl ethyl methyl ethyl carbinol. The thresholds are determined using a modified single-staircase procedure. The geometric mean of the first four staircase reversal points following the third staircase reversal is used to determine the threshold value.

Nasal resistance is measured for each side of the nose with anterior rhinomanometry.

Taste evaluation begins with suprathreshold whole-mouth testing for quality, intensity, and pleasantness perception for sucrose, citric acid, sodium chloride, and caffeine. Threshold testing is performed when indicated. Suprathreshold tongue quadrant testing and electrogustometry are performed to detect regional deficits.

There is much in the literature that indicates that anosmic individuals are depressed. Using the Beck Depression Inventory, patients with dysosmia or dysgeusia are shown to be particularly prone to depression.

DIAGNOSIS

Disorders of the sense of smell are caused by interference with the access of odorant molecules to the olfactory neuroepithelium, damage to the olfactory neuroepithelium, and damage to the central olfactory pathways. Disease processes that interfere with odorants reaching the olfactory receptors can be thought of as transport causes, while damage to the olfactory neuroepithelium and central pathways can be thought of as sensorineural causes.

Transport olfactory losses may result from obstruction of the nasal cavity because of swollen mucous membrane, as in acute upper respiratory infections, sinusitis, and allergic rhinitis; structural changes such as deviations of the nasal septum, polyps, and masses; and abnormalities of the mucus in which the olfactory knobs project.

We do not have psychophysical methods for differentiating sensory from neural olfactory losses. Sensory olfactory losses are caused by viral infections, inhalation of toxic chemicals, some forms of head injury, drugs that affect cell injury, and radiation therapy to the head. Neural olfactory losses occur with head trauma, neoplasms of the anterior cranial fossa, neurosurgical procedures, multiple sclerosis and other demyelinating diseases, Korsakoff's syndrome and other degenerative central nervous system diseases, and the administration of neurotoxic agents.[10]

Disturbances of the sense of taste are caused by conditions that interfere with the access of tastant molecules to the receptor cells in the taste bud (transport causes), that injure the receptor cells (sensory causes), or that damage gustatory afferent nerves and their central pathways (neural causes).

Transport gustatory losses result from xerostomia, heavy metal intoxication, and bacterial colonization of the taste pore.

Sensory gustatory losses result from inflammatory and degenerative diseases in the oral cavity, drugs that affect cell turnover, radiation therapy to the oral cavity and pharynx, viral infections, endocrine disorders, neoplasms, and trauma.

Neural gustatory losses result from neoplasms, trauma, and operations in which the gustatory afferents are injured.

The leading causes of olfactory disorders are head trauma and viral infections, and both of these causes are related to age and gender. Head trauma is a relatively more frequent cause of sensorineural olfactory losses in children and young adults. Men are more frequently injured than women. Viral infections are a more important cause of sensory olfactory losses in older adults. Women are more frequently affected than men.

TREATMENT

Treatment of patients with most transport olfactory losses (bacterial rhinitis and sinusitis, allergic rhinitis, polyps, neoplasms, and structural abnormalities in the nasal cavities) can be undertaken rationally and with optimism at any age. Allergic management, antibiotic therapy, systemic corticosteroid therapy, topical corticosteroid therapy (beclomethasone or flunisolide), and operations for structural abnormalities of the nasal cavities, nasal polyps, chronic hyperplastic sinusitis, and neoplasms are effective in restoring the sense of smell when the problem is attributable to interference with the odorant reaching the olfactory neuroepithelium. At the present time, we know little about alterations in the mucus environment of the receptor cells, but this important theoretic possibility must not be overlooked in the study of olfactory disorders.

Treatment of patients with sensorineural olfactory losses is a problem. Evaluation of therapy is confounded by spontaneous recovery, and any therapeutic approach may appear to have merit in some patients. Zinc and vitamin therapy have their advocates, but lack validation of their efficacy. Currently, we lack reasonable therapeutic strategies for the sensorineural olfactory losses.

Treatment for gustatory losses remains limited. Artificial saliva benefits some patients with an abnormal salivary milieu. Treatment for bacterial and fungal infections of the oral cavity and pharynx is appropriate and helpful in some patients, particularly in the elderly. Withdrawal of drugs affecting cell turnover is usually helpful if the patient's general condition permits. No reasonable therapeutic strategies exist for sensorineural gustatory losses.

From the Department of Otorhinolaryngology and Human Communication and the Smell and Taste Center, University of Pennsylvania School of Medicine, Philadelphia, PA 19104. Supported in part by the National Institute of Neurological and Communicative Disorders and Stroke Grant number 16365.

References

1. Monti Graziadei GA, Graziadei PPC. Neurogenesis and neuron regeneration in the olfactory system of mammals: II. Degeneration and reconstitution of the olfactory sensory neurons after axotomy. J Neurocytol 1979; 8:197–213.
2. Norgren R. The gustatory system in mammals. Am J Otolaryngol 1983; 4:234–237.
3. Nakashima T, Kimmelman CP, Snow JB. Structure of human fetal and adult olfactory neuroepithelium. Arch Otolaryngol 1984; 110:641–646.
4. Naessen R. An inquiry on the morphological characteristics and possible changes with age in the olfactory region in man. Acta Otolaryngol 1971; 71:49–62.
5. Doty RL, Shaman P, Applebaum SL, Giberson R, Sikorski L, Rosenberg L. Smell identification ability: changes with age. Science 1984; 226:1441–1443.
6. Nakashima T, Kimmelman CP, Snow JB. Effects of olfactory nerve section and hemorrhage on the olfactory neuroepithelium. Surgical Forum Volume 1984; XXXV:562–564.
7. Nakashima T, Kimmelman CP, Snow JB. Immunohistopathologic analysis of olfactory degeneration caused by ischemia. Otolaryngol Head Neck Surg 1985; 93:40–47.
8. Doty RL, Shaman P, Dann M. Development of the University of Pennsylvania Smell Identification Test: a standardized microencapsulated test of olfactory function. Physiol Behav (Monograph) 1984; 32:489–502.
9. Doty RL, Newhouse MG, Azzalina JD. Internal consistency and short-term test-retest reliability of the University of Pennsylvania Smell Identification Test. Chem Senses 1985; 10:297–300.
10. Doty RL, Snow JB. Age-related alterations in olfactory structure and function. In: Margolis F, Getchell TV, eds. Molecular neurobiology of the olfactory system. New York: Plenum, 1988.

Chapter Sixteen

AGE-RELATED ALTERATIONS IN TASTE AND SMELL FUNCTION

RICHARD L. DOTY, Ph.D.

INTRODUCTION

The chemical senses protect us from such environmental hazards as leaking natural gas, spoiled food, and smoke, and provide the primary basis for the perception of the flavor of foods and beverages. Furthermore, these important senses contribute immensely to the overall quality of life and, in dysfunction, serve as a warning for a number of pathologic conditions. Therefore, an understanding of age-related changes in chemosensation is of considerable significance to the layman and medical practitioner alike.

Although advances have been made in documenting the nature of age-related changes in taste and smell perception, causal relations have yet to be demonstrated between the psychophysical alterations and the underlying pathologic mechanisms. Furthermore, because only a fraction of the available stimuli and psychophysical testing procedures have been employed, it is possible that many such changes have yet to be elucidated. Nevertheless, as indicated in this chapter, considerable progress has been made in understanding the anomalies that occur in chemosensory function during the later years. The present monograph reviews this progress and provides a perspective for future research endeavors in this emerging area of geriatric otolaryngology.

OLFACTION

Odor Detection

Impairment in the ability to detect low concentrations of odorants is found in later life. An example of the nature of the change in detection thresholds across the age-span is presented in Figure 16-1.[1] Although these curves represent sensitivity to only one odorant (the rose-like smelling compound phenyl ethyl alcohol), their general shape is likely representative of the curves of many compounds since olfactory thresholds typically correlate with one another. It should be noted that, on the average, the decline in sensitivity (i.e., rise in thresholds), while present in both sexes, begins at an earlier age in men than in women.

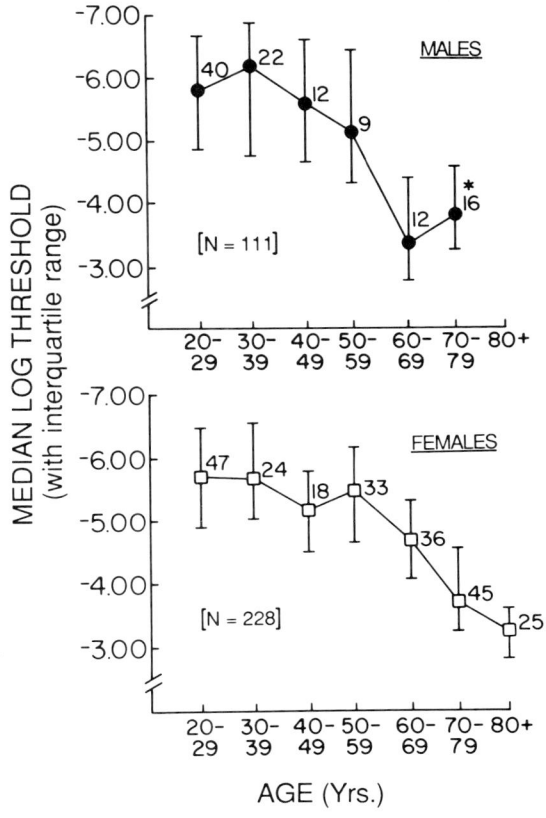

Figure 16-1 Log phenyl ethyl alcohol odor detection threshold values as a function of age and gender in non-smoking subjects. Numbers by data points indicate sample sizes. Note that concentration values are plotted inversely on the Y axis. * The 7 men over age 79 have been included in the 70 to 79 year age group. Reproduced with permission from Deems DA, Doty RL. Age-related changes in the phenyl ethyl alcohol odor detection threshold. Trans Pa Acad Ophthalmol Otolaryngol 1987; 39:646-650.

Odor Identification

As with odor detection, there is an age-related decrease in the ability to identify or recognize odorants.[2] This decrease, exemplified by scores on the University of Pennsylvania Smell Identification Test (UPSIT, Fig. 16-2), is strikingly similar to that noted for phenyl ethyl alcohol thresholds (see Fig. 16-1), thus suggesting the possibility that the odor identification deficit may be secondary to the odor detection deficit, at least in some cases. As can be observed in Figure 16-2, peak performance in odor identification ability occurs in the third through fifth decades of life and markedly declines after the seventh decade, with women generally outperforming men at all ages. Using the criterion of an UPSIT score of 19 or less as major impairment, more than half of the subjects between the ages of 65 and 80 years, and over three-quarters of those older than 80 years, evidence such impairment.[2] The poor scores in the older age range are likely not attributable to losses in memory as such, since (1) the memory load on the UPSIT does not exceed the span of immediate attention and (2) UPSIT scores of elderly subjects do not significantly correlate with scores on the Wechsler Memory Scale.[3] Interestingly, the sex difference shown in Figure 16-2 is present to the same relative degree in several cultural groups, including American Blacks, American Caucasians, American Koreans, and Native Japanese.[4]

Odor Intensity Perception

Several procedures have been developed for assessing the perceived intensity of odorants at suprathreshold concentrations, including tests of whether odor intensity increases appropriately with increments in odorant concentration. In one procedure (termed magnitude estimation), subjects assign numbers proportionate to the relative intensity of different concentrations of an odorant. In a related

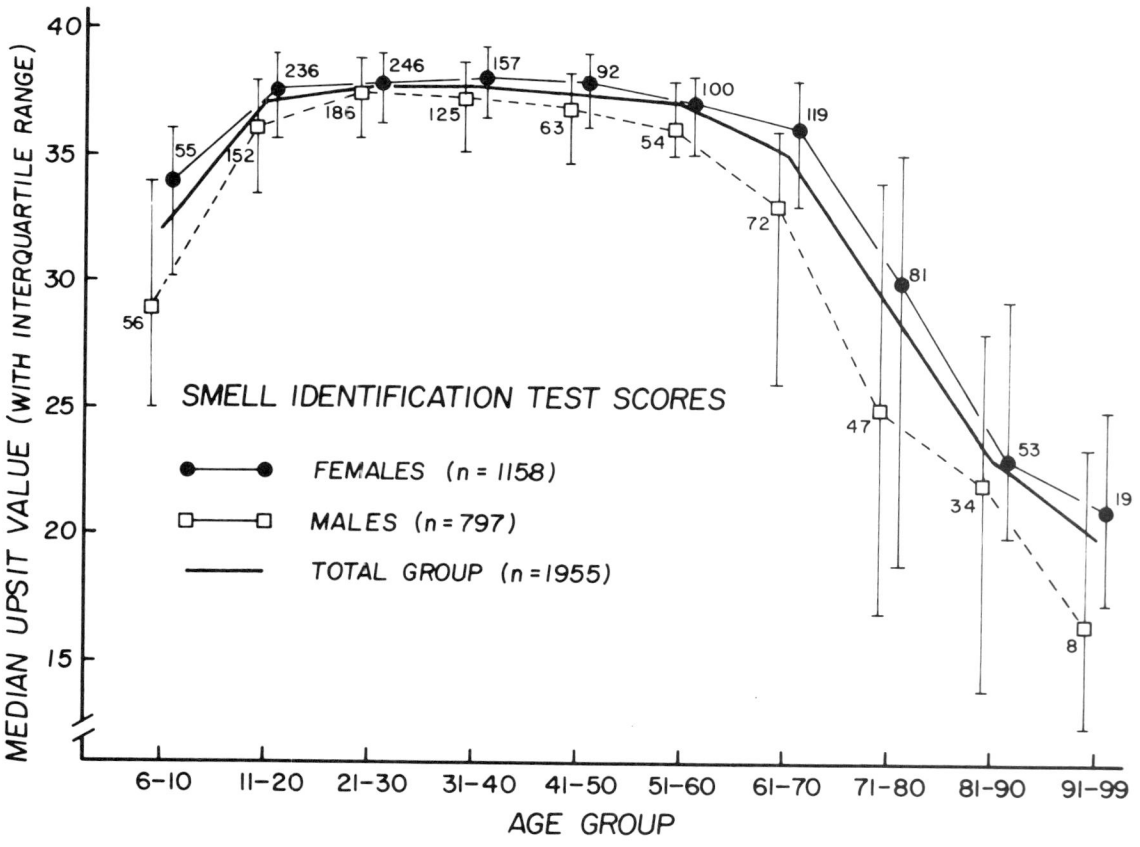

Figure 16-2 Scores on the University of Pennsylvania Smell Identification Test (UPSIT) as a function of age in a large heterogeneous group of subjects. Numbers by data points indicate sample sizes. Reproduced with permission from Doty RL, Shaman P, Applebaum SL, Giverson R, Sikorski L, Rosenberg L. Smell identification ability: changes with age. Science 1984; 226:1441-1443. Copyright 1984 by the American Association for the Advancement of Science.

procedure (termed cross-modal matching), subjects signify such magnitudes by using another sensory dimension, such as linear extent (by pulling a tape measure a distance proportionate to the perceived intensity). In still another procedure (termed magnitude-matching), stimuli from two modalities (e.g., olfaction and audition) are presented in interspersed trials and judged on a common scale of perceptual magnitude. Assuming that individuals or groups are alike in the way they perceive the intensities of one of these modalities (e.g., low frequency tones), the judgments of the other modality can be normalized to allow for a more accurate assessment of the interindividual differences.

Murphy,[5] using the method of magnitude estimation, reported that the average rate of growth of the perceived intensity of menthol across a suprathreshold concentration range was twice as great for 10 young adults (18 to 26 years of age) than for 10 elderly ones (66 to 93 years of age). Such an increase was not observed by Rovee et al[6] using a similar procedure for the odorant propanol.

Stevens et al,[7] using a cross-modal matching procedure, found that the standardized magnitude estimation functions of young (18 to 25 years) and old (65 to 83 years) persons for isoamyl butyrate (which they report is a relatively nonirritating odorant) and carbon dioxide (a trigeminal stimulus with minimal or no odor qualities) did not differ significantly in slope. However, the function of the older subjects for both odorants was displaced downward (i.e., evidenced a lower y-intercept), thus suggesting that older persons have a proportional loss of smell function across a broad range of stimulus concentrations. A similar finding was reported by Stevens and Cain[8] for isoamyl butyrate, benzaldehyde, d-limonene, pyridine, ethanol, and isoamyl alcohol, implying that the deficit is present for odorants ranging widely in chemical structure, psychological quality, and hedonic tone. Interestingly, this age-related decrement in the perceived intensity of odors is present when the odors are presented retronasally (i.e., to the olfactory receptors from inside the oral cavity, as during chewing and swallowing).[9] Since the intensity of retronasal odor perception is influenced by mouth movements that occur during deglutition,[10] some age-related alterations in flavor perception could result from alterations in pressure and/or flow relations within the nasopharynx caused, for example, by changes in the speed and amount of chewing and swallowing.

Odor Discrimination

If threshold and suprathreshold measures of odor detection and perceived intensity are altered by aging processes, then it is likely that the ability to distinguish qualitatively among odorants is also impaired. This is indeed the case, as exemplified by the pioneering study of Shiffman and Pasternak.[11] These investigators had 16 19- to 25-year-olds and 16 72- to 78-year-olds rate 91 pairs of 14 commercial food flavors on a 5-inch "same-different" rating scale. The data were subjected to a statistical procedure (termed multidimensional scaling) that places the responses in two-dimensional space relative to the perceived similarities of the stimuli. The multidimensional spaces obtained for a number of elderly subjects, unlike those obtained for the younger ones, grouped stimuli of different psychological quality in proximate regions, implying that the older persons had difficulty discriminating the qualitative differences.

Odor Hedonics

Historically, the measurement of the pleasantness or unpleasantness of odorants has been a popular undertaking. This is attributable in part to the fact that humans spontaneously use hedonic descriptors when judging odors (e.g., "good," "bad," "pleasant," "unpleasant"),[12] and conceivably reflects the olfactory system's intimate association with the determination of flavor, the monitoring of foodstuffs, and, at least in the case of many nonhuman animals, sexual behavior.[13] Anatomically, olfactory pathways are closely related to limbic regions and structures known to influence, if not regulate, emotional and pleasurable events.

Albeit limited, there is evidence that elderly subjects do not derive the same degree of enjoyment or displeasure as younger persons from olfactory stimulation. This may be closely related to their decreased smell sensitivity. Thus, if an odorant is perceived as less intense by an elderly person than by a younger one, its perceived pleasantness (or unpleasantness) would also be expected to be correspondingly altered, depending on the form of the intensity/pleasantness relationship for the odorant in question.[14] Therefore, it is not surprising that increases in menthol concentration produce larger increments in estimates of odor pleasantness by young subjects than by elderly subjects[5] and that diesel fumes are less offensive to older than to younger persons.[15]

Odor Perception in Age-Related Diseases

It is noteworthy that a number of age-related diseases (some of which have been suggested as being models for early aging) are accompanied by alterations in olfactory function. The analysis of the pathologic substrates involved in these diseases may provide clues as to the basis for age-related olfactory deficits. Although there is recent evidence that patients with Down's syndrome and Huntington's chorea suffer decrements in smell function,[16,17] the most extensive evidence for smell loss in age-related diseases comes from studies of patients with Alzheimer's disease (AD) and parkinsonism. While there is circumstantial evidence that such dysfunction may be related to specific biochemical and structural alterations in olfactory-related brain regions, cause and effect relations have yet to be elucidated.

Alzheimer's disease has been suggested by some as having its genesis within the olfactory system.[18] The basis of such thinking stems primarily from neuropathologic studies that find the distribution of neurofibrillary tangles and neuritic plaques (the neuropathologic hallmarks of this disease) disproportionately present within limbic structures associated with olfactory function. Thus, Pearson et al[19] state,

> "The invariable finding of severe and even maximal involvement of the olfactory regions in Alzheimer's disease is in striking contrast to the minimal pathology in the visual and sensorimotor areas of the neocortex and cannot be without significance. In the olfactory system, the sites that are affected—the anterior olfactory nucleus, the uncus, and the medial group of amygdaloid nuclei—all receive fibers directly from the olfactory bulb. These observations at least raise the possibility that the olfactory pathway is the site of initial involvement of the disease."

Such findings gain even more significance in the context of theories that some dementia-related diseases may be related to environmental toxins or viruses and of observations that (1) the olfactory system is a major conduit of such materials into the central nervous system[20] and that (2) inoculation of rodents with some viruses results in necrosis of the olfactory neuroepithelium, the olfactory bulbs and tracts, and the prepyriform cortex.[21]

The evidence for deficits in odor perception in Alzheimer's disease patients is overwhelming; marked decrements in both odor identification and detection ability have been noted in a number of studies (Fig. 16-3), although total anosmia is rarely present.[22] Such alterations appear to occur early in the disease process and to be unrelated to disease stage. Interestingly, most AD patients are initially unaware of an olfactory dysfunction.[22]

Patients with Parkinson's disease (PD), a disorder that shares a number of clinical, neuropathologic, and neurochemical features with AD, also evidence decrements in odor identification, detec-

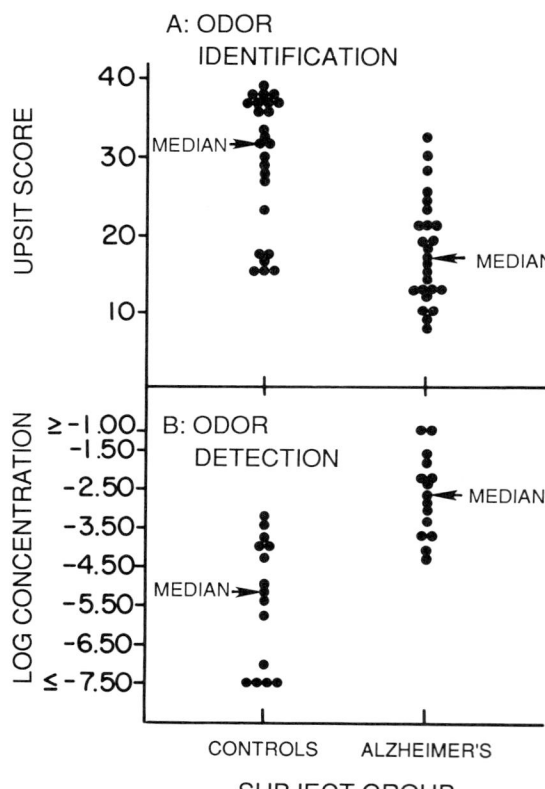

Figure 16-3 *A*, University of Pennsylvania Smell Identification Test (UPSIT) scores for patients with Alzheimer's disease and for age-, gender-, and race-matched controls. *B*, Detection threshold values for phenyl ethyl alcohol for patients with Alzheimer's disease and for matched controls. Each dot signifies an individual subject's data point. Although some overlap appears between the Alzheimer's disease and control subject data when plotted in this manner, very few of the Alzheimer's disease subjects performed better than their matched controls. Reproduced with permission from Doty RL, Reyes P, Gregor T. Presence of both odor identification and detection deficits in Alzheimer's disease. Brain Res Bull 1987; 18:597-600.

tion, and discrimination.[23-25] Their olfactory deficit, as measured by the UPSIT and the phenyl ethyl alcohol detection threshold test (Figure 16-4), appears to be indistinguishable from that of Alzheimer's disease when the degree of dementia is statistically equated using analysis of covariance.[24] Furthermore, the olfactory disorder appears to be independent of neurologic ratings of motoric symptoms of the disease, as well as independent of various neuropsychological, cognitive, and motor measurements.[26]

The olfactory dysfunction of parkinsonism appears to be unrelated to the severity of the disease symptoms, and no relationship is apparent between the magnitude of the UPSIT or threshold deficits and the duration of the disease (Figs. 16-5 and 16-6).[24] This lack of an association between disease duration and the degree of the olfactory dysfunction is supported by longitudinal testing; no significant differences in UPSIT test scores were observed in 24 PD patients retested after intervals ranging from 5 months to 3 years.[24]

The olfactory deficit of PD rarely reflects total anosmia. Thus, in the Doty, Deems, and Stellar study,[24] only 13 percent of the 38 patients who received detection threshold testing were unable to detect the highest odorant concentration presented in a threshold test, a figure in close correspondence to a 17 percent anosmia rate reported in an earlier study by Ward et al.[25] This observation is further supported by the finding that all but one of 41 PD patients who were asked whether or not an odor was present on each UPSIT item answered affirmatively to 35 or more of the items, even though the majority were unable to identify most of the odors or felt that the perceived sensation did not correspond to the response alternatives.[24]

TASTE

Despite the fact that many studies that explore taste perception in the elderly suffer from methodologic problems (e.g., lack of forced-choice responses, failure to rinse between stimulus presentations), most arrive at the general conclusion that some alterations in taste sensation occur as a function of age. However, as subsequently noted, the magnitude of such effects are small, and few studies have addressed the issue of confounding influences from gender, oral hygiene, cigarette smoking, and other variables. Interestingly, earlier reports that the number of taste buds decrease with age have been recently challenged.[27,28]

Taste Detection

Age-related decrements in taste sensitivity, as measured by detection or recognition threshold tests, have been noted for standard sweet, sour, bitter, and salty tastants, as well as for amino acids and artificial sweeteners. In addition, age-related alterations in lingual sensitivity to low electrical current (which is assumed to stimulate taste afferents, rather than trigeminal ones) have also been reported. However, loss of taste function as a result of advancing age appears to be less robust than loss of smell function, and some well-controlled studies fail to document such changes for all tastants.

Most studies indicate that older persons are less sensitive than younger ones to sodium chloride,[29,30] although the age-related decrements are not large. For example, Grzegorczyk et al[29] found the mean sodium chloride detection threshold to be 3.0 mM in a group of 20 subjects ranging in age from 20

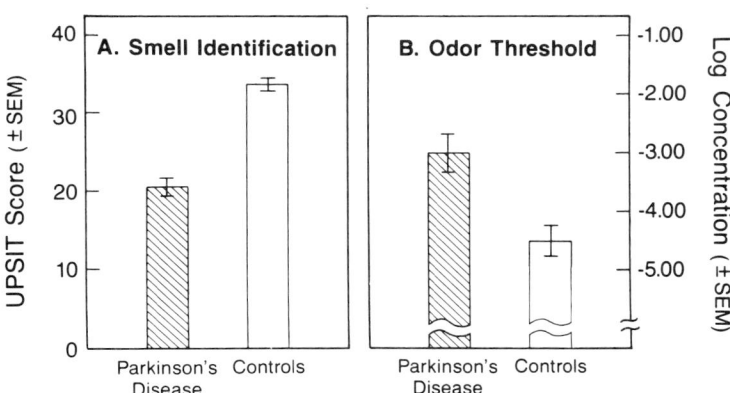

Figure 16-4 Mean University of Pennsylvania Smell Identification Test (UPSIT) scores, *A*, and phenyl ethyl alcohol odor detection threshold values, *B*, for Parkinson's disease patients and matched normal controls. Reproduced with permission from Doty RL, Deems D, Stellar S. Olfactory dysfunction in Parkinson's disease: a general deficit unrelated to neurologic signs, disease stage, or disease duration. Neurology 1988; 38:1237-1244.

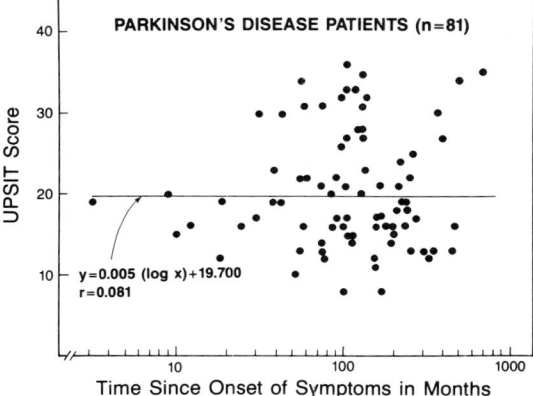

Figure 16–5 University of Pennsylvania Smell Identification Test (UPSIT) scores of Parkinson's disease patients as a function of disease duration. Reproduced with permission from Doty RL, Deems D, Stellar S. Olfactory dysfunction in Parkinson's disease: a general deficit unrelated to neurologic signs, disease stage, or disease duration. Neurology 1988; 38:1237–1244.

to 39 years, and 6.3 mM in 28 subjects ranging in age from 65 to 95 years. This relatively definitive study employed a forced-choice procedure and water rinses between stimulus presentations.

Like sodium chloride, thresholds for bitter and sour compounds also evidence an elevation in the later years.[30–33] There is some controversy as to whether such elevation is due to age, per se, or to cumulative influences of smoking. Thus, Glanville, Kaplan, and Fischer[32] initially reported that taste thresholds for 6-n-propylthiouracil (PROP, a phenylthiocarbimide- or PTC-like compound) and

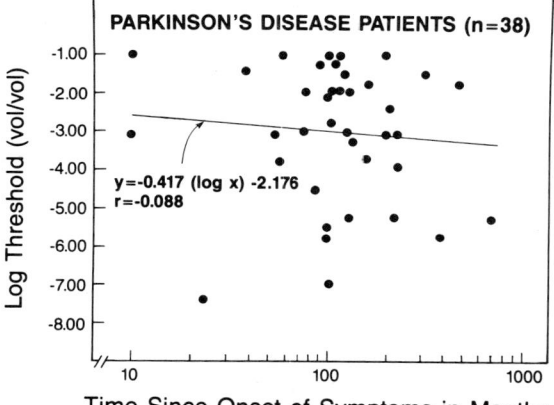

Figure 16–6 Phenyl ethyl alcohol odor detection threshold values of Parkinson's disease patients as a function of disease duration. Reproduced with permission from Doty RL, Deems D, Stellar S. Olfactory dysfunction in Parkinson's disease: a general deficit unrelated to neurologic signs, disease stage, or disease duration. Neurology 1988; 38:1237–1244.

quinine increase with age, with males exhibiting a greater increase than females. However, in a later study in which only nonsmokers were tested, these authors found no influence of either age or sex on such taste thresholds (n = 268, ages ranging from 16 to 55 years).[33] These investigators concluded:

> "...aging within the 16- to 55-year age span did not seem to be associated with a significant deterioration in taste sensitivity unless combined with smoking. The sex difference sometimes observed in population surveys seemed to be an artifact associated with differential smoking habits of men and women."

Of all the classic taste modalities, that of sweet appears to be the most robust. Thus, statistically-significant age-related alterations in sucrose sensitivity have not been observed by every investigator (e.g., Weiffenbach[30]), and those who have observed such alterations report they are small and often occur only in the later years.[34] It is of interest that the magnitude of the age-related effects seen by some investigators is similar (on a molar basis) to that observed for nonsweet tastants. For example, Moore et al[35] reported a mean sucrose threshold of 3.6 mM in 30 subjects who ranged in age from 20 to 45 years, compared to a mean sucrose threshold of 8.0 mM in 29 subjects who ranged in age from 60 to 88 years. These molar values are similar to those reported by Grzegorczyk et al[29] for sodium chloride.

In summary, while most studies find age-related changes in taste sensitivity to at least some tastants, the magnitude of such changes is small. Furthermore, the role of variables such as previous smoking history, gender, and oral hygiene is rarely systematically addressed. As noted by Bartoshuk et al,[36] it is conceivable that age-related decreased taste sensitivity at low concentrations reflects the presence of a "masking" background taste or a mild dysgeusia that results in poor discrimination between the water control and the tastant. This hypothesis is supported by observations that improvement of oral hygiene results in the lowering of taste thresholds.[37,38] Langan and Yearick[38] found, for example, that elderly persons who received professional oral hygiene therapy three times weekly for 5 weeks evidenced a lowering of thresholds for sucrose and sodium chloride relative to a control group who were similarly visited by an oral hygienist who only inspected and swabbed the teeth. Whether or not improvement of oral hygiene would influence the taste thresholds of cigarette smokers has yet to be determined.[39]

Taste Intensity Perception

Age-related differences in the perceived intensity of suprathreshold concentrations of tastants have been reported. For example, Schiffman et al[40] and Schiffman and Clark[41] found that, compared to young college students, elderly individuals provided less steep group slopes of magnitude estimates for 10 artificial sweeteners and 23 amino acids. More recently, Bartoshuk et al,[36] using the method of magnitude matching, assessed the perceived intensities of sodium chloride, sucrose, citric acid, and quinine hydrochloride in 18 elderly subjects (16 females and 2 males; mean age = 82.8) and in 18 young controls (16 females and 2 males; mean age = 24.4). Assuming that sounds (the matching modality) were equivalently loud to elderly and to young adults, these authors found that moderate and strong tastes were equivalently strong to these two age groups. However, the lower concentrations were rated as more intense by the elderly subjects, and the highest concentrations as less intense, resulting in a flattening of the psychophysical functions.

In an extensive recent study, Weiffenbach, Cowart, and Baum[42] had 91 men and 79 women between the ages of 23 and 88 years extend a tape measure in proportion to the perceived relative intensity of various suprathreshold concentrations of sucrose, sodium chloride, citric acid, and quinine sulfate. There were no dramatic differences in group functions reflecting taste intensity judgments for any of the age groups or for any taste quality. Nevertheless, other measures did reflect age-related and quality-specific decreases. For example, intraclass correlation coefficients were significantly lower in older, than in younger, subjects for sodium chloride, citric acid, and quinine sulfate, but not for sucrose.

Taste Hedonics

Surprisingly few studies have examined taste hedonics in older subjects. One notable exception is the study by Enns et al,[43] which found no significant differences in hedonic ratings given to a series of sucrose solutions by 21 fifth-grade students, 27 college students, and 12 older persons with an average age of 71 years. Interestingly, the males in each age category gave the most concentrated solution (1.0 M) significantly higher pleasantness ratings than did the females.

GENERAL CONCLUSIONS

It is clear from the aforementioned review that nearly all psychophysical measures of taste and smell perception are altered in elderly individuals. However, the basis of such changes is poorly understood. Thus, it is not presently known whether most cases of decreased taste or smell function in older persons are attributable to aging processes themselves or to phenomena correlated with aging, such as the culmination of repeated insults from viral infections, the onset of age-related diseases, poor oral hygiene, and the use of medications commonly prescribed for the elderly.

Despite these etiologic uncertainties, it is apparent that the age-related deficits observed in olfaction are larger than those observed in taste, and that the majority of elderly persons have significant loss of smell function. Even though older persons have a higher frequency of taste complaints than younger persons (e.g., sour and bitter dysgeusias),[44] it must be kept in mind that many of their reports of "taste loss" are referrable to their decrement in olfactory function, which is known to attenuate food flavor.[45] In this regard, it is important to note that xerostomia (which is more prevalent in aged populations) has little influence on human taste thresholds.[46]

Supported by Grant NS 16365 from the National Institute of Neurological and Communicative Disorders and Stroke, the Hoffman Fund, and the Jennie F. Isermann Memorial Fund for Parkinson's Disease Research at the St. Barnabas Medical Center, Livingston, New Jersey.

References

1. Deems DA, Doty RL. Age-related changes in the phenyl ethyl alcohol odor detection threshold. Trans Pa Acad Ophthalmol Otolaryngol 1987; 39:646–650.
2. Doty RL, Shaman P, Applebaum SL, Giberson R, Sikorski L, Rosenberg L. Smell identification ability: changes with age. Science 1984; 226:1441–1443.
3. Doty RL, Brugger WE, Jurs PC, Orndorff MA, Snyder PJ, Lowry LD. Intranasal trigeminal stimulation from odorous volatiles: psychometric responses from anosmic and normal humans. Physiol Behav 1978; 20:175–185.
4. Doty RL, Applebaum SL, Zusho H, Settle RG. A cross-cultural study of sex differences in odor identification ability. Neuropsychologia 1985; 23:667–672.
5. Murphy C. Age-related effects on the threshold, psychophysical function and pleasantness of menthol. J Gerontol 1983; 38:217–222.
6. Rovee CK, Cohen RY, Shlapack W. Life-span stability in olfactory sensitivity. Dev Psychol 1975; 11:311–318.

7. Stevens JC, Plantinga A, Cain WS. Reduction of odor and nasal pungency associated with aging. Neurobiol Aging 1982; 3:125–132.
8. Stevens JC, Cain WS. Age-related deficiency in the perceived strength of six odorants. Chem Senses 1985; 10:517–529.
9. Stevens JC, Cain WS. Smelling via the mouth: effect of aging. Percept Psychophys 1986; 40:142–146.
10. Burdach K, Doty RL. The effects of tongue movements, swallowing and spitting on retronasal odor perception. Physiol Behav 1987; 41:353–356.
11. Schiffman S, Pasternak M. Decreased discrimination of food odors in the elderly. J Gerontol 1979; 34:73–79.
12. Harper R, Bate-Smith EC, Land DG. Odour description and odour classification. New York: American Elsevier, 1968.
13. Doty RL. Odor-guided behavior in mammals. Experientia 1986; 42:257–271.
14. Doty RL. An examination of relationships between the pleasantness, intensity and concentration of 10 odorous stimuli. Percept Psychophys 1975; 17:492–496.
15. Engen T. The perception of odors. New York: Academic Press, 1982.
16. Warner MD, Peabody CA, Berger PA. Olfactory deficits and Down's syndrome. Biol Psychiat 1988; 23:836–839.
17. Moberg PJ, Pearlson GD, Speedie LJ, Lipsey JR, Strauss ME, Folstein SE. Olfactory recognition: differential impairments in early and late Huntington's and Alzheimer's diseases. J Clin Exp Neuropsychol 1987; 9:650–664.
18. Harrison PJ. Pathogenesis of Alzheimer's disease—beyond the cholinergic hypothesis. J R Soc Med 1986; 79:347–352.
19. Pearson RCA, Esiri MM, Hiorns RW, Wilcock GK, Powell TPS. Anatomical correlates of the distribution of the pathological changes in the neocortex in Alzhemier disease. Proc Natl Acad Sci USA 1985; 82:4531–4534.
20. Shipley MT. Transport of molecules from nose to brain: transneuronal anterograde and retrograde labeling in the rat olfactory system by wheat germ agglutin-horseradish peroxidase applied to the nasal epithelium. Brain Res Bull 1985; 15:129–142.
21. Goto N, Hirano N, Aiuchi M, Hayashi T, Fujiwara K. Nasoencephalopathy of mice infected intranasally with a mouse hepatitis virus, JHM strain. Japanese Journal of Experimental Medicine 1977; 47:59–70.
22. Doty RL, Reyes P, Gregor T. Presence of both odor identification and detection deficits in Alzheimer's disease. Brain Res Bull 1987; 18:597–600.
23. Anasari KA, Johnson A. Olfactory function in patients with Parkinson's disease, J Chronic Dis 1975; 28:493–497.
24. Doty RL, Deems D, Stellar S. Olfactory dysfunction in Parkinson's disease: a general deficit unrelated to neurologic signs, disease stage, or disease duration. Neurology 1988; 38:1237–1244.
25. Ward CD, Hess WA, Calne DB. Olfactory impairment in Parkinson's disease. Neurology 1983; 33:943–946.
26. Doty RL, Riklan M, Deems DA, Reynolds C, Stellar S. The olfactory and cognitive deficits of Parkinson's disease are independent. 1988 submitted.
27. Arvidson K. Location and variation in number of taste buds in human fungiform papillae. J Dent Res 1979; 87:435–442.
28. Miller IJ Jr. Human taste bud density across adult age groups. J Gerontol 1988; 43:B26–B30.
29. Grzegorczyk PB, Jones SW, Mistretta CM. Age-related differences in salt taste acuity. J Gerontol 1979; 34:834–840.
30. Weiffenbach JM. Taste and smell perception in aging. Gerodontology 1984; 3:137–146.
31. Falconer DS. Sensory thresholds for solutions of phenyl-thiocarbamide. Ann Eugen Camb 1947; 13:211–222.
32. Glanville EV, Kaplan AR, Fischer R. Age, sex, and taste sensitivity. J Gerontol 1964; 19:474–478.
33. Kaplan AR, Glanville EV, Fischer R. Cumulative effect of age and smoking on taste sensitivity in males and females. J Gerontol 1965; 20:334–337.
34. Dye CJ, Koziatek DA. Age and diabetic effects on threshold and hedonic perception of sucrose solutions. J Gerontol 1981; 36:310–315.
35. Moore LM, Nielson CR, Mistretta CM. Sucrose taste thresholds: age-related differences. J Gerontol 1982; 37:64–69.
36. Bartoshuk LM, Rifkin B, Marks LE, Bars P. Taste and aging. J Gerontol 1986; 41:51–57.
37. Hyde RJ, Feller RP, Sharon IM. Age effects on taste and smell. J Dent Res 1981; 60:1730–1734.
38. Langan MJ, Yearick ES. The effect of improved oral hygiene on taste perception and nutrition of the elderly. J Gerontol 1976; 31:413–418.
39. Krut LH, Perrin MJ, Bronte-Stewart B. Taste perception in smokers and non-smokers. Br Med J 1961; 1:384–387.
40. Schiffman SS, Lindley MG, Clark TB, Makino C. Molecular mechanism of sweet taste: relationship of hydrogen bonding to taste sensitivity for both young and elderly. Neurobiol Aging 1981; 2:173–185.
41. Schiffman SS, Clark TB. Magnitude estimates of amino acids for young and elderly subjects. Neurobiol Aging 1980; 1:81–91.
42. Weiffenbach JM, Cowart BJ, Baum BJ. Taste intensity perception in aging. J Gerontol 1986; 41:460–468.
43. Enns MP, van Itallie TB, Grinker JA. Contributions of age, sex, and degree of fatness on preference and magnitude estimations for sucrose in humans. Physiol Behav 1979; 22:999–1003.
44. Cohen T, Gitman L. Oral complaints and taste perception in the aged. J Gerontol 1959; 14:294–298.
45. Deems DA, Doty RL, Moore-Gillon V, Settle RG, Shaman P, Snow JB Jr. Smell and taste disorders: analysis of patient data from the University of Pennsylvania Smell and Taste Center (1981–1986). 1988, submitted.
46. Weiffenbach JM, Fox PC, Baum BJ. Taste and salivary function. Proc Natl Acad Sci 1986; 83:6103–6106.

IMMUNOLOGY

AGE-RELATED IMMUNE DEFICIENCY

RICHARD A. MILLER, M.D., Ph.D.

INTRODUCTION

With increasing age, the immune system becomes progressively worse at protecting us from infectious and neoplastic illness. In the last 5 years, our understanding of the cellular and molecular bases of the immune reaction has greatly improved, and these fresh perspectives have begun to trickle down to influence the immunogerontologic literature as well. My goal here is to describe the current consensus, and to suggest research areas from which new insights seem likely to emerge.

Invading microbes, and probably many kinds of nascent tumors, elicit a series of reactive changes aimed at confining and destroying the foreign materials. T and B lymphocytes, each armed with surface receptors specific for foreign chemical determinants, are triggered by contact with these immunogens to proliferate, thus increasing the numbers of specific cells able to participate in the defensive reaction. The clones of responding cells eventually differentiate into effector cells: B cells into antibody-secreting plasma cells, and T lymphocytes into lymphokine-secreting or cytotoxic effectors. The lymphokines produced by T cells include some that promote B cell growth and maturation, others that recruit and activate less specific effectors including mononuclear and polynuclear phagocytes, and still others that support the activation of the T cells themselves in an "autocrine" fashion. Although B lymphocytes are able to bind intact antigens, free in solution, the T cells only recognize fragments of antigens that have been processed (via proteolysis) and presented, together with human leukocyte antigen (HLA) histocompatibility molecules, on the surface of other cells. This "antigen-presenting" role can be played by macrophages, several kinds of reticular dendritic cells, and even by B lymphocytes.

Immune function in humans can be tested either in vitro, by examining the responsiveness of cells in culture, or in vivo, by injection of a test antigen that can elicit antibody production, delayed hypersensitivity, or some other quantifiable evidence of immune response. Animal models permit, in addition, tests for the ability of the host to deal with inoculations of pathogens and tumor cells. Most of these tests show a decline in the average strength of the immune reaction with an increase in age of the subject. There is usually great variation in the responsiveness shown by members of random population samplings, particularly among elderly subjects, and for most tests some old subjects score as well as the average young individual. The prevalence, within the aged cohort, of diseases that themselves lead to reduced immunity greatly complicates the interpretation of findings. Many measures of immune function, however, decline gradually throughout adult life, even in age groups where illness is rare, and show declines even among groups of elderly volunteers selected for apparent good health. Despite a few hints[1] that depressed immune function, even in apparently healthy old people, is a powerful predictor of imminent decline, there is a lamentable paucity of studies attempting to define the relationships—causal or even correlative—between immune status and clinical risk.

AGE-ASSOCIATED IMMUNE DYSFUNCTION: AREAS OF CURRENT CONSENSUS

What, then, goes wrong? Why don't lymphocytes work well in old people? Studies of humans and of animal models have produced a small area of general agreement and a number of provocative new results, the implications of which researchers are now actively exploring. Let me first discuss five areas of consensus.

1. Small changes do occur in the numbers of different kinds of T and B cells and in immunoglobulin concentrations, but these do not seem large enough to account for the observed functional declines. The development of antibodies able to discriminate T from B lymphocytes and to delineate separate cell subsets within these two major populations has made it possible to ask whether aging leads to alterations in the proportions of different cell types. "Helper" T cells that tend to initiate and support both cellular and humoral immune reactions tend to express the CD4 (CD = cluster-of-differentiation) marker molecule on their surface, whereas a complementary subset that expresses CD8

determinants seems specialized for cytotoxic and suppressive functions. CD4-positive cells make up about two-thirds of the T cells in human blood. Most, though not all, studies of CD4 and CD8 expression in aging humans and rodents have demonstrated a small (5 percent to 15 percent) shift toward an increasing proportion of the CD8 cell type with increasing age. Functional studies, however, usually show a much more substantial decline, with age, in measures of both helper and cytotoxic T cell activity, and it does not seem likely that the small changes in relative cell number can account for the accompanying functional losses.

2. Deficits in T cell function seem more dramatic than changes in the function of either B lymphocytes or antigen-presenting cells (APC). Many experiments have been done in which mixtures of T, B, and antigen-presenting cells taken from donors of various age groups have been tested in vitro, usually for ability to proliferate in response to polyclonal activators (e.g., mitogenic plant lectins like phytohemagglutinin or lipopolysaccharide), or for ability to produce antibody. In general, the strength of the ensuing responses seems to depend largely on the age of the T cell donor, rather little on the age of the B cell donor, and little or not at all on the age of the APC donor. Careful study often can demonstrate declines in B cell function with age, but these are typically much less striking than tests for T cell dysfunction.

This disparity may reflect the different developmental biology of these cell types. B cells, and most APCs, arise constantly from bone marrow precursors throughout adult life, and are for the most part fairly short-lived. Although some T lymphocytes are also short-lived, others may (in humans) survive as "memory cells" years or decades after their initial stimulation. It is possible, though unproven, that these long-lived memory cells might gradually undergo structural changes that lead to disordered function.

3. The thymus gland involutes with age—but does this matter? In humans and rodents, the thymus gland, beginning around the time of puberty, gradually shrinks and, at the same time, becomes progressively infiltrated with connective and adipose tissue at the expense of functional parenchyma. Indices of function, including measures of the numbers of T cells exported per day and of the production of so-called thymic "hormones" (see subsequently), also diminish in parallel with the morphologic involution. The transplantation studies of Hirokawa[2] have also suggested that the ability of thymic tissue to support production of mature T cells from bone marrow-derived pro-thymocytes declines rapidly, in mice, in the months surrounding sexual maturation. It has therefore seemed reasonable to ascribe some portion of the blame for age-related declines in T cell responsiveness to a loss of thymic function.

There may well be some truth to this idea, but in my opinion a stronger and more detailed case still needs to be made. Although neonatal thymectomy of mice leads to profound impairments in the immune response, the effect of this intervention declines dramatically within the first few days of life,[3] and functional deficits in mice that undergo thymectomy as adults, though demonstrable, are more subtle. Attempts have also been made to show immune restoration by injection of candidate hormones derived from thymic tissue. Occasional successes have been reported, but the greater number of unimpressive results[4] and the recent finding that at least some of these substances are also produced by nonthymic tissues have left many immunologists still unconvinced that the nominated thymic hormones play important physiologic roles in T cell development. Much more needs to be learned about age-associated alterations in thymus function and their contribution to loss in immune responsiveness.

4. Experimental transplantation protocols have been used to test the ability of mature lymphocytes from old mice to work in young recipients. In general, these studies have shown that the defective responses of T and B cells from old mice are intrinsic, in the sense that the responses are not repaired simply by placing the lymphocytes within a young recipient.[5] The immune responses of old mice can, however, be largely restored by grafting both syngeneic bone marrow and newborn thymus tissue,[6] thus suggesting that lymphocytes, once generated by marrow stem cells within a thymic microenvironment, are not then critically dependent on any age-sensitive host function. Prethymic stem cells, however, require a period of intrathymic maturation, and do not develop into mature T cells when inoculated into old hosts unless the old hosts also receive a transplanted thymic gland from an extremely young donor.

5. In addition to quantitative declines in immune function (e.g., diminished proliferation, lower antibody production), older individuals often show defects in the quality of the immune response that may be of equal clinical significance. These include a decline in the amount of IgG antibody produced, a lower production of high affinity antibodies, an abnormal secretion of antibody with autoimmune specificity, and alterations in the specific variable region genes used by both T and B cells activated by the foreign antigens. Some of these effects of age

could be expected to have dangerous consequences. Only high affinity antibodies, to take one example, are able to detect antigens present at low concentrations (e.g., at the very start and at the end of an infection). The relatively low production of high affinity antibodies by old people could leave them particularly vulnerable to infectious illness. One experimental study of antitumor immunity[7] has suggested that alterations in the specific clones of T cells that participate in the antitumor response may lead to a critical decline in resistance to tumor growth.

CURRENT RESEARCH INITIATIVES

With this survey as background, let us next consider a few of the areas in which ongoing research work has been most productive and from which additional progress seems likely to emerge. I will talk about four main problems: the role of interleukin-2, mosaic models for T cell senescence, defects in gene expression, and abnormalities in T lymphocyte activation.

Interleukin-2

Interleukin-2 (IL-2), a 15,000 dalton glycoprotein made by helper T cells, is required for the growth of most T lymphocytes and also plays a role in the growth and maturation of activated B lymphocytes and natural killer cells. Within the first 12 to 24 hours after activation, T cells begin both to secrete IL-2 and to express on their surface high affinity receptors for IL-2; the binding of IL-2 to the IL-2 receptor delivers a key signal that prepares the cells to begin deoxyribonucleic acid (DNA) synthesis and to progress towards mitosis. Many laboratories[8] have now shown that T cells from old humans and rodents produce less IL-2 than do cells from young controls. Indeed, addition of purified IL-2 to in vitro culture media can cure (at least partially) many of the deficient responses of old lymphocytes, and injection of IL-2 along with antigen can, in some cases, substantially improve in vivo immune responses of old mice.

Although these results certainly suggest that deficient production of IL-2 is an important aspect of immunosenescence, one must be cautious not to oversimplify, to assume that IL-2 generation is the key to the problem. For one thing, many workers also find a decline, with age, in expression of the IL-2 receptor by T cells exposed to activating agents. Assays that estimate the number of cells able to respond to IL-2 consistently show age-related deficits.[9] Even demonstrations that high doses of IL-2 can restore youthful levels of T cell proliferation may reflect a pharmacologic effect of saturating levels of growth factor working on abnormally small numbers of reactive cells. Helper T cells also make many other active lymphokines, including myeloid colony stimulating factors, interferon, lymphotoxin, at least three different B cell-stimulating factors, and many others; it seems almost certain that defective production of these factors by aged T cells has physiologic consequences still to be defined. Furthermore, too little is yet known about age-associated deficits in responses to lymphokines by various cell types within and outside the immune system. At least some T cell reactions, moreover, seem not to be mediated by stable soluble factors, but instead require direct cell contact between the T cell and its target; the study of senescent change in these so-called "cognate" interactions is in its infancy.

Mosaic Model

Many lines of evidence support a picture of the aging immune system as a mosaic of functional and nonfunctional cells, with the latter becoming more frequent at older ages. Studies using cell sorter methods, for example, have shown a decline with age in the number of T cells that can, when exposed to mitogen, leave their usual resting state and begin to progress towards DNA synthesis.[10] Limiting-dilution culture methods, that can estimate the proportion of cells that can participate in a particular immune reaction, show in agreement that age leads to a decrease[9] in the fraction of T cells that can make IL-2, generate killer effector cells, or proliferate in response to IL-2. The old T cells that do respond, however, seem to produce just as strong a response, per cell, as do T cells from young mice. Diminished responder frequencies have also been demonstrated, at least for some antigens, for B lymphocytes.[11]

Thus, one can view the immune system of an old subject as containing an increasing number of cells that look like normal lymphocytes, but that do not function appropriately. This formulation suggests a number of key problems. Can one find a surface marker or some other chemical property that distinguishes the "good" from the "bad" cells? Where do the bad cells come from? That is, are they newly formed by a defective developmental scheme, or are they cells produced long ago that have only recently become dysfunctional? And what is the molecular basis, or potential bases, for the activation defect? Do all of the nonfunctional cells become stuck at the same step of the activation process, or are there

Gene Expression

Methods for the study of specific gene expression have only recently been applied to the question of immune dysfunction in aging, and a great deal of additional work is needed in this area. It seems likely now, from work either published or in press, that aging leads to a decline in the production, by mitogen-treated T cells, of messenger ribonucleic acid (mRNA) that is specific for IL-2, IL-3 (another lymphokine), at least one chain of the two-chain IL-2 receptor, and the c-myc protooncogene thought to play a key role in the preparation of resting cells for entry into the cell cycle. It is not as clear whether defective mRNA production reflects disorders in gene transcription (i.e., synthesis of the earliest mRNA precursors from the DNA code), as suggested by some laboratories, or alterations in intranuclear processing of the primary transcripts, as our own work on c-myc suggests. Nor can it safely be assumed that translation of the mRNA that is produced will proceed with equal efficiency in old and young cells.

Future exploration of this area will be highly rewarding. Many basic questions need to be answered. Are defects in gene expression limited to some genes, or only to a subset? Are the characteristic defects those of disordered transcription, of intranuclear processing, or of mRNA stability and translation? Lymphocytes can be activated by a variety of physiologic and pharmacologic agents, and it remains to be determined whether equivalent defects of gene expression are associated with these various pathways. Studies of the myc, fos, and IL-2 genes, among others, are now revealing how gene expression is controlled by chromatin configuration, inducible DNA-binding proteins, and specific promoter and enhancer sequences within and around the coding sequences themselves. Application of these insights to the problems of aging should prove extremely fruitful.

A second, related issue concerns age-related changes in immunoglobulin and T cell receptor gene selection. Each T and B cell, early in its life, chooses and expresses two receptor genes from a much larger library. The result of these choices by individual cells determines the repertoire of receptors, and hence the antigenic recognition pattern, of the organism at any point in its life. Although solid proof is still lacking, there are tantalizing hints that the pattern of gene utilization may vary systematically as the animal ages. Such a shift could contribute to age-related declines in both response strength and qualitative effectiveness. The explanation for such a shift would require much hard work by developmental and molecular biologists.

Activation Defects

T cells respond to mitogens by a sequence of molecular events whose interelations are still being worked out. Table 17–1 presents a selected list of some of the key transitions. Later events are thought to depend, through links that are still unclear, on earlier ones. A similar cascade mediates B lymphocyte activation as well. Our laboratory, like many others, is attempting to learn whether T cells from aging animals and humans exhibit deficits at one or more of these stages. We have good evidence, at least for mice, that aging leads to a decline in the ability to increase intracellular calcium concentration after stimulation with the plant lectin Concanavalin A (Con A)[12] or with antibodies to the T cell receptor (a stimulus thought to mimic antigen exposure.) There are published reports[13] that two other extremely early steps, translocation of protein kinase C (PK-C) and production of inositol phosphates from phospholipid precursors, are also diminished in T cells from old mice. Our own data (Lerner and Miller, in preparation), however, suggest that there is little, if any, change in inositol phosphate production in old mice, and a consensus has yet to emerge about these and other elements of the earliest activation processes. Further, almost nothing is yet known about the links between these early steps and the activation of new genes, or about age-related changes in later events, e.g., the

TABLE 17–1 Early Events in T Lymphocyte Activation

0 to 5 minutes	Increased Ca^{2+} concentration
0 to 5 minutes	Increased production and hydrolysis of inositol phospholipids
0 to 5 minutes	Increased protein kinase C function
15 minutes	Transcription of c-fos gene
30 minutes	Transcription of c-myc gene
4 hours	Expression of IL-2, IL-2 receptor, IL-3, and so on
18 hours	DNA synthesis
24 hours	First mitosis

IL-2-induced progression towards DNA synthesis.

Some insight can be gained from attempts to stimulate cell division by agonists that act, not on extracellular receptors, but at intracellular sites. Phorbol esters (e.g., phorbol myristic acetate [PMA]), which stimulate PK-C, and the calcium ionophore ionomycin can in concert induce T and B cell proliferation by bypassing the ligand-mediated signalling steps that usually lead to increases in cellular calcium and PK-C function. We have shown[14] that optimal doses of ionomycin can, with PMA, induce a proliferation from old T cells that is nearly equivalent to that seen in young T cells and that is much higher than that induced in old T cells by the strongest extracellular mitogens. Although the perturbations induced by PMA and ionomycin are admittedly far stronger and more enduring than those generated by physiologic stimuli, the results suggest that T cells from old mice may be relatively successful at recognizing and responding to intracellular signals once these are produced, and that defects in proliferation may result largely from inability to generate the appropriate intracellular signals in response to extracellular stimuli.

What goes wrong in the signalling process? One obvious hypothesis is that the signal transduction apparatus is itself defective in T cells from old mice. T cell receptors are linked, possibly via a guanosine nucleotide binding (G) protein, to intracellular enzymes and may also be directly coupled to calcium channels. Each of these postulated links needs careful dissection to see if it functions appropriately in T cells from old mice. Our most recent data, however, have suggested that one need not postulate any problems in the signal transduction pathway to explain the observed alteration in calcium ion concentrations. We have used ionomycin, at very small doses, to challenge the ability of T cells from old and young mice to regulate their internal calcium concentrations when confronted with an abrupt increase in calcium entry from the cell's exterior. We find (Miller et al, submitted) that equal doses of ionomycin lead to greater changes in free calcium concentration in young T cells than in T cells from old mice. Since ionomycin carries calcium across cell membranes without involvement of specific ligands or receptor-linked signals, it seems likely that the age-related difference in response to calcium influx is caused by some alteration in the cell's intrinsic calcium buffering mechanism. Intracellular calcium ion concentrations are known to be fine-tuned by several cellular systems, including a plasma-membrane extrusion pump and intracellular sequestering pumps in the mitochondria endoplasmic reticulum. We postulate that the diminished calcium concentrations seen in old T cells that are challenged by limiting doses of ionomycin may reflect changes in these pumps or in their regulation that result in abnormally high sensitivity to small changes in free calcium ion concentration.

Other Considerations

This necessarily brief review has had to omit detailed consideration of several important threads of research into age-related immune decline that are now receiving experimental attention, and areas that should be receiving such attention but are not. T and B lymphocytes regulate one another by a network of complementary specificities whose contribution to the overall regulation of immune response strength is a matter of intense controversy. Some work has suggested that aging leads to a shift in the repertoire of controlling, receptor-specific cells and antibodies. Studies of age-related changes in suppressive T and non-T cells are also underway in many laboratories, although the difficulty of designing reproducible assay systems and the lack of cloned suppressor cells and suppressive factors has impeded progress here. We have not considered the evidence that aging leads to an increase in autoimmune antibody production (though not of classic autoimmune diseases!), nor the idea that autoreactions may contribute to the development of degenerative diseases, including atherosclerosis and adult-onset diabetes. It seems perfectly reasonable that age-related changes in neural and endocrine function may have immunologic sequelae, and indeed a recent study[15] of immune rejuvenation in rats bearing a hormone-secreting tumor is likely to stimulate much more attention to this key area. The suggestion that the loss of immune function leaves elderly patients more vulnerable to infection and to neoplasia, while compelling general assent, remains unfortunately more an article of faith than a conclusion derived from a cadre of detailed mechanistic studies.

A CONCLUDING ADVERTISEMENT

The immune system presents certain major advantages to a scientist who wants to study the biology, basic or applied, of aging. Immune systems can be taken out of the body, modified, and reassembled either in culture or in vivo, and will then function more or less normally in response to physiologically pertinent challenges. Immune function declines with age, is of undoubted clinical relevance, and depends on cells, factors, and genes that are, to an increasing extent, available in clonal forms. Since immunology is a "hot" field, it is both intellectually exciting and reasonably well-funded. The gerontologist who masquerades as an immunologist will benefit by finding him- or herself surrounded by hundreds of real immunologists all turning out new reagents and ideas that they are perfectly willing to let him or her try out on old people or old mice.

Supported in part by grants AG-03978 and AG-07114 from the National Institutes of Health, by a Scholar Award from the Leukemia Society of America, and by a Research Career Development Award from the National Institute on Aging.

References

1. Roberts-Thomson IC, Whittingham S, Youngchaiyud U, Mackay IR. Aging, immune response, and mortality. Lancet 1974; 2:368-370.
2. Hirokawa K, Makinodan T. Thymic involution: effect on T cell differentiation. J Immunol 1975; 114:1659-1664.
3. Miller JFAP, Marshall AHE, White RG. The immunological significance of the thymus. Adv Immunol 1962; 2:111-162.
4. Hiramoto RN, Ghanta VK, Soong SJ. Effect of thymic hormones on immunity and life span. In: Goidl E, ed. Aging and the immune response. New York: Marcel Dekker, 1987:177.
5. Callard RE, Basten A. Immune function in aged mice. IV. Loss of T cell and B cell function in thymus-dependent antibody responses. Eur J Immunol 1978; 8:552-558.
6. Hirokawa K, Albright JW, Makinodan T. Restoration of impaired immune functions in aging animals. I. Effect of syngeneic thymus and bone marrow grafts. Clin Immunol Immunopathol 1976; 5:371-376.
7. Flood PM, Urban JL, Kripke ML, Schreiber H. Loss of tumor-specific and idiotype-specific immunity with age. J Exp Med 1981; 154:275-290.
8. Gillis S, Kozak R, Durante M, Weksler ME. Immunological studies of aging. Decreased production of and response to T cell growth factor by lymphocytes from aged humans. J Clin Invest 1981; 67:937-942.
9. Miller RA. Age-associated decline in precursor frequency for different T cell-mediated reactions, with preservation of helper or cytotoxic effect per precursor cell. J Immunol 1984; 132:63-68.
10. Staiano-Coico L, Darzynkiewicz Z, Melamed MR, Weksler ME. Immunological studies of aging. IX. Impaired proliferation of T lymphocytes detected in elderly humans by flow cytometry. J Immunol 1984; 132:1788-1792.
11. Zharhary D, Klinman NR. Antigen responsiveness of the mature and generative B cell populations of aged mice. J Exp Med 1983; 157:1300-1308.
12. Miller RA, Jacobson B, Weil G, Simons ER. Diminished calcium influx in lectin-stimulated T cells from old mice. J Cell Physiol 1987; 132:337-342.
13. Proust JJ, Filburn CR, Harrison SA, Buchholz MA, Nordin AA. Age-related defect in signal transduction during lectin activation of murine T lymphocytes. J Immunol 1987; 139:1472-1478.
14. Miller RA. Immunodeficiency of aging: restorative effects of phorbol ester combined with calcium ionophore. J Immunol 1986; 137:805-808.
15. Kelley KW, Brief S, Westly HJ, Novakofski J, Bechtel PJ, Simon J, Walker EB. GH3 pituitary adenoma cells can reverse thymic aging in rats. Proc Natl Acad Sci USA 1986; 83:5663-5667.

Chapter Eighteen

HISTOCOMPATIBILITY ANTIGENS, SENSORINEURAL HEARING DISORDERS, AND SENESCENCE

JOEL M. BERNSTEIN, M.D., Ph.D.
THOMAS C. SHANAHAN, Ph.D.
DANIEL AMSTERDAM, Ph.D.

INTRODUCTION

A basic question in medicine is why some people develop certain diseases and others do not. Since the discovery of the human leukocyte antigen (HLA) system in the 1960s, a great deal of attention has been focused on the HLA system and its role in transplantation immunity.[1] However, the association of HLA alleles with particular diseases is one of the most intriguing aspects of the major histocompatibility complex (MHC), which is located on the short arm of chromosome 6 in the human.[2] The most remarkable associations have been with autoaggressive and inflammatory diseases, such as lupus erythematosus (SLE), and with diseases in which a receptor abnormality is implicated, such as myasthenia gravis and Graves' disease.[3] The purpose of this presentation is to briefly outline three areas for discussion. One is a description of the major histocompatibility complex in man as it relates to immune function, immune recognition, and its possible relationship to senescence. Secondly, new studies will be presented from our tissue typing laboratory that suggest a relationship between certain HLA antigens and disorders of the temporal bone, including Meniere's disease, otosclerosis, metabolic presbycusis, and sensorineural hearing loss in general. Finally, because this is a symposium on the aging process, the potential relationship of the HLA antigens associated with sensorineural hearing loss to those of the aging process will be considered.

THE MAJOR HISTOCOMPATIBILITY COMPLEX

Although the MHC was originally identified by its role in transplant rejection, it is now recognized that proteins coded for by this region are involved in many aspects of immunologic recognition, including interaction between lymphoid cells as well as between lymphocytes and antigen presenting cells.[4]

A genetic map of the region of chromosome 6 in the human that shows the HLA gene complex appears in Figure 18–1. Regions B, C, and A encode Class I molecules. Class I molecules are found on all nucleated cells of the body. Region D and region DR encode for alpha- and beta-chains of the Class II proteins that are found on more restricted cells: macrophages, other antigen-presenting cells such as Langerhans cells of the skin, B cells, and activated T cells. In between the B and D loci is a third group of genes that code for proteins of both the classic and alternative complement pathway, including C4A, C4B, C2, and Factor B. The Class I and Class II proteins are schematically represented in Figure 18–2. Class I protein consists of two polypeptides; the large peptide is encoded by the MHC and noncovalently associated with the polypeptide beta-2-microglobulin, which is encoded outside the MHC on chromosome 15.[5] Class II proteins consist of two noncovalently associated peptides referred to as alpha- and beta-chains, both of which are en-

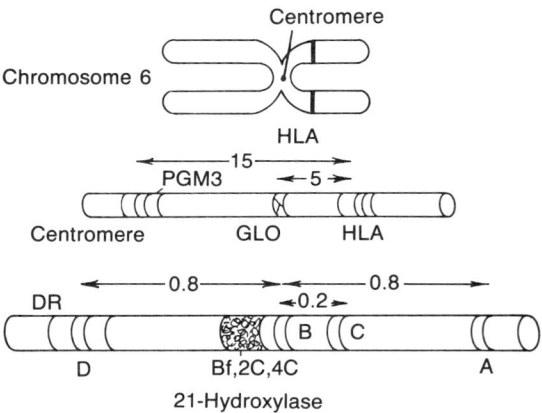

Figure 18–1 A schematic drawing of the short arm of chromosome 6 that demonstrates the relative locations of the genes that code for the Class I antigens (A, B, C), the genes that code for the Class II antigens (D, DR), and the genes that code in between B and D for the complement proteins, C2, C4A, C4B, and Factor B (Class III antigens).

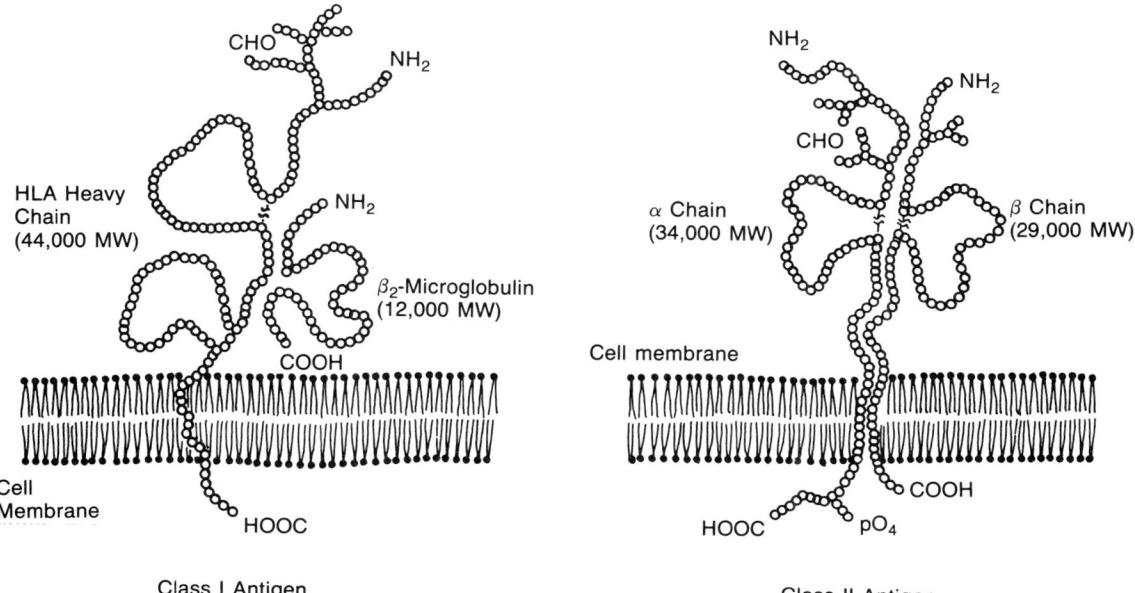

Figure 18-2 A schematic representation of the Class I antigen. On the left there is an alpha-chain that consists of a glycoprotein with three portions; one portion lies outside the membrane, a second portion lies within the lipid layer of the membrane, and the third portion, which is the carboxylic terminal, is inside the cell membrane. This alpha-, or heavy chain, which is approximately 44,000 daltons in size, is noncovalently linked with a beta-2-microglobulin, which is only present on the outer surface of the cell membrane and which has a molecular weight of 12,000. On the right of the diagram is a schematic representation of the Class II antigen, which corresponds to the gene product of the DR locus and consists of both an alpha- and a beta-chain. These chains have a variable region at the amino terminal end and have a constant region in the cell membrane. Class II antigens are found on macrophages, other antigen-presenting cells, B cells, and activated T cells, whereas Class I antigens are present on the plasma membrane of all nucleated cells of the body.

coded by the MHC. If the antigens of a particular MHC region from different patients are examined, they are found to have similar basic structures, but the fine structure of each antigen differs in each individual. These fine differences may be assessed by employing antisera against the antigens. The structure of the alpha- and beta-chains of the A, B, C, and DR antigens are similar to immunoglobulins in that they consist of two polypeptide chains with constant and variable regions. These variable regions, which consist of differences in amino acid sequences, therefore, make up a tremendous variety of possible gene products. It has been estimated that there are as many as 2,000 genes that may exist between the A and B loci in chromosome 6.[6] Furthermore, examination of the HLA antigens in many diverse populations has emphasized the extraordinary polymorphism of the A, B, C, and DR loci. More than 300,000,000 genetically different individuals could be expected on the basis of the existing HLA alleles. Of these, 30,000,000 individuals would be antigenically distinguishable. Thus, HLA typing is one of the most powerful tools for the study of population genetics. This is attributable to the highly polymorphic nature of HLA, as well as to the linkage disequilibrium characteristics of HLA.

At the present time the HLA-A locus contains 23 alleles, the B locus 47, the C locus 8, the DR locus 14, the DQ locus 3, and the DP locus 6. This polymorphism also extends to the genes that code for the four different complement proteins where different alleles have been identified for C2, Factor B, C4A, and C4B. In addition to the histocompatibility antigens just mentioned, there are other genes within the HLA complex, including genes for determining disease susceptibility, structural genes for red cell enzymes and antigens, regulatory genes, and genes for various types of receptor or binding proteins.[7]

More recently, it has been suggested that the MHC might play a significant role in aging. Table 18-1 suggests that there are several genes closely related to the MHC that may be related to the process of senescence. The structural gene for superoxide dismutase-2 is located on the same chromosome in man as is the MHC.[8] Superoxide dismutase con-

TABLE 18-1 Relationship of Major Histocompatibility Locus (MHC) to Aging

Controls all aspects of thymus-dependent immunity
    Antibody production (T helper cells)
    Down regulation of immune response (T suppressor cells)
    Delayed hypersensitivity
    Cell-mediated immunity (cytotoxic cells)
Superoxide dismutase (structural gene)
cAMP levels (involved in many cell functions, especially in lymphocytes)
DNA repair capacity

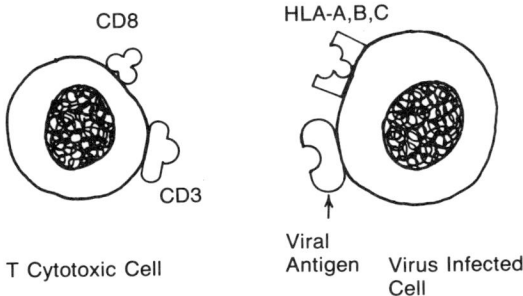

Figure 18-3 A schematic and hypothetical representation of cytotoxic killing of a virally-infected somatic cell. The cytotoxic T cell recognizes the viral antigen only in the context with the transplantation antigens HLA A, B, and C. CD3 (cluster-of-differentiation-3) is a T cell antigen present on both T suppressor and T helper cells. It is responsible for recognizing specific viral antigens. CD8, which is an antigenic determinant on the surface of the T cytotoxic cell, is recognized by Type I antigen HLA A, B, and C. In this way, the cytotoxic T cell recognizes viral antigen.

verts the highly toxic radical superoxide, formed in the course of normal metabolism, to hydrogen peroxide and oxygen. Evidence has been cited in the literature for a so-called free-radical theory of aging.[9] Levels of mixed functions of oxidase have been correlated inversely with species life span. The level of cyclic adenosine monophosphate (AMP) is intimately involved in many cell functions, and in particular, lymphocytes may show age-related alterations and may be MHC regulated.[10] Evidence exists of a preliminary nature that the MHC may influence deoxyribonucleic acid (DNA) repair capacity and may thus have a profound effect on the ability of DNA in the aging process.[11] While this review will largely concern the relationship between MHC and sensorineural hearing loss, the overall evidence cannot fail to suggest that the MHC and MHC-linked genes may constitute a multigene family that exerts a multifactorial influence on the aging process, a family that includes and goes beyond immune function to comprise a major life support homeostatic system.

There are two aspects of the major histocompatibility complex that will be briefly mentioned. First is the presentation of antigens to T helper cells and T cytotoxic cells, and second is the existence of immune response genes that may play a critical role in the qualitative and quantitative response of an individual to an antigen both extrinsic to the body and to autoantigens.

FUNCTION OF THE MAJOR HISTOCOMPATIBILITY COMPLEX

The HLA antigens on the surface of T lymphocytes are essential for reactions of immune recognition. HLA antigens are recognized by T cell subpopulations and are summarized in Figure 18-3. Cytotoxic T cells involved in recognition and rejection of virally-infected cells recognize HLA A, B, and probably C on the infected cells, and, in cooperation with T helper cells, cause destruction of these infected cells. Most virally-infected cells display viral antigens on the surface of their plasma membrane with the HLA, A, B, and C antigens present on the surface of this infected cell. In this way, cytotoxic T cells are primed to kill cells infected with that virus. However, they will not kill cells of a different HLA haplotype infected by the same virus. This phenomenon is referred to as haplotype-restricted killing.[12] Thus, cytotoxic T cells recognize both the viral antigen and the MHC antigen independently, or a combination of the viral antigen and the MHC antigen associated with the cell surface may produce an altered conformation of the MHC molecule. This condition may be recognized as altered self and is an example of physiologic autoimmunity.

Similar principles of haplotype restriction apply to T helper cells, which recognize antigens on macrophages, and to B cells in association with HLA-D or HLA-DR antigens. This is described in Figure 18-4. Activation of T cells by antigen cannot occur by interaction between the antigen and the T cell alone. Instead, the antigen is somehow processed by an antigen-presenting cell and then appropriately presented to the T cell in conjunction with the DR molecule on the surface of the antigen-presenting cell. Thus, the T cell must appropriately view the antigen in conjunction with the DR molecule expressed on the surface of the antigen-presenting cell. Therefore, it has been hypothesized that the mechanism by which DR molecules control immune reac-

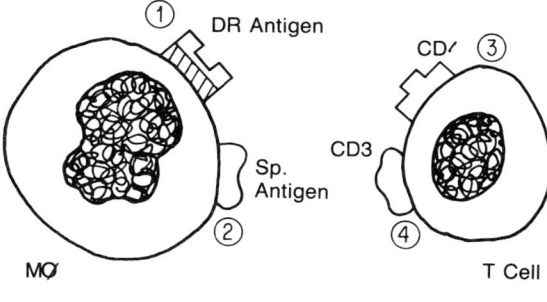

Figure 18-4 This schematic and hypothetical diagram represents haplotype restriction related to antigen recognition by a T helper cell. A T helper cell recognizes a specific antigen only in conjunction with the Type II antigen coded for by the DR region of chromosome 6. CD3 or cluster-of-differentiation-3 antigen is found on both T helper and T suppressor cells and recognizes specific antigens. CD4, or cluster-of differentiation-4, is a specific helper-inducer antigen that is present on T helper cells and that recognizes the Class II antigen on macrophage. In this way, the T helper cell recognizes specific antigens only in conjunction with a specific Class II antigen on the macrophage.

tivity is dictated by the way in which the T cell appropriately or inappropriately reviews the antigen.

Once it became known that the HLA-D and DR loci appeared to represent the human equivalent of the rodent immune response (Ir) genes and that the product of these genes were DR molecules, several groups of investigators have attempted to show a demonstration or an association between specific HLA antigens and specific clinical disorders in an attempt to implicate a specific immunologic reactivity with the expression of that clinical disorder. However, in order to do that, it was necessary to distinguish the HLA antigen molecules on the surface of the cells of one individual from those on the surface of another individual.

It is possible to distinguish HLA antigens in the population by utilizing serologic reagents.[13] These serologic reagents are derived from the sera of multiparous women, which contains, through repeated sensitization during pregnancy, the antibodies against paternal HLA molecules. Once this serotyping became available, it was relatively easy to go through the population and determine if there was a special association between HLA serotypes and a clinical disorder. For example, it has been shown that, in multiple sclerosis, there is a high incidence of the DR2 molecule in patients.[14] The percentage of occurrence of this antigen in patients with multiple sclerosis is about 50 percent compared to about 30 percent in the control population without the disease. This computes to a relative risk of five. Similarly, patients with autoimmune diseases such as myasthenia gravis, Graves' disease, chronic active hepatitis, systemic lupus erythematosus, celiac disease, and dermatitis herpetiformis seem to have a high incidence of DR3 that may range anywhere from a relative risk of three in myasthenia gravis to 14 in chronic active hepatitis. In rheumatoid arthritis the expression of the DR4 molecule is present in about 60 percent of patients, whereas it is present in 20 percent of the normal population; this computes to a relative risk of five.

Given the fact that the human immune response genes may be associated with certain human diseases, an important question to ask is, "What role do the immune response genes play in the expression of that disease?" It has been hypothesized that a specific immune response contributes to the expression of human disease. However, this has not really been absolutely demonstrated in any clinical disease. Two diseases, however, that come close to this might be the association of HLA B27 with ankylosing spondylitis and the association of HLA A3 with hemochromatosis. However, an association has been noted between certain HLA DR antigens and an increase in immune responsiveness. This is particularly true with the DR3 antigen.[15] It appears that the DR3 antigen is related to a turning on or turning up of the immune response. This is particularly noted with patients who also have the B8/DR3 haplotype. The B8/DR3 haplotype seems to be associated with the presence of increased autoantibodies, increased autoimmune diseases, and increased incidence of circulating immune complexes. Such a turning on of the immune response may, therefore, be detrimental to the individual in that it not only produces disease, but these diseases are related to a decrease in survival. It has been found that DR3 individuals have both increased cell-mediated and humoral antibody immune responses. Furthermore, there is evidence that they have decreased clearance of immune complexes in their circulation.

HLA ANTIGENS AND DISORDERS OF THE TEMPORAL BONE

With these thoughts in mind, a discussion of the possible role of HLA antigens and sensorineural hearing loss will now be considered. We have recently completed a study of 85 patients with different disorders of the temporal bone, including Meniere's disease, otosclerosis, metabolic presbycusis, and other types of sensorineural hearing loss. Lymphocytes were obtained from 52 normal control subjects for DR typing. Of these, 30 were typed for the Cw series antigens. An additional 100 normal subjects were typed for HLA A and B antigens.

The techniques used for the lymphocyte cytotoxic tests for HLA A, B, C, and DR have been thoroughly described.[16] These will be briefly reviewed.

Materials and Methods

Cell suspensions prepared in phosphate buffered saline (PBS) from the buffy coat portion of centrifuged blood were underlaid with 3 ml of Isolymph (Gallard-Schlesinger Corp., Carle Place, NY) density gradient and centrifuged for 15 minutes at 300 times gravity. Lymphocytes harvested from the resulting interface were treated with 0.8 ml Lymphokwik T/B (One Lambda Inc., Los Angeles, CA) cell isolation reagent in 1 ml Fisher tubes for 30 minutes at 37°C. Following a 0.2 ml overlay with Hank's buffered salt solution (HBSS) (M.A. Bioproducts, Walkersville, MD), the tubes were spun for 2 minutes at 2,000 times gravity, using a Fisher centrifuge, and the viable cells located in the pellet were collected.

HLA A, B, Cw Typing

The cell count was adjusted to 2 to 5 × 10^6 cells per milliliter. Using a 50 μL Hamilton syringe, 1 μL of the cell preparation was added to each cell of preloaded typing trays for HLA A, BR, and DR typing (Gen-Trak, Inc., Wayne, PA) and HLA Cw typing (Pel-Freeze Inc., Brown Deer, WI). After a half hour of incubation, 5 μL of rabbit complement was added to each well. The trays were then incubated for 1 hour at room temperature. This was followed by the addition of 5 μL of eosin, and approximately 5 minutes later, an equal volume of 37 percent formalin was added. The trays were read at 160 times magnification, using a Zeiss inverted phase contrast microscope. Eosin uptake served as an indicator of cell death.

DR Typing by One Color Fluorescence

Peripheral blood lymphocytes were prepared as described in the previous section, but the cells were adjusted to a concentration of 15 to 20 × 10^6 cells per milliliter, and 1 μL was added to each well on the HLA-DR typing tray. The trays were then incubated for 35 minutes at room temperature on a rotator. Prescreened rabbit complement was added to the trays (5 μL per well) and incubated for 1 hour at room temperature. This was followed by the addition of 2 μL of ethidium bromide (4 μg per milliliter) in HBSS with 5 percent ethylenediaminetetraacetic acid (EDTA) to each well. The cells were allowed to settle, and the trays were observed at 160 times magnification, using a Zeiss fluorescent microscope equipped with rhodamine filters. The trays were scored for cell death, which was indicated by the uptake of ethidium bromide and its subsequent intracellular fluorescence following ultraviolet stimulation.

Results

The relative risk was calculated for each antigen and selected haplotypes using the formula:

$$RR = \frac{\text{patients antigen-positive} \times \text{controls antigen-negative}}{\text{controls antigen-positive} \times \text{patients antigen-negative}}$$

Eighty-five patients with sensorineural hearing loss included 27 patients with Meniere's disease, 38 patients with otosclerosis, 9 patients with congenital or hereditary deafness, 7 patients with metabolic presbycusis, and 4 patients with progressive sensorineural hearing disorder. The percentage of HLA antigens for the entire group of sensorineural hearing loss is shown in Table 18–2. There is a significant increase in the percentage of patients with the A1/B8, B8/DR3 and particularly with the A1/B8/DR3 haplotype. A relative risk of three or more is considered to be significant. There was no evidence of an increased percentage of Cw 7. Table 18–3 reviews the data for otosclerosis and Meniere's disease. B8 was significantly elevated in patients with otosclerosis. B18 was significantly elevated in patients with Meniere's disease. The haplotype A1/B8 was elevated in patients with otosclerosis, and the haplotypes B8/DR3 and A1/B8/DR3 were significantly elevated in patients with both otosclerosis and Meniere's disease. Table 18–4 shows the

TABLE 18–2 HLA Frequencies in Controls and Sensorineural Hearing Loss Patients

Haplotype	P *	C †	RR ‡
A1/B8	20%	8	2.5
B8/DR3	20%	4	5.2
A1/B8/DR3	14%	2	7.1

* Patients
† Control population
‡ Relative risk
n = 85

TABLE 18-3 HLA Antigens and Haplotypes in Otosclerosis and Meniere's Disease

Antigen and Haplotype	Controls	Meniere's	Otosclerosis
B8	12%	21% (1.9)*	42% (3.1)
B18	8%	25% (3.8)	15% (2.0)
DR3	17%	21% (1.3)	21% (1.2)
A1/B8	8%	13% (1.8)	24% (3.5)
B8/DR3	4%	13% (3.9)	21% (6.5)
A1/B8/DR3	2%	8% (4.3)	15% (8.8)

* Relative Risk

HLA antigens and haplotypes in metabolic presbycusis. Although the population studied is relatively small, it is interesting to note that the same HLA antigens are significantly elevated in the population with metabolic presbycusis. The B8/DR3 haplotype has a relative risk of 10, which was the highest in all groups studied. A small group of patients with congenital or hereditary deafness have also been evaluated, and again, B8 and B18 appear to be increased in frequency in this small group of patients (data not shown).

Discussion

The fact that the frequency of the haplotype A1/B8/DR3 and B8/DR3 occurred in 20 percent of patients with sensorineural hearing loss, but in only 4 percent of the control population, is striking. The abnormal HLA frequencies might suggest a possible immunogenetic predisposition to the development of sensorineural hearing loss. It is also interesting that the B8/DR3 is a haplotype present in patients with autoimmune diseases that are related to certain immune complexes. In a previous report from our laboratory,[17] we suggested that patients with Meniere's disease, otosclerosis, and other sensorineural hearing disorders have a higher incidence of circulating immune complexes than a control population and, furthermore, have a higher incidence of autoantibodies, including thyroid antibody, antismooth muscle antibodies, and also antibodies to Type II collagen (Table 18-5). Type II collagen is found in various parts of the inner ear, as described by T.J. Yoo,[18] and may be an important antigen related to certain types of inner ear disorders such as otosclerosis and Meniere's disease. It is possible that the B8/DR3 haplotype, when present with other environmental triggers and possibly with other anatomical factors, is linked to a series of events that may produce autoimmunity in the inner ear and to the eventual development of such diseases as otosclerosis, Meniere's disease, and metabolic presbycusis. Alternatively, the inheritance of B8/DR3 may be linked to other genes that are responsible for these disorders.

It has recently been suggested by Bowman and Nelson[19] that the Class I antigen, Cw7, occurred in a high percentage of patients with sensorineural deafness, compared to a healthy age and race matched control. However, in our study we found that Cw7 was present in almost a third of the normal population, and even though our patients had a slightly higher incidence of Cw7, it was not significantly greater than the control group. In population studies that have been published, it appears that Cw7 occurs in over 40 percent of the normal population.[20] Thus, the study reported by Bowman and Nelson showing 50 percent distribution of Cw7 in their sensorineural hearing loss group may not be significant.

To our knowledge, this is the first report of the relationship of the haplotype B8/DR3 among patients with disorders of the temporal bone, including Meniere's disease, otosclerosis, and metabolic presbycusis. Therefore, the last topic that we would like to emphasize is the significance of the B8/DR3 haplotype. As mentioned previously, this haplotype appears to be related to a number of autoimmune diseases associated with circulating immune complexes and autoantibodies. These diseases include Graves' disease, myasthenia gravis, Type I or insulin-dependent diabetes, celiac disease, dermatitis herpetiformis, and systemic lupus erythematosus. There is a great body of literature on the relationship of the B8 and B8/DR3 haplotype and immunologic dysregulation (Table 18-6). For example, some patients with these haplotypes have defective immune adherence receptors on erythrocytes.[21] Erythrocytes with C3b receptors may serve in the disposal of serum immune complexes formed either physiologically or as a result of immunopatho-

TABLE 18-4 HLA Antigens and Haplotypes in Metabolic Presbycussis

Antigen and Haplotype	P*	C†	RR‡
B8	43%	12%	5.5
B18	43%	8%	8.6
DR3	29%	17%	1.9
A1/B8	29%	8%	4.6
B8/DR3	29%	4%	10.0
A1/B8/DR3	14%	2%	8.5

* Patients
† Control population
‡ Relative risk
n = 7

TABLE 18-5 Immune Complexes and Autoantibodies in Sensorineural Hearing Disorder

Disease	# of Cases	Immune Complexes #	%	Rf #	%	Thyr. #	%	Micros. #	%	ANA #	%	AMA #	%	SMA #	%	Type II Collagen #	%
Meniere's Disease	16	11	69	1	6	3	19	4	25	6	38	0	0	8	50	1	6
Otosclerosis	7	5	71	0	0	1	14	2	29	2	29	0	0	4	57	2	14
Progressive sensorineural hearing loss	23	16	70	0	0	0	0	0	0	6	26	0	0	11	48	5	22
Sudden deafness	13	9	70	0	0	0	0	0	0	4	31	0	0	3	23	4	31
Miscellaneous	18	10	56	0	0	0	0	0	0	5	28	0	0	7	39	4	22
Noise-induced hearing loss	21	4	19	0	0	0	0	0	0	2	9	0	0	0	0	0	0
Totals	98	55	56	1	1	4	4	6	6	25	26	0	0	33	34	16	16

Rf, rheumatoid factor; Thyr, thyroglobulin antibodies; Micros, microsomal antibodies; ANA, antinuclear antibodies; AMA, antimitochondrial antibodies; SMA, smooth muscle antibodies. From Bernstein JM. The immunobiology of autoimmune disease of the inner ear. In: Bernstein JM, Ogra PL, eds. Immunology of the ear. New York: Raven Press, 1987:419-426.

logic processes. Defective C3b receptors, therefore, could lead to the maintenance of immune complexes in the circulation. Furthermore, defective Fc receptor functions associated with the HLA B8/DR3 haplotype have been seen in patients with dermatitis herpetiformis and also in normal subjects with the HLA B8/DR3 haplotype.[22] Again, since removal of immune complexes from the circulation may depend on the Fc receptor function of tissue macrophages, it might be concluded that patients with HLA B8/DR3 haplotype have increased amounts of circulating immune complexes. The occurrence of impaired Fc function in a high percentage of both diseased and normal persons with the specific HLA haplotype B8/DR3 documents the existence of an immunologic deficit that is generally linked to commonly occurring histocompatibility antigens. That HLA B8/DR3 antigens are frequently linked to diseases with immunologic dysfunction is especially intriguing. This observation raises the possibility that those patients with the HLA B8/DR3 haplotype have a defective expression of Fc receptors on a number of circulating and fixed cells. It may be that the Fc receptor defect renders it likely that IgG-containing immune complexes are not cleared and destroyed normally, but remain in that circulation and are deposited in tissues, thus producing tissue damage. This concept is somewhat similar to the theory that Walford[23] presented over 20 years ago in which he suggested that aging may be related to persistent low levels of circulating immune complexes that eventually lead to the development of tissue injury.

It has been reported that impaired lymphocyte response to suboptimally-stimulating concentrations of phytohemagglutinin (PHA) in Sjögren's syndrome may be associated exclusively in patients with HLA B8.[24] This decreased proliferation is also apparent in the response to suboptimal concentrations of concavalin.

Lymphocyte proliferation in vitro to wheat glutinin has been reported to be significantly more frequent in HLA B8-positive normal subjects than in those without this antigen.[25] Finally, a study by Greenberg and Yunis[26] found a decreased PHA response by lymphocytes from normal women with HLA B8. Since the response to a suboptimal concentration of PHA is highly dependent on cellular interaction, it has been suggested that a specific subclass of T cells, namely the helper-inducer cell, is involved in response to suboptimal concentrations of mitogens.

These findings in general in regard to HLA B8/DR3 take on an added dimension in view of the fact that susceptibility and resistance to disease and the regulation of immune responsiveness are related to survival. Interestingly, therefore, that it has been shown that B8 is associated with decreased survival in women.[27]

TABLE 18-6 Immunologic Abnormalities Associated With the Haplotype B8/DR3

Defective immune adherence (C3b) receptor on erythrocytes
Defective Fc receptor density on macrophages
Decreased T cell function and decreased survival in women
Increased immunoglobulin synthesis and decreased Con A-induced suppression of T cells
Increased incidence of circulating autoantibodies
Decreased lymphocyte response to suboptimal concentrations of PHA
Increased response of HLA/B8 positive persons to wheat gluten antigen

SUMMARY

One of the most important developments in clinical immunology in the past decade has been the demonstration that increased frequencies of specific histocompatibility antigens occur in individuals with a variety of diseases. This implies that genes predisposing to these disorders reside in or near the major histocompatibility complex. The increased prevalence of antigens HLA B8/DR3 in a number of organ-specific autoimmune diseases suggests that a gene or genes in the HLA region associated with these alleles may predispose to the development of autoimmunity. It is therefore of great interest that the haplotype HLA B8/DR3 is often associated with a number of disorders of the temporal bone, including Meniere's disease, otosclerosis, and metabolic presbycusis. It is also interesting that this haplotype is present in a number of patients with congenital or hereditary sensorineural hearing loss. The son of one patient who had Meniere's disease and Hashimoto's disease had Type I diabetes, thus suggesting that the haplotype was involved in two autoimmune diseases as well as Meniere's disease in one family.

Inasmuch as this haplotype is associated with a turned on immune system that leads to the development of autoantibodies, circulating immune complexes, decrease in immune complex clearance, and depressed T cell function, it is certainly reasonable to hypothesize that patients who have this genetic HLA haplotype may be more prone to develop autoantibodies directed against Type II collagen. Inasmuch as there seems to be evidence from more than one laboratory that Type II bovine collagen can cause lesions that resemble the osteolytic lesions of otosclerosis and can produce hydrops in experimental animals, and because patients with Meniere's disease and otosclerosis have serum antibody directed against Type II collagen, it is interesting to speculate that patients who have the A1/B8/DR3 haplotype have a predisposition to develop autoantibodies directed against Type II collagen. Antigen-antibody complexes comprised of Type II collagen and its antibody may fix complement and deposit nonspecifically in the stria vascularis to produce strial atrophy over a long period of time. Furthermore, it is possible that patients with this haplotype may also develop circulating immune complexes that may deposit in the subepithelial layer of the endolymphatic sac or that a situ immune complex might occur in this area and ultimately cause dysfunction of the sac or fibrosis of obstruction of the endolymphatic duct with eventual endolymphatic hydrops. It is interesting in this regard that relapsing polychondritis is associated with a high incidence of auditory and vestibular dysfunction in the inner ear, and it has been quite well established now that this disease is the result of autoimmunity, in which antibodies are directed against Type II collagen in the nasal cartilage, auricular cartilage, and other anatomical sites where Type II collagen is present.[27]

Finally, because these patients have disorders of immunoregulation and have a higher tendency to develop autoimmune diseases, such as Graves' disease, Hashimoto's disease, and systemic lupus erythematosus, the longevity or survival rate of these patients would be significantly impaired. Thus, we have tried to suggest that there may be a relationship between histocompatibility antigens that are seen in sensorineural hearing loss and the aging process. This wide range of immunologic perturbations may lead to a decrease in survival. An immunologic theory of aging had been proposed by Walford[23] over 20 years ago, which rests on the thesis that autoimmune damage to the cells and tissues contributes to the actual process of aging. Thus, it is possible that genes of the major histocompatibility complex can influence the rate of immune senescence by altering the immunologic reactivity of the patient.

In conclusion, it is suggested that patients who have certain HLA antigens may have a predisposition to develop sensorineural hearing loss. It is striking that the haplotype that is most commonly found in these patients with sensorineural hearing loss is one that is associated with an increased rate of senescence. This is particularly found in such diseases as Type I diabetes, Down's syndrome, and systemic lupus erythematosus. Both Type I diabetes and systemic lupus erythematosus have a high incidence of A1/B8/DR3 haplotype. These two diseases are characterized by accelerated aging. It is thus possible that patients with A1/B8/DR3 have an increased rate of aging, and this may be related to the development of certain sensorineural hearing disorders. Obviously, further research is necessary in this exciting area, and a much larger number of patients with these disorders must be studied to determine whether or not this hypothesis exists.

References

1. vanRood JJ, vanLeeuwen A. Leukocyte grouping; a method and its application. J Clin Invest 1963; 42:1382–1390.
2. Schaller JG, Hansen J. HLA relationships to disease. Hosp Pract 1981; 16:41–49.
3. Meredith PJ, Walford RL. Autoimmunity, histocompatibility and aging. Mech Ageing Dev 1979; 9:61–77.
4. Weksler MR. The senescence of the immune system. Hosp Pract 1981; 16:53–64.

5. Snary D, Barnstable CJ, Bodmer WF, Goodfellow PM, et al. Cellular distribution, purification and molecular nature of human Ia antigens. Scand J Immunol 1977; 6:439–452.
6. Bodmer FW, Bodmer JG. Evolution and function of HLA system. Br Med Bull 1978; 34:309–316.
7. Sneel GD. Recent advances in the histocompatibility immunogenetics. Adv Genet 1979; 20:291–355.
8. Smith GS, Walford RL. Influence of the main histocompatibility complex on aging in mice. Nature 1977; 270:727–729.
9. Harman D. Free radical theory of aging; nutritional implications. Age Ageing 1978; 1:143–150.
10. Tam CF, Walford RL. Cyclic nucleotide levels in resting and mitogen stimulated cell suspensions from young and old mice. Mech Ageing Dev 1978; 7:309–320.
11. Walford RL, Bergmann K. Influence of genes associated with the main histocompatibility complex of desoxyribonucleic acid excision repair capacity and bleomycin sensitivity in mouse lymphocytes. Tissue Antigens 1979; 14:336–342.
12. Roitt I, Brostoff J, Male D. Genetic control of immunity. In: Immunology. St. Louis, MO: CV Mosby, 1985:13.1–9.
13. Eguro SY, Dorf ME, Amos DB. Cross reactions of HLA antibodies VI. Dissection of a complex serum. Tissue Antigens 1973; 3:195–203.
14. Roitt I, Brostoff J, Male D. Autoimmunity and autoimmune diseases. In: Immunology. St. Louis, MO: CV Mosby, 1985:23.1–11
15. Ambinder JM, Chiorazzi N, Gibofsky A, et al. Special characteristics of cellular immune function in normal individuals of the HLA-DR3 type. Clin Immunol Immunopathol 1982; 232:269–274.
16. Shanahan TC, Grybel MB, Cohen E, et al. Evaluation of HLA-DR typing by ethidium bromide fluorescence. Ann Clin Lab Sci 1987; 17:236–240.
17. Bernstein JM. The immunobiology of autoimmune disease of the inner ear. In: Bernstein JM, Ogra PL, eds. Immunology of the ear. New York: Raven Press, 1987:419.
18. Yoo TJ, Floyd RA, Kitano H. Animal model of autoimmune ear disease. In: Bernstein JM, Ogra PL, eds. Immunology of the ear. New York: Raven Press, 1987:463.
19. Bowman CA, Nelson RA. Human leukocytic antigens in autoimmune sensorineural hearing loss. Laryngoscope 1987; 97:7–9.
20. Bauer MP, Neugebauer M, Albert ED. Reference tables of two-locus haplotype frequencies for all MHC marker loci. In: Albert ED, Bauer MP, Mayr WR, eds. Histocompatibility Testing 1984. New York-Tokyo: Springer-Verlag Berlin Heidelberg, 1984:677.
21. Miyakawa Y, Yamada A, Kosaka K. Defective immune adherence (C3b) receptor on erythrocytes from patients with systemic lupus erythematosus. Lancet 1981; 2:493–497.
22. Lawley TJ, Hall RP, Fauci AS, Katz SI, et al. Defective Fc receptor functions associated with HLA B8/DR3 haplotype. N Engl J Med 1981; 304:185–192.
23. Walford RL. The immunologic theory of aging. Copenhagen: Munksgaard, 1969.
24. McCoombs CC, Michalski JP. Lymphocyte abnormality associated with HLA-B8 in healthy young adults. J Exp Med 1982; 156:936–941.
25. Cunningham-Rundles S, Cunningham-Rundles C, Pollack MS, et al. Response to wheat antigen in in vitro lymphocyte transformation among HLA-B8-positive donors. Transplant Proc 1978; 10:977–979.
26. Greenberg LJ, Yunis EJ. Histocompatibility determinants, immune responsiveness and aging in man. Fed Proc 1978; 37:1358–1362.
27. Pearson CM. Relapsing polychondritis: clinical and immunological features. In: Parker CW, ed. Clinical immunology. Vol. 2. Philadelphia: WB Saunders, 1980.

PRESBYPHAGIA

INTRODUCTION

HASKINS K. KASHIMA, M.D.

Neither the criteria or severity categories for dysphagia in the elderly nor, therefore, the prevalence of this disorder has been established. Swallowing performance in the elderly can be termed "presbyphagia". It may be useful to designate *primary presbyphagia* as deglutition modified by physiologic changes that accompany aging. *Secondary presbyphagia* designates dysphagia in the elderly attributable to specific disorders—neurologic, iatrogenic, or other comorbidities.

PREVALENCE OF DYSPHAGIA

Ambulatory Elderly

According to figures from the National Center for Health Statistics, "dysphagia" was ranked 174th among reasons for office visits to physicians during 1977 and 1978; "symptoms referable to the throat" was ranked 3rd and "cough" was ranked 5th on the same list.[1] In a survey of office-based ambulatory care for patients 75 years or older, swallowing related disorders failed to be ranked among the top 25 diagnoses.[2] A 1975-76 survey of office visits to otolaryngologists does not list dysphagia among the top 10 complaints or among the top 10 diagnoses.[3] On the other hand, 2 percent of the population 65 years and older and having difficulty with activity of daily living also have difficulty with eating.[4]

These inconstant estimates of dysphagia prevalence reflects, in part, the recognition and/or designation failure by physicians.

Hospitalized Patients

M. Groher and R. Bukatman (1986) reviewed the prevalence of swallowing disorders among adult patients in two major hospitals.[5] Twelve percent of 462 patients in one hospital and 13 percent of 610 patients in another were evaluated as having swallowing dysfunction. The highest percentage of dysphagia patients (33 percent and 34 percent) were observed in the neurology-neurosurgery services at each hospital. Dysphagia rates of 6 to 15 percent were reported from other estimates in acute care general hospitals; 30 to 50 percent dysphagia rate occurred among patients after head injury, neurologic disorder, or head and neck resections for cancer.[5]

Nursing Home Elderly

Siebens et al in a study of 240 residents in a skilled nursing facility designated 47 percent as requiring physical assistance during meals.[6] The elderly in nursing homes have multiple comorbidities and increased likelihood of dysphagia. Other estimates of feeding dependency in nursing homes run as high as 50 percent (Elliott[7]).

SWALLOWING EVALUATION IN THE ELDERLY

Deglutition performance is evaluated by (1) clinical history, physical, and endoscopic examination; (2) radiographic studies, (3) manometric measurements, and (4) electromyographic techniques.

Dynamic imaging, by cine or video, is the current state-of-the-art radiographic study of oropharyngeal deglutition; the multiple and simultaneously occurring components of deglutition are recorded and examined at full and slow speed and by stop-frame in order to evaluate their individual performances. O. Ekberg and L. Walgren[8] reviewed cine-radiographic examinations performed for dysphagia in 854 patients and found evidence of pharyngeal dysfunction in 67 percent of males and 57 percent of females. The proportion of patients with pharyngeal dysfunction increased with age. In a related study of 101 dysphagic subjects over 80 years old, radiographic documentation of pharyngeal abnormality was found in 80 percent of patients; the abnormalities were more marked and multiple dysfunctions were more common than among 60-year-old dysphagic patients.[9]

B. Sonies et al[10] measured the duration of the oral phase of swallowing by using ultrasound to record the time lapse from swallow initiation to maximum hyoid elevation and to the return of the tongue to normal position and configuration. The oral phase duration was significantly shorter in young (less than 26 years) than in older (over 55 years) adults. Oral phase duration changed little after 55 years.

To date, studies documenting swallowing pattern changes associated with advancing age have been lacking; most current concepts are derived from findings in a subset of elderly dysphagic patients whose radiographic findings are so-called "normal".

CONCLUSIONS

An indeterminate proportion of oropharyngeal dysphagia masquerades under a variety of misleading symptoms, and detection of swallowing impairment may be delayed. Occult dysphagia, mislabeled as postnasal drip, excess mucus, or nervous cough, may be the earliest symptom of neurologic and systemic disorders.

Dysphagia at any age poses difficult problems for recognition, evaluation, and management. Among elderly citizens, dysphagia is a dilemma whose numbers and severity may be underestimated. Improved detection and development of objective severity assessment, combined with knowledge of aging effects on swallowing physiology, should lead to better estimates as to the prevalence of dysphagia in the elderly and improved management to achieve optimum benefit for the elderly dysphagic.

In the panel to follow, Dr. Jeff Palmer describes the technique and value of electromyogram (EMG) in swallow evaluation; Dr. Andrew Blitzer reviews the clinical problem of aspiration, and Dr. Leslie Malmgren describes findings in aging peripheral nerves. The titles have been chosen to demonstrate the breadth of the clinical and research challenge and opportunities.

The assistance of Ms. Joanna Chen Lin, librarian at the Gerontology Research Center, NIA, Baltimore, and Ms. Deborah Gustin, librarian at the Loch Raven Veterans Administration Hospital, Baltimore is gratefully acknowledged.

References

1. Patients' reasons for visiting physicians. National Ambulatory Medical Care Survey, United States, 1977-78. Vital and Health Statistics. DHHS Publication No. (PHS) 82-1717, December, 1981.
2. Koch H, Smith MC. Office-based ambulatory case for patients 75 years old and over. National Ambulatory Medical Care Survey, 1980 and 1981. NCHS Advancedata 110. August 21, 1985.
3. Koch H. Office visits to otolaryngologist. National Ambulatory Medical Care Survey, United States, 1975-76. Advancedata 34. August 30, 1978.
4. La Croix AZ. Determinants of health—exercise and activities of daily living. Health Statistics on Older Persons. United States, 1986. Analytical and Epidemiological Studies. Series 3, No. 25.
5. Groher M, Bukatman R. The prevalence of swallowing disorders in two teaching hospitals. Dysphagia 1986; 1:3-6.
6. Siebens H, Trupe E, Siebens A, et al. Correlates and consequences of eating dependency in institutionalized elderly. JAGS 1986; 34:192-198.
7. Elliott JL. Swallowing disorders in the elderly: a guide to diagnosis and treatment. Geriatrics 1988; 95-100.
8. Ekberg O, Walgren L. Dysfunction of pharyngeal swallowing. A cine radiographic investigation in 854 dysphagial patients. Acta Radiol Diagn 1985; 26:389-395.
9. Borgstrom PS, Ekberg O. Pharyngeal dysfunction in the elderly. J Med Imaging 1988; 2:74-81.
10. Sonies BC, Stone M, Shawker T. Speech and swallowing in the elderly. Gerodontology 1984; 3:115-123.
11. Campbell-Taylor I, Fisher RH. The clinical case against tube feeding in palliative care of the elderly. The American Geriatrics Society 1987; 35:1100-1104.

SWALLOWING DISORDERS AND ASPIRATION IN THE ELDERLY

ANDREW BLITZER, D.D.S., M.D.

INTRODUCTION

Life-threatening pulmonary disease may be produced by intermittent or persistent or acute or chronic aspiration. Aspiration is the soiling of the tracheobronchial tree, which may produce cough, intermittent fever, recurrent tracheobronchitis or pneumonia, atelectasis, and/or empyema. Weight loss, cachexia, and dehydration may accompany the pulmonary symptoms in a patient with long-standing aspiration. In many cases, the soilage of the airway is secondary to pooling in the hypopharynx from a mechanical or neuromuscular disability of phase I and/or phase II of swallowing, and from a disability of phase III of swallowing (cricopharyngeal achalasia, esophageal dysmotility or immotility, esophageal obstruction and/or reflux). In addition, laryngeal incompetence allows for swallowed material to enter the airway and produce a soilage of the tracheobronchial tree. In many conditions, there is simultaneous laryngeal and swallowing dysfunction producing severe aspiration and disability. The elderly population are particularly prone to the ravages of aspiration since mechanical impairment from muscle weakness and neurologic dysfunction are more common in this age group. Since our population is gradually aging, aspiration and swallowing disorders will become an increasingly common cause of disease and death. A better understanding of the pathophysiology of these disorders, an approach to the evaluation and management of these disorders, and an attempt to address the remaining questions should increase the quality and quantity of life and decrease some of the cost of medical care.

NEUROLOGIC IMPAIRMENT, ASPIRATION, AND SWALLOWING DISORDERS

Neurologic disorders related to vascular or degenerative disease are more common in the elderly. Many of these changes produce a wide spectrum of disabilities of swallowing and aspiration.

Neurologic disorders may cause aspiration and/or swallowing disorders and include those causing changes in the cerebral cortex, such as stroke, drugs, epilepsy, tumors, infection, or trauma. Diffuse brain lesions can cause increased intracranial pressure that results in stupor or coma (neoplasia, hematoma, abscess, massive infarction; infection such as meningitis, encephalitis, or cerebritis; degenerative disorders such as Jacob-Creutzfeldt disease or adrenoleukodystrophy; excess ingestion of alcohol, narcotics or barbiturates; or elevated or low levels of calcium, glucose or sodium). Aspiration syndromes can also be found in patients with changes in the subcortical gray matter as seen in extrapyramidal syndromes of Parkinson's disease, Huntington's disease, myoclonus, and tardive dyskinesias. Motor neuron disorders can also produce aspiration and swallowing disorders and include progressive spinal muscular atrophy (PSMA), progressive bulbar palsy (PBP), amyotrophic lateral sclerosis (ALS), and poliomyelitis (now rare).

Pharyngeal and esophageal dysfunction can also be produced from diseases that affect the neuromuscular junction such as myasthenia gravis, and the Eaton-Lambert syndrome. Peripheral nerve disorders, such as Guillain-Barré syndrome, or injury to the nerves can produce dysfunction. Primary muscle disorders such as polymyositis, muscular dystrophy, and metabolic myopathies can also produce aspiration and swallowing disorders.[1]

PULMONARY CONSEQUENCES OF CHRONIC ASPIRATION

Slight soilage of the airway can be found even in normals during sleep, but aspirated bacteria and foreign material are cleared. Viral infections, ethanol ingestion, and altered states of consciousness can increase the quantity of material aspirated, decrease the response, and therefore increase the severity of the consequences. As the level of consciousness and/or mechanical impairment (including tracheostomy) and/or neurologic impairment increases, the quantity and frequency of the aspiration increases.[2-5]

The effects of aspiration depend on the quantity of the aspirate, the pH, and the status of the pulmonary system. Aspiration of solid material may obstruct the airway, which may cause asphyxia and death. Smaller particles may obstruct bronchi, thus causing a secondary pneumonia and a possible empyema. If a large quantity of low pH material is aspirated, an intense bronchospasm occurs, as well as severe injury to the pulmonary capillary endothelium and the epithelium of the distal airways. This reaction was best described by Mendelson in 1946[6] when he reported mortalities during obstetric anesthesia. This damage results in hypotension, hypoxia, and hypercarbia secondary to the pulmonary edema. Fever, bronchopneumonia, and/or atelectasis is produced if there is a smaller quantity of aspirate. Chest roentgenograms often reveal scattered, irregular densities. The lower lobes are more often involved, as is the right side. The upper lobes may be involved in patients who are supine.[7] Chronic aspiration is caused by a neuromuscular or mechanical inability to swallow feedings or secretions while protecting the airway. Chronic intermittent soilage of the airway produces chronic pulmonary disease. Evaluation of these patients with clarification of the etiology should be expeditious, and a treatment plan should be based on the disability.[8-11]

PHASE I AND II OF SWALLOWING

The swallowing mechanism depends on each event taking place in a precisely coordinated effort. If the events are unsynchronized, there will be nasal reflux, choking, aspiration, or regurgitation.

Phase I swallowing is the oral phase in which the tongue prepares the bolus for swallowing. The tongue mixes the food with saliva and sorts out the large particles to be chewed again. The tongue then forms a bolus against the palate and coats it with mucous. The tongue presses against the palate, thus squeezing the bolus into the oropharynx. The soft palate elevates, sealing the nasopharynx and preventing nasal reflux. When the bolus reaches the vallecula, the larynx is elevated.[12]

Phase II of swallowing is the pharyngeal phase and occurs after the bolus has passed the faucial pillars. This phase is completely involuntary, and respiration is inhibited during this phase. As the base of the tongue has moved posteriorly, the epiglottis has tipped posteroinferiorly at the same time as the larynx has been raised by the supraglottic musculature. The bolus is deflected posterolaterally away from the larynx by the epiglottis. As the bolus descends toward the hypopharynx, the airway is protected by the epiglottis and aryepiglottic folds and, more importantly, by the closure of the glottis.[8,12-14]

Phase III is the esophageal phase and may fail because of failure to open the upper esophageal sphincter (the cricopharyngeus muscle) or failure of the contraction of the esophagus itself. The upper esophageal sphincter or cricopharyngeus muscle was studied by Kirchner in 1958.[15] He studied the function of this muscle in dogs by utilizing endoscopy, x-ray studies, and pressure recordings. He found that the cricopharyngeus was in the state of contraction during the resting phase. The horizontal fibers of the cricopharyngeus muscle were behaviorally different from the oblique fibers and the thyropharyngeus, collectively called the inferior constrictor. The skeletal muscle is innervated by the vagus nerve, which provides tonic stimulation for contraction via lower motor neuron activity.[16,17] During swallowing, the muscle relaxes and then contracts to a pressure equal to or greater than the resting pressure. The nerve to the cricopharyngeus muscle arises in the vagal nuclei and passes without synaptic interruption to the motor end plates via the vagus nerve. These motor end plates are cholinergically mediated through nicotinic junctions. The maintained contraction of rest is neurogenic, and central inhibition is responsible for the relaxation on swallowing.[18] Conditions such as basilar artery thrombosis that damage vagal function interfere with relaxation of the cricopharyngeus and cause cricopharyngeal achalasia and dysphagia with aspiration. Neuropathic and myopathic conditions may produce a relative cricopharyngeal achalasia or a dysynchrony. A pharyngeal pressure of 15 to 23 mm Hg is normally exerted by the cricopharyngeus and must be overcome by pharyngeal pressure to induce opening of the sphincter.

Evaluation of Swallowing

Evaluation of these phases of swallowing is complex, but is necessary in order to accurately find the etiology of the swallowing disorders. After the physical examination, the best test is a modified barium swallow or "cookie swallow." In this procedure, a video recording is made so that the swallowing effort can be studied at slow speed. Small amounts of barium and different consistencies of barium are given to best assess all aspects of phase I and II of swallowing. The patients are also kept upright in their natural swallowing position. The patients' positions can also be changed to see which one allows for the best swallowing results. Aspiration assessment can be made for consistency, position, and the associated dysfunction.[19,20]

Other tests have successfully been used for swallowing analysis. Ultrasonography has been valuable in studying the oral phase of swallowing, but cannot be used for the pharynx or larynx because of the interference of the cervical spine.[21] Manometry is also useful in detecting subtle failures in pressure generation. Generally, this procedure is performed by utilizing an apparatus that measures pressure at the cricopharyngeus, the body of the esophagus, and the lower esophageal sphincter. The pressure sensors can be altered to measure pharynx, cricopharyngeus, and esophageal body. Manometry cannot, however, give information about aspiration. For this reason, McConnel et al[22] have devised a method of assessment using manofluorography, combining both manometry and fluoroscopy. With this method, they report accurate information about swallowing disorders with aspiration.

Evaluation of patients should include fiberoptic laryngoscopy, which offers a better functional assessment of the swallowing effort than other types of laryngoscopy. A modified barium swallow with cine is important in the assessment of a disability in phase I, II, and/or III of swallowing. Frame by frame in anteroposterior and lateral projections, the swallowing effort can be analyzed for adynamic areas, relative obstructions, and dysynchrony. Manometric studies are also useful in the evaluation of functional disabilities in swallowing, including relative cricopharyngeal achalasia.[23] The two techniques can be combined as manofluorography, as described by McConnel et al.[22]

Therapy for Swallowing Disorders

Treatment should be aimed at dealing with the defect causing the system failure. Patients with a unilateral hypoglossal nerve paralysis usually do not have any noticeable functional deficit in the swallowing effort. If both hypoglossal nerves are injured or if the patient has a central disease, such as a cerebral vascular accident (CVA) or ALS, or a myopathic process, swallowing and speech may be severely limited. Swallowing therapy sometimes can improve the situation, or patients can be taught to feed by gavage, thereby bypassing the oral phase. In patients with velopharyngeal insufficiency and nasal reflux, the soft palate or posterior pharyngeal wall can be augmented, prosthetic devices can be fabricated, or a pharyngeal flap may be used to eliminate the failure. The epiglottis is helpful in swallowing, but is not crucial. Many patients can be taught to swallow again after epiglottectomy or supraglottic resection. Treatment of phase I and II swallowing disorders may include feeding by gavage (with a bulb syringe and rubber tube) or by nasogastric tube. However, patients with nasogastric tubes often have reflux around the tube and/or continue to aspirate saliva.[19,20,24] In these cases, other measures may be necessary, such as gastrostomy, tracheostomy, and other laryngeal and pharyngeal procedures.

A cricopharyngeal myotomy often helps correct the dysphagia or aspiration where there is true cricopharyngeal achalasia or relative cricopharyngeal achalasia. Some authors have cited cricopharyngeal myotomy as the treatment of choice for dysphagia attributable to various neurologic conditions; however, cricopharyngeal myotomy is only a treatment for true and relative cricopharyngeal achalasia. Those conditions that produce a cricopharyngeal achalasia benefit from a myotomy. Those patients with more generalized mechanical failure who have failure in all the phases of swallowing, such as in ALS, brain stem stroke, or myopathies, have limited or no benefit from such a procedure.[25-34]

Peristalsis of esophageal striated muscles is also mediated by vagal cholinergics. The peristaltic action can be reduced or abolished by curare and succinylcholine in the proximal esophagus and by atropine in the distal esophagus. Pharmacologic agents can be used to modify esophageal motility. Most of the research of pharmacologic agents has been in patients with gastroesophageal reflux and has been aimed at increasing pressures at the lower esophageal sphincter and increasing peristaltic contractions. The two most commonly used agents are bethanechol (which increases esophageal contractility, but also increases the gastric acid secretions) and metoclopramide (a potent antiemetic that has been found to increase contractility without increasing gastric acidity).[35,36]

Patients with parkinsonism have a tremulous and/or breathy voice, but also may have difficulty swallowing. Parkinson patients have been found to have a lengthened phase I attributable to lingual motility disorders, a lengthened phase II with vallecular stasis, and a lengthened phase III. These findings are not seen in patients with benign essential tremor. Patients with diabetes display weak peristaltic action and poor sphincter pressure.[35]

Acute and chronic changes from caustic ingestion can also severely disrupt phase III of swallowing. Changes from caustic ingestion may lead to aspiration because of a decrease in sensation, fibrosis, and a dysynchronous swallowing effort. The damage from caustic ingestion may be irreversible and difficult to treat. Patients with severe damage from caustic ingestion may need an esophageal bypass, using mobilized stomach or small or large bowel. This may be the only way to allow swallowing and to prevent aspiration.

Swallowing therapy can be planned, based on swallowing studies and individual observation. The consistency of the food, the head position, the neck position, the method of food introduction, the quantity of food, and other parameters can be used to help patients develop a method of adequate alimentation.

Dental prostheses can also be of benefit to some patients with phase I swallowing defects. Certain types of obturators or guide bar appliances can be used to guide food away from nonfunctional areas to allow functional areas to deal with the injested food. Before and after modified barium swallow studies are excellent methods of achieving optimum function from these disabled patients.[37,38]

ASPIRATION AND LARYNGEAL INCOMPETENCE

Swallowing disorders have been described in the previous section. Many of these disorders also promote aspiration, even in patients who have normal laryngeal function. In phase II of swallowing, the larynx is elevated, the glottis and supraglottis close to protect the airway, and the bolus is propelled into the food passage. If the swallowing is impaired, material may remain in the hypopharynx at the end of the swallow. When the larynx descends to its normal position and the glottis and supraglottis open, residual material in the hypopharynx may reflux into the now open glottic chink and descend into the airway.

Aspiration may also occur if the laryngeal function is impaired. As the portal of the airway, the larynx must maintain its competency as the sphincter to prevent aspiration. Voluntary closure of the larynx occurs when phonating, swallowing, coughing, or during a valsalva. Involuntary closure occurs with tactile stimulation of the supraglottic structures. The reflex adduction of the vocal cords is triggered through the sensory afferents of the superior laryngeal nerve. Unilateral stimulation produces a bilateral response. If there is interference with the sensory afferents, foreign material in the supraglottic and glottic areas may escape detection and fail to trigger laryngeal closure. Without closure, swallowed material then descends through the glottis until it is detected by sensory fibers of the recurrent laryngeal nerve, which innervates the undersurface of the vocal cord and subglottis. These fibers initiate a cough response to clear the foreign material. When the sensory fibers of the vagus are disabled, a cough is not produced until there is stimulation of the vagal fibers of the trachea, where there is considerable crossover.

Neuromuscular or mechanical impairment of the larynx also allows aspiration. A unilateral vocal cord paralysis may produce incomplete glottic closure, thereby allowing soilage of the airway. Recurrent laryngeal nerve damage from tumor, trauma, or infection may produce vocal cord impairment, thus leaving an open glottic chink. Medialization of the paralyzed cord and hyperadduction of the contralateral vocal cord may allow patients to accommodate for a vocal cord paralysis. Posterior glottic closure is most important for the prevention of aspiration. Many patients can have part or all of a vocal cord resected for cancer, thereby producing an anteriorly-open glottic chink, and have little or no aspiration. If an arytenoid cartilage is removed or if there is damage to the posterior commissure, aspiration may become overwhelming unless reconstruction is done.

The mechanical disability markedly increases as the injury to the vagus moves proximally. Base of skull lesions or trauma to the vagus nerve produce dysfunction of both the superior and recurrent laryngeal nerves, thus causing greater sensory and motor disability than the recurrent laryngeal nerve alone. Central lesions, such as brain stem strokes, produce disabilities far worse than vagal lesions alone.

An open glottic chink can be attributable to a mechanical disability alone, such as congenital, traumatic, or surgical deficiencies. Mechanical changes in vocal cord volume or position, either uniform or segmental, may allow for aspiration. Traumatic dislocation of the cricoarytenoid joint may leave the vocal cord fixed in a relatively open position.[39,40]

Evaluation of Laryngeal Dysfunction

An etiologic evaluation should be performed on patients found to have an open glottic chink, hoarseness, and intermittent aspiration secondary to decreased activity of a vocal cord. Indirect laryngoscopy and fiberoptic laryngoscopy allows for careful inspection of the vocal apparatus at rest and during function. The movement of the vocal cords and the coordination of the activity can be evaluated visually. Tremors, twitches, and other unusual movements can also be detected. In addition, the use of a stroboscope allows rapid, unusual movements or an uncoordinated movement to be seen. Laryngeal electromyography can also be helpful in understanding the nature of a laryngeal dysfunction, because early neuromuscular changes can be detected electrically. Electromyography can easily find patterns of denervation, reinnervation, tremor, myoclonus, and myopathy.[41] Electroglottography is another method of studying the characteristics of the vocal cord movement. It is based on the change in potentials of the vocal cords as measured by surface electrodes. Electroencephalography, brain stem evoked response audiometry, computed tomography (CT), and magnetic resonance imaging (MRI) are also important in cases where a brain stem or central cause of laryngeal dysfunction is theorized.

Treatment of Aspiration and Laryngeal Incompetence

Once the etiologic evaluation is complete, a therapeutic plan can be fabricated, based on the etiology.

Tracheotomy

Patients with copious, chronic secretions and laryngeal and/or pharyngeal disabilities may have intractable aspiration. These patients may warrant a separation of the airway and the food passages. Tracheotomy is the most commonly used method of dealing with this situation. Utilizing a cuffed tracheostomy tube, the airway can be secured with an independent external portal. Secretions or food substances that pass through the larynx are kept above the tracheotomy tube cuff. Access for good pulmonary toilet is also provided through the tracheotomy tube. Since the cuff should periodically be deflated to prevent acute injuries to the tracheal mucosa, careful suctioning of secretions above the cuff before deflation is necessary to prevent soilage of the airway on cuff deflation. Tracheotomy is, however, only a short-term solution since, with time, pressure from the cuff will produce tracheomalacia and an inability to obtain an effective seal, thereby allowing continued airway soilage. Therefore, other solutions are necessary for long-term disability.[42-45]

Vocal Cord Augmentation

An open glottic chink may be caused by anatomical deficiency, mechanical impairment, or a neuromuscular disability that is not compensated for by the contralateral cord and should be corrected if symptomatic. In 1911[46] Bruning reported medializing a paralyzed vocal cord by using an injection of paraffin. When it was found that the paraffin produced granulomas, other materials were tested, including glycerine, cartilage, bone dust, and tantalum. Arnold,[47] in 1962, reported medializing a vocal cord by utilizing tantalum and glycerine and then Teflon and glycerine. Lewy and others[48-50] have since used Teflon and have corroborated Arnold's results.

Teflon is injected into the larynx during a direct laryngoscopy. The needle is placed as far laterally as possible in the middle area of the vocal cord. The procedure is best performed under local anesthesia so that the airway can constantly be assessed. Small quantities of Teflon can be injected, medially displacing a paralyzed vocal cord. If too much Teflon is injected, the airway may be diminished, producing stridor or obstruction. Judicious use of the Teflon is imperative since Teflon is difficult to remove from the larynx. Teflon should not be placed in the vocalis muscle for medialization since this produces an irregularly-shaped vocal cord and changes the resonant characteristics of the cord. Some anatomical deficiencies of the vocal cord can be augmented with small amounts of Teflon.[51-53]

In situations where there is some hope of return of function (such as in brain stem strokes or recurrent laryngeal nerve trauma), glycerine or gelfoam injection can be used for medialization where necessary. Medialization can be accomplished for a limited time until the material is resorbed, thus allowing for return of function or for conversion with a permanent material. Vocal cord injection can also be performed in selected patients percutaneously via the cricothyroid membrane, as recently reported by Ward.

In larger defects where a large quantity of Teflon is necessary, augmentation with cartilage implants or alloplastic materials may be more effective and safe. Autogenous costochondral, nasal septal, or thyroid cartilage is easily placed submucosally through a midline thyrotomy. This technique was described by Meurmann in 1952, and was later refined by others.[54-58]

Glottic Prosthesis

Several authors have reported the use of a glottic stent in an attempt to separate the food and air passages without the use of an inflated cuffed tracheotomy tube. The theory behind this technique is like a cork in a bottle. This can be a prefabricated or custom made prosthesis that is placed in the larynx endoscopically, and is usually held in place with transcutaneous sutures. The insertion technique is simple, the patient has a tracheotomy for an airway, and the procedure is easily reversible. The problems are related to local inflammation, discomfort, scarring at the glottic level, and the leak of fluid around the prosthesis because of inefficient seal.[59] Recently a new type of stent has been described by Eliachar et al[60] that allows phonation. It is made of silicone, is inserted through the tracheostomy site below the glottis, and extends through the cords. It is a tube with a slit in a dome, much like a large Blom-Singer tube. According to the authors, this adequately occludes the larynx to prevent aspiration, yet allows phonation through the slit in the tube.

Laryngectomy

For the better part of this century, many patients with aspiration were offered a total laryngectomy for treatment of their chronic aspiration. This provides a permanent cutaneous tracheostoma and a permanent separation of the airway and food passage. It eliminates phonation and the possibility of reversal in patients who might recover some or all of their function. It also adds the morbidity of an extensive surgical procedure.[61] Some suggest that laryngectomy is still indicated in patients with poor prognoses, associated medical problems, and evidence of impaired wound healing.[62] A wide field laryngectomy need not be performed on patients who aspirate and who are not deemed candidates for the other procedures listed in this chapter. The author has accomplished the goal of total laryngectomy in several patients by utilizing a modified small field laryngectomy. The strap muscles are preserved, and the resection includes the hyoid to the lower border of the cricoid cartilage. The mucosa of the postcricoid region and that covering the arytenoid cartilages is preserved. Closure is accomplished with a narrow suture line covered with a second layer of strap muscle.

Glottic and Supraglottic Laryngeal Closure

Several procedures were designed to surgically close the larynx in an attempt to provide an adequate separation of the food and air passages, to avoid the tracheal damage from a constantly inflated cuffed tracheotomy tube, and to create a potentially reversible situation. These procedures can be done electively after tracheotomy and stabilization of the patient.

Montgomery in 1975[63] described a glottic closure procedure. His technique was performed through a median thyrotomy. The mucosa of the vocal cords was stripped bilaterally, and a figure-of-eight suture was placed to close the glottis and allow fibrous union of the vocal cords. This technique allows adequate separation of the air and food passages with a permanent tracheotomy. If the vocal cords are functional preoperatively, the seal occasionally pulls apart before healing and leaks posteriorly. The patient cannot phonate. The procedure is potentially reversible, but laryngeal webs are difficult to remove, and the vocal cords themselves may not function well because of scarring. For this reason, the Montgomery procedure was modified by Sasaki et al.[64] They added a sternocleidomastoid muscle flap interposed into the subglottic region to provide a better seal. When the larynx opens and leaks, however, the muscle flap also leaks. This added flap also makes reversal more difficult.

Habal et al in 1972[65] described a two-layered horizontal closure of the supraglottis. A pharyngotomy is performed, and an incision is made around the perimeter of the epiglottis, the aryepiglottic folds, the arytenoids, and the interarytenoid area. The glossoepiglottic ligaments are severed, and the tip of the epiglottis is then folded over the arytenoids. The mucosa is sutured closed, and the mucosa from the pyriform sinus is rotated over the epiglottis as a second layer. Patients breathe through a noncuffed tracheotomy tube. The patients cannot phonate, but the procedure is potentially reversible. Strome and Fried[66] reported such a reversal by using a sequential enlargement of an epiglottic window with a CO_2 laser in 1983. In some cases, perhaps attributable to the spring of the epiglottic cartilage, the suture line opens posteriorly, thus allowing recurrent aspiration.

Biller et al in 1983[67] described a vertical supraglottic closure that left a small opening at the epiglottic tip. With an opening at the level of the tip of the epiglottis, aspiration does not occur, but phonation is possible in some patients. The technique consists of a pharyngotomy, an incision along the edge of the epiglottis, the aryepiglottic folds, the arytenoids, and the interarytenoid area. The epiglottic cartilage can be scored in a vertical direction to break the spring. The supraglottis is then closed in two layers as a vertical tube with a several-millimeter opening at the tip of the epiglottis to allow potential phonation. A permanent tracheotomy is necessary. The procedure is potentially reversible. The procedure was originally described as an alternative to total laryngectomy in patients undergoing total glossectomy. This author has used this closure successfully in several patients with intractable aspiration, with excellent results. Patients often can eat again, and some can speak.

Laryngeal Diversion

In 1975, Lindeman[68] described a procedure to separate the air and food passage in a reversible fashion without damage to the laryngeal structures. In this procedure, the subglottic trachea is severed at the third or fourth tracheal ring and the distal portion is brought out and sewn to the neck skin. A small opening is made in the esophagus at the level of the proximal tracheal stump and larynx. The edges of the esophageal opening are then sewn to the proximal trachea in an end-to-side anastomosis. This system allows all material entering the larynx to exit into the esophagus and provides complete separation of the airway. Phonation cannot occur following this treatment. If the patient recovers function, the procedure is reversible. Lindeman reported two such reversals of his procedure. Closure is obtained by separating the proximal trachea from the esophagus, and the esophageal opening is closed primarily. The distal trachea is separated from the skin, and an end-to-end anastomosis is accomplished. This again allows phonation, respiration, and swallowing in a normal fashion. This author has used this technique many times with success.[69,70]

Lindeman reported two cases who had high tracheostomies. In these patients, he did not attempt a tracheoesophageal (T-E) fistula, but rather closed the proximal segment on itself and brought the distal segment out to the skin as a permanent stoma. Pooling of secretions in the blind end pouch was not found to be a problem.

Baron and Dedo[71] adapted the blind pouch technique to three patients. The first and second tracheal rings were separated. The first ring was split anteriorly in the midline, and the two cartilaginous halves were sewn together, thus closing off the trachea. The second ring was brought out as a stoma. They suggest that this technique is less complicated with less surgical time than the tracheoesophageal diversion procedures. They also noted that pooling of secretions was not a problem.

Tucker[72] devised an alternative diversion technique in which both the proximal and distal trachea stumps are diverted to the anterior cervical skin, thereby creating a double-barrelled tracheostome. The proximal trachea is brought out to the skin through a split in the sternocleidomastoid muscle; this maneuver supposedly compresses the trachea, thus minimizing leakage of aspirated material to the skin. This procedure has the obvious disadvantage of draining corrosive substances to the cervical skin.

Krespi et al,[73] described a modification of the Lindeman procedure in patients who had had previous high tracheostomies. In this procedure, an incision is made at the superior aspect of the previous tracheostome and carried down to the trachea. The mucosal lining of the cricoid cartilage and the first and second tracheal rings are dissected from the cartilage and preserved as a superiorly-based mucosal flap. A submucosal resection of the inferior half of the cricoid and proximal tracheal rings is performed. An esophagotomy is made at the level of the first tracheal ring, and the tracheal mucosal flap is sutured to the esophagotomy. A sternocleidomastoid flap is rotated between the trachea and esophagus and serves as a second layer of closure for the tracheoesophageal suture line. The distal trachea is sutured to the cervical skin as a permanent tracheostome.

Partial Cricoid Resection

Krespi et al[74] recently have described a technique for use in patients who have had head and neck cancer resections and who develop postoperative aspiration. At the time of surgery, a submucosal dissection of the posterior aspect of the cricoid is performed. A large segment of the center of the posterior cricoid lamina is removed. This, in conjunction with a cricopharyngeal myotomy, leaves a large hypopharyngeal portal for secretions and food and decreases the anteroposterior diameter of the larynx. Aspiration is therefore abolished or markedly decreased. Phonatory capability remains. Patients require a permanent tracheotomy. This procedure may be useful in other patients who aspirate, although the collapse of the subglottic airway is reversible. More work is necessary to assess the future role of this innovative procedure.

FUTURE DIRECTIONS

Nerve Grafting

For a long time surgeons and neurologists have been concerned with treatment for damage to motor nerves. Early in the century, surgeons began to treat severed motor nerves by suturing them back together and hoping that they would heal and function again. As techniques became more sophisticated, magnification and better lighting became available, and fine suture material, microsurgical instruments, and antibiotics were developed, the possibility of successful nerve repair and grafting became a reality. In facial reanimation, cable grafting has been used from the proximal facial nerve or from the contralateral facial nerve to the distal facial nerve by using the greater auricular or sural nerves. In situations where the proximal facial nerve is damaged or not available for grafting, other nerves are used to connect to the distal facial nerve to provide tone and facial function.[75] The most success has been achieved by using the ipsilateral hypoglossal nerve sewn to the distal facial nerve trunk.[76] This allows for tone and function without a great loss of function of the tongue. Other nerves that have been used are the phrenic nerve and the ansa hypoglossi.[77] These techniques have recently been applied to denervated muscles of the larynx to allow for reinnervation, particularly of the abductor muscles in cases of bilateral vocal cord paralysis.[78,79]

An extension of this desire to reinnervate muscles has been performed by several authors by using a nerve implantation or a neuromuscular pedicle. In these procedures, a nerve (either part or all of the vagus, the ansa hypoglossi, the phrenic, or the accessory) has been directly implanted into laryngeal muscle or has been transferred with muscle and motor end plates and grafted into muscle. Both of these techniques show some limited success, and hopes for their improvement continue. Presently, these techniques have been used for restoration of abductive functions of the larynx in respiration. There is reason to believe that they could also be used for adductive functions for swallowing and phonation.[80,81]

In addition, regional muscle transfers have been used to reanimate denervated areas, especially in the face. Several authors[82] have popularized the use of the masticator muscles with a different nerve supply to be surgically transposed in order to allow restoration of facial tone and function. Such techniques are theoretically possible in the larynx and pharynx by utilizing other ipsilateral or contralateral deep neck muscles. Distant muscles have also been brought to a new region by use of microvascular surgery. The arterial and venous supply are reanastomosed, and nerve supply is obtained from the contralateral nerves or other regional nerves. This technique also may be useful in reanimating the paralyzed or paretic larynx and pharynx.

Electrical Pacing

The newest of techniques for allowing restoration of function is laryngeal pacing.[83-86] Although it has been known for a long time that one could electrically stimulate a muscle to contract, it is the advent of microprocessors that allows for coordinated and directed muscle stimulation. Sensors can be placed in the pharynx that can detect pressure, liquid, and distortion, and that then can be used to send a variable response signal to the laryngeal muscles implanted. This allows for an appropriate response for each encounter. At the moment, the microprocessors for such a function are not small enough. However, there is little doubt that they will be shortly. Multichannel electrodes will allow for implantation in each of the laryngeal muscles that are not functional, and the microprocessor will be able to address each of these muscles independently, thus allowing for a more physiologic response to stimulation. The afferent supply can come from connections to the contralateral laryngeal nerves or from small receptors of the microprocessor. This work seems to be most promising and should be encouraged with funding on a larger scale.

Stabilization or Reversal of Neural Degeneration

Certainly, a method of preventing, stabilizing, or reversing central or peripheral neural degeneration is the best treatment of all. Increased knowledge of the central diseases is allowing for the detection of chemical changes within the brain. Replacement of depleted neurotransmitters, necessary metallic ions, or enzyme precursors may allow for continued normal function or reversal of impeded function. The future use of nerve growth factors and implantation of fetal neural tissues may allow for the reversal of centrally-damaged functions and eliminate the need for elaborate local rehabilitation.[87,88]

CONCLUSION

Chronic recurrent aspiration and swallowing disorders occur in patients with a diverse group of disabilities. Many techniques have been developed to allow thorough evaluation for identification of the underlying disability. There is an eclectic group of therapeutic possibilities to provide better laryngeal function and swallowing and to avert the often fatal course of continued aspiration. Many innovative surgical procedures are available to compensate for severe functional deficits. Some of these can be reversed if the patient recovers from his underlying disability. In the future, it may be possible to use more sophisticated nerve grafting or electronic microcomputerized laryngeal pacing in order to allow return of laryngeal and pharyngeal function. Continued research in these areas will allow otolaryngologists to better treat those patients afflicted with these disorders.

References

1. Brin MF, Younger D. Neurologic disorders and aspiration. Otolaryngol Clin North Am in press.
2. Bonano PC. Swallowing dysfunction after tracheostomy. Ann Surg 1970; 174:29–33.
3. Nahum AM, Harris JP, Davidson TM. The patient who aspirates—diagnosis and management. J Otolaryngol 1981; 10:10–16.
4. Bartlett JG, Gorbach SL. The triple threat of aspiration pneumonia. Chest 1975; 68:560–566.
5. Huxley EJ, Viroslav J, Gray WR, Pierce AK. Pharyngeal aspiration in normal adults and patients with depressed consciousness. Am J Med 1978; 64:564–568.
6. Mendelson CL. Aspiration of stomach contents into lungs during obstetrical anesthesia. Am J Obstet Gynecol 1946; 52:191–205.
7. Hawkins DB. Noninfectious disorders of the lower respiratory tract. Bluestone CD, Stool SE, eds. Pediatric otolaryngology. Philadelphia: WB Saunders, 1983:1265.
8. Ardan GM, Kemp FH. The protection of laryngeal airway during swallowing. Br J Radiol 1952; 25:406–416.
9. Buchin PJ, Jahn AF. Medical management of disorders of swallowing. Otol Clin North Am 1984; 17:713–724.
10. Cameron JL, Reynolds J, Zuidema GD. Aspiration in patients with tracheostomies. Surg Gynecol Obstet 1973; 136:68–70.
11. Awe WC, Fletcher WS, Jacob SW. The pathophysiology of aspiration pneumonitis. Surgery 1966; 60:232–239.
12. Didio LJA, Anderson MC. The "sphincters" of the digestive system. Baltimore: Williams & Wilkins, 1968.
13. Atkinson M, Kramer P, Wyman SM, Ingelfinger FJ. The dynamics of swallowing. I. Normal pharyngeal mechanisms. J Clin Invest 1957; 36:581–595.
14. Negus JE. The second stage of swallowing. Acta Otolaryngol (Suppl) 1949; 78:78–82.
15. Kirchner JA. The motor activity of the cricopharyngeus muscle. Laryngoscope 1958; 68:1119–1159.
16. Van Overbeck JJ, et al. Cricopharyngeal myotomy in pharyngeal paralysis, cineradiographic and manometric indications. Ann Otol Rhinol Laryngol 1979; 88:596–602.
17. Yoshida Y. Localization of efferent neurons innervating the pharyngeal constrictor muscles and the cervical esophagus muscle in the cat by means of horseradish peroxidase method. Neurosci Lett 1981; 10:91–95.
18. Christenson J. Innervation and function of the esophagus. Stipa S, Belsey RHR, Moraldi A, eds. Medical and surgical problems of the esophagus. London: Academic Press, 1981:14.
19. Logemann JA, Bytell DE. Swallowing disorders in three types of head and neck surgical patients. Cancer 1979; 44:1095–1105.
20. Logemann J. Evaluation and treatment of swallowing disorders. San Diego: College Hill Press, 1983.
21. Shawker T, Sonies B, Stone M. Real-time ultrasound visualization of tongue movement during swallowing. J Clin Ultrasound 1983; 11:485.
22. McConnel FMS. Analysis of pressure generation and bolus transit during pharyngeal swallowing. Laryngoscope 1988; 98:71–78.
23. Blonsky ER, Logemann JA, Boshes B, Fisher HB. Comparison of speech and swallowing function in patients with tremor disorders and in normal geriatric patients: a cinefluorographic study. J Gerontol 1975; 30:299–303.
24. Shedd DP, Scatliff JA, Kirchner JA. A cineradiographic study of post-resectional alterations in oropharyngeal physiology. Surg Gynecol Obstet 1960; 110:69–89.
25. Stevens KM, Newell RC. Cricopharyngeal myotomy in dysphagia. Laryngoscope 1971; 81:1616–1620.
26. Mills CP. Dysphagia in pharyngeal paralysis treated by cricopharyngeal sphincterotomy. Lancet 1973; 1:455–457.
27. Lebo CP, Sang K, Norris FH. Cricopharyngeal myotomy in amyotropic lateral sclerosis. Laryngoscope 1976; 86:862–868.
28. Calcaterra TC, Kadell BM, Ward PH. Dysphagia secondary to cricopharyngeal muscle dysfunction: surgical management. Arch Otolaryngol 1975; 101:726–729.
29. Seaman WB. Cineroentgenographic observations of the cricopharyngeus. Am J Roent 1966; 96:922–931.
30. Montgomery W, Lynch JP. Oculopharyngeal muscular dystrophy treated by inferior constrictor myotomy. Trans Am Acad Ophthal Otolaryngol 1971; 75:986–993.
31. Wilkins SA. Indications for the section of the cricopharyngeus muscle. Am J Surg 1964; 108:533–538.
32. Begley MD. Cricopharyngeal achalasia. J Coll Radiol (Aust) 1962; 6:138–141.
33. Ross ER, Green R, Auslander MD, Biller HF. Cricopharyngeal myotomy: management of cervical dysphagia. Otolaryngol Head Neck Surg 1982; 90:434–441.
34. Asherson N. Achalasia of the cricopharyngeal sphincter. J Laryngol Otol 1950; 64:747–758.
35. Schulze-Delrieu K. Esophageal pharmacology. In: Cohen S, Soloway RD, eds. Diseases of the esophagus. New York: Churchill Livingstone, 1982:35.
36. Diamant NE. Normal esophageal physiology. In: Cohen S, Soloway RD, eds. Diseases of the esophagus. New York: Churchill Livingstone, 1982:1–33.
37. Wurster CF, Krespi YP, Davis JW. Combined functional oral rehabilitation after radical cancer surgery. Arch Otolaryngol 1985; 111:530–533.
38. Chalian VA, Drane JB, Standish SM. Maxillofacial prosthetics: multidisciplinary approach. Baltimore: Williams & Wilkins, 1971.
39. Sessions DG, Ogura JH, Cralsky RH. Late glottic insufficiency. Laryngoscope 1975; 85:950–959.
40. Litton WB, Leonard JR. Aspiration after partial laryngectomy: cineradiographic studies. Laryngoscope 1969; 79:887–908.
41. Blitzer A, Lovelace RE, Brin MF, Fahn S, Fink ME. Electromyographic findings in focal laryngeal dystonia (spastic dysphonia). Ann Otol Rhinol Laryngol 1985; 94:591–594.
42. Bryant LR, Tinkle JK, Dubiler L. Tracheal damage from cuffed tracheostomy tubes. JAMA 1971; 215:625–628.
43. Thilenius OG, Vial CB. Chronic tracheotomy in dogs. J Appl Physiol 1963; 18:439–440.
44. Fee WE, Ward PA. Permanent tracheostomy: a new surgical technique. Ann Otol Rhinol Laryngol 1977; 86:635–638.
45. Fearon B, McDonald RE, Smith C. Airway problems in children following prolonged endotracheal intubation. Ann Otol Rhinol Laryngol 1966; 75:975–986.
46. Bruning W. Uber eine neue behandlungsmethode. Verh Deutche Laryngol 1911; 18:151.
47. Arnold GE. Vocal rehabilitation of paralytic dysphonia. Arch Otolaryngol 1962; 76:358–368.
48. Lewy RB. Glottic rehabilitation with Teflon injection—the return of voice, cough, and laughter. Acta Otolaryngol 1964; 58:214–220.
49. Rontal E, Rontal M, Morse G, Brown EM. Vocal cord injec-

tion in the treatment of acute and chronic aspiration. Laryngoscope 1976; 86:625-634.
50. Schramm VL, May M, Lavorato AS. Gelfoam paste injection for vocal cord paralysis: temporary rehabilitation of glottic competence. Laryngoscope 1978; 88:1268-1273.
51. Dedo HH, et al. Intracordal injection of Teflon in the treatment of 135 patients with dysphonia. Ann Otol Rhinol Laryngol 1973; 82:661-667.
52. Rubin HJ. Intracordal injection of silicone in selected dysphonias. Arch Otolaryngol 1965; 81:604-607.
53. Rubin HJ. Misadventures with injectable polytef (Teflon). Arch Otolaryngol 1975; 101:114-116.
54. Meurmann Y. Operative mediofixation of the vocal cord in complete unilateral paralysis. Arch Otolaryngol 1952; 55:544-553.
55. Opheim O. Unilateral paralysis of the vocal cord. Acta Otolaryngol 1955; 45:226-230.
56. Waltner JG. Surgical rehabilitation of voice following laryngofissure. Arch Otolaryngol 1958; 67:99-101.
57. Levine HL, Tucker HM. Surgical management of the paralyzed larynx. In: Bailey B, Biller HF, eds. Surgery of the larynx. Philadelphia: WB Saunders, 1985:117.
58. Smith GW. Aphonia due to vocal cord paralysis corrected by medial positioning of the affected vocal cord with a cartilage autograft. Can J Otolaryngol 1972; 1:295-298.
59. Weisberger EC, Huebsch SA. Endoscopic treatment of aspiration using a laryngeal stent. Otolaryngol Head Neck Surg 1982; 90:215-222.
60. Eliachar I, Roberts JK, Hayes JD, Tucker HM. A vented laryngeal stent with phonatory and pressure relief capability. Laryngoscope 1987; 97:1264-1268.
61. Montgomery WW. Total laryngectomy. In: Montgomery WW, ed. Surgery of the upper respiratory system. Philadelphia: Lea & Febiger, 1973:484.
62. Cannon CR, McLean WC. Laryngectomy for chronic aspiration. Am J Otolaryngol 1982; 3:145-149.
63. Montgomery WW. Surgical laryngeal closure to eliminate chronic aspiration. N Engl J Med 1975; 292:1390-1391.
64. Sasaki CT, Milmoe G, Yanagisawa EJ, Berry K, Kirchner JA. Surgical closure of the larynx for intractable aspiration. Arch Otolaryngol 1980; 106:422-423.
65. Habal MB, Murray JE. Surgical treatment of life endangering chronic aspiration pneumonia. Plast Reconstr Surg 1972; 49:305-311.
66. Strome M, Fried MP. Rehabilitative surgery for aspiration. Arch Otolaryngol 1983; 109:809-811.
67. Biller HF, Lawson W, Baek S-M. Total glossectomy: a technique of reconstruction eliminating laryngectomy. Arch Otolaryngol 1983; 109:69-73.
68. Lindeman RA. Diverting the paralyzed larynx: a reversible procedure for intractable aspiration. Laryngoscope 1975; 85:157-180.
69. Yarington CT, Linderman RC, Sutton D. Clinical experience with the tracheoesophageal anastomosis for intractable aspiration. Ann Otol Rhinol Laryngol 1976; 85:609-612.
70. Blitzer A. Evaluation and management of chronic aspiration. NY State J Med 1987; 87:154-160.
71. Baron BS, Dedo HH. Separation of the larynx and trachea for intractable aspiration. Laryngoscope 1980; 90:1927-1932.
72. Tucker HM. Management of the patient with an incompetent larynx. Am J Otolaryngol 1979; 1:47-56.
73. Krespi Y, Quatela VC, Sisson GA, Som ML. Modified tracheoesophageal diversion for chronic aspiration. Laryngoscope 1984; 94:1298-1301.
74. Krespi Y, Sisson G. Management of chronic aspiration by subtotal and submucosal cricoid resection. Ann Otol Rhinol Laryngol 1985; 94:580-583.
75. Crumley RL. Rehabilitation of the facial nerve. In: Otolaryngology-head and neck surgery. Cummings CW, et al, eds. St. Louis: CV Mosby, 1986:1071.
76. Conley J, Baker DC. Hypoglossal-facial nerve anastomosis for re-innervation of the paralyzed face. Plast Reconstr Surg 1979; 63:63-72.
77. Hardy R, Perret G, Myers R. Phrenicofacial anastomosis for facial paralysis. J Neurosurg 1957; 14:400-404.
78. Crumley R. Phrenic nerve graft for bilateral vocal cord paralysis. Laryngoscope 1983; 93:425-428.
79. Rice D. Laryngeal reinnervation with the ansa cervicalis. Arch Otolaryngol 1983; 109:480-481.
80. Tucker HM. Selective reinnervation of paralyzed facial muscles by the neuro-muscular island pedicle technique: new concepts in rehabilitation of the longstanding facial paralysis. In: Fish U, ed. Facial nerve surgery. Birmingham: Aesculapius, 1977:251.
81. Tucker HM. Neurologic disorders. In: Tucker HM, ed. The larynx. Stuttgart: Thieme Med Publ, 1987:235.
82. May M. Muscle transposition for facial reanimation: indications and results. Arch Otol Head Neck Surg 1984; 110:184-189.
83. Broniatowski M, Ilyes LA, Jacobs GB, Nose Y, Tucker HM. Artificial reflex arc: a potential solution for chronic aspiration. A canine study based on a laryngeal prosthesis. Laryngoscope 1988; 98:235-237.
84. Broniatowski M, Ilyes LA, Jacobs G, Stepnick DW, Nose Y, Tucker HM. Artificial reflex arc: a potential solution for chronic aspiration I. Neck skin stimulation triggering strap muscle contraction in the canine. Laryngoscope 1987; 97:331-333.
85. DeVilliers R, Nose Y, Meier W, et al. Long term continuous electrostimulation of a peripheral nerve. Trans Am Soc Artif Intern Organs 1964; 10:357-365.
86. Tobey DN, Sutton D. Contralaterally elicited electrical stimulation of paralyzed facial muscles. Otolaryngol Head Neck Surg 1978; 87:812-818.
87. Bowden REM, Gutmann E. Denervation and reinnervation of human voluntary muscle. Brain 1944; 67:20-72.
88. Diamond J, Cooper E, Turner C, et al. Trophic regulation of nerve sprouting. Science 1976; 183:371-377.

Chapter Twenty

TECHNIQUES FOR EXAMINING PHARYNGEAL SWALLOWING

JEFFREY B. PALMER, M.D.

INTRODUCTION

Swallowing is a dynamic process. Static methods can be used to evaluate pharyngeal anatomy, but examination of the mechanism of swallowing demands dynamic techniques. Numerous methods have been applied for analyzing the fluid dynamics, kinematics, and neurophysiology of normal and abnormal pharyngeal swallowing.[1] Three of the most important, videoradiography, manometry, and electromyography, will be discussed in this brief review.

VIDEORADIOGRAPHY

Dynamic radiographic imaging of pharyngeal swallowing is essential to its evaluation.[2-4] A common study paradigm is the swallowing of liquid barium while fluoroscopic images of the bolus and the neighboring structures are recorded on videotape, a method known as videoradiography. This is a kinematic technique for analyzing functional anatomy and physiology. It reveals pharyngeal motions, but not necessarily the effector mechanisms that produce them.

Videoradiography demonstrates normal and abnormal events of pharyngeal swallowing, such as motions of the tongue, palate, hyoid bone, and larynx, changes in the contour of the pharyngeal wall, progression of the bolus into the esophagus, and penetration of contrast material into the larynx or trachea.[5] It is a sensitive screening test for pharyngeal dysfunction, although etiologic diagnosis generally requires additional studies. Videoradiography is also invaluable for rehabilitation, where it is used to determine empirically the therapeutic efficacy of altering bolus consistency, patient posture, or other factors associated with feeding.[6]

Some weaknesses of videoradiography are that it is limited in temporal and spacial resolution, difficult to quantify, limited to a two-dimensional view of a three-dimensional performance, and fails to show the details of pharyngeal wall motion, particularly motion that is parallel to the wall.[7]

MANOMETRY

A manometer is a device for measuring the pressure in a fluid. Manometry has proven utility in the evaluation of esophageal motor dysfunction,[8] but its use in the pharynx is controversial. Manometry is used to study the mechanical pumping action of the pharynx. The amplitude of pressure spikes on the recording is believed to reflect the adequacy of pharyngeal constriction, and their absence signals motor dysfunction. There is widespread agreement about the general appearance of manometric recordings from the normal pharynx and pharyngoesophageal (PE) segment (Fig. 20-1). However, the details of these complex wave forms are poorly understood because of numerous technical problems. There have been difficulties in designing appropriate manometers, and motions of the pharynx relative to the manometer complicate this problem.[9] There is confusion over the difference between a true hydrodynamic pressure and the force

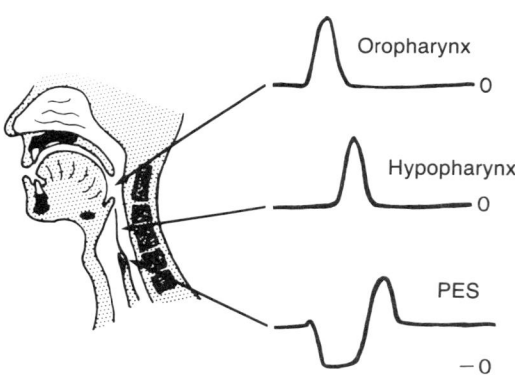

Figure 20-1 Schematic representation of pharyngeal manometric recording. During resting conditions, the pharynx is open (via the nasal airway) and is at atmospheric pressure ("0" pressure on this figure), whereas a high pressure zone is maintained in the pharyngoesophageal segment (PES) by virtue of the wall contracting tonically around the manometer. Swallowing elicits a wave of contraction that propagates through the pharynx, whereas the PES undergoes a brief cessation of contraction. With permission from Dodds WJ, Kahrilas PJ, Dent J, Hogan WJ. Considerations about pharyngeal manometry. Dysphagia 1987; 1:209-214. Courtesy of Springer Verlag, New York.

of the pharyngeal wall squeezing the transducer. The latter circumstance arises whenever the device is in a potential space, e.g., the pharyngoesophageal segment between swallows.[10] Accurate manometric recordings may someday provide a reliable quantitative method for assessing pharyngeal motor dysfunction, but there are substantial technical limitations at present.

ELECTROMYOGRAPHY

Electromyography (EMG) is the recording of electrical activity from muscle. Two major types of EMG have been utilized to study pharyngeal swallowing. The first type is analysis of individual myoelectric potentials, usually recorded with intramuscular needle electrodes, to evaluate the integrity of the motor unit (Fig. 20-2). This is the usual procedure in diagnostic clinical EMG studies. The second type of EMG, usually performed with surface electrodes or with fine wire intramuscular electrodes, is analysis of the timing and quantity of electrical activity in specific muscles during swallowing (Fig. 20-3). This method is useful for studying the biomechanics of swallowing. Since the quantity of myoelectric activity is directly related to the force of muscle contraction, EMG provides insight into the specific effector mechanisms underlying normal and pathologic swallowing. If a muscle is electrically active during a motion, it may play a role in producing the motion.[11,12]

Reliable techniques have been developed for the positioning of EMG electrodes to examine many of the muscles of pharyngeal swallowing. Seven of these have been examined in our laboratory: the genioglossus, the geniohyoid, the palatopharyngeus, the thyroarytenoid, the pharyngeal constrictors, and the cricopharyngeus (Table 20-1).[13,14] We use a functional component model to describe the kinesiology of pharyngeal swallowing. The six component functions are oral transport, closure of the velopharyngeal isthmus, elevation of the larynx and pharynx, closure of the larynx, opening of the pharyngoesophageal segment, and propulsion of the bolus into the esophagus. The actions of each of the seven muscles have been analyzed in relation to each component function (Table 20-2).

Clinical applications for pharyngeal EMG include differentiation of nerve from muscle disease and of upper from lower motor neuron disease, localization of the site of cranial nerve pathology, detection of subclinical disease, and differentiation of weakness from anatomic fixation (e.g., by adhesions).

Several technical problems impede pharyngeal EMG.[14] There is difficulty in positioning electrodes in deeply-placed muscles. Motion artifacts may obscure myoelectric signals. Controlling the force of contraction is extremely difficult in some of these muscles. The presence of EMG electrodes may alter myoelectric activity patterns, and the scarcity of normative data makes it difficult to interpret clinical findings. In spite of these difficulties, clinically useful data can be obtained by the experienced electromyographer.

CONCLUSIONS

It is clear that many technical problems remain in the diagnostic examination of pharyngeal swallowing. Current research includes improvement of recording techniques for EMG and manometry, development of quantitative methods for measuring pharyngeal motion, assessment of the changes in pharyngeal function associated with normal aging, and a combination of the various approaches in order to permit simultaneous measurement of displacements, pressures, and muscle activity. The goal is

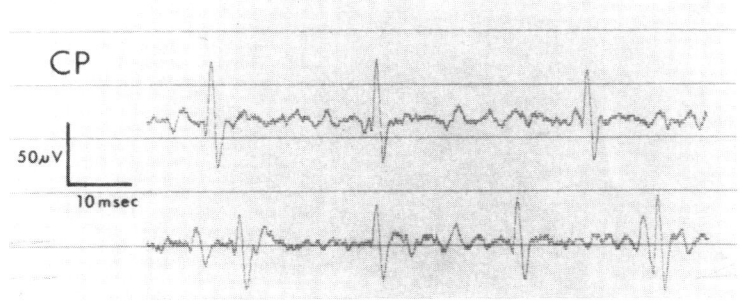

Figure 20-2 Individual myoelectric potentials (motor unit action potentials) recorded in the tonically-contracting cricopharyngeus (CP) muscles by using bipolar suction electrodes. With permission from Tanaka E, Palmer JB, Siebens AA. Bipolar suction electrodes for pharyngeal electromyography. Dysphagia 1986; 1:39-40. Courtesy of Springer Verlag, New York.

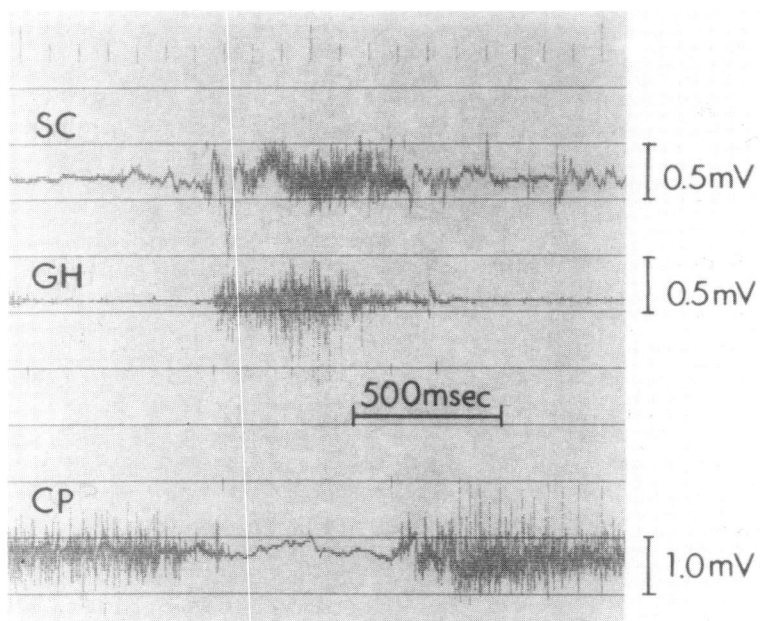

Figure 20–3 Myoelectric activity during a water swallow, recorded simultaneously in the superior constrictor (SC), geniohyoid (GH), and cricopharyngeus (CP) muscles by using hooked wire electrodes. With permission from Palmer JB, Tanaka E, Siebens AA. Electromyography of the pharyngeal musculature: technical considerations. Arch Phys Med Rehabil, in press.

TABLE 20–1 Actions of Seven Muscles of Pharyngeal Swallowing

Muscle	Action
Genioglossus	Depresses and protrudes tongue
Geniohyoid	Pulls hyoid bone ventrad
Tongue intrinsics	Change shape of tongue surface
Palatopharyngeus	Approximates palatopharyngeal folds, elevates pharynx and larynx
Thyroarytenoid	Tenses vocal folds
Pharyngeal constrictors	Constrict the pharynx on its contents
Cricopharyngeus	Compresses the pharyngoesophageal segment against the cricoid cartilage

TABLE 20–2 Muscles that Contribute to Each Component Function

Function	GG	GH	IT	PP	TA	PC	CP
Oral transport	+	+	+				
Close velopharyngeal isthmus				+		+	
Elevate larynx and pharynx		+		+			
Close larynx				+		+	
Open pharyngo-esophageal segment		+		+			(−)*
Propel bolus				+		+	+

* Inhibiting the tonic contraction of the cricopharyngeus muscle contributes to opening the pharyngoesophageal segment.
Genioglossus=GG, Geniohyoid=GH, Intrinsinc tongue=IT, Palatopharyngeus=PP, Thyroarytenoid=TA, Pharyngeal constrictor=PC, Cricopharyngeus=CP

the development of a biomechanical model for pharyngeal swallowing. It is our belief that many of the technical problems will be solved within the next few years and that substantial body of knowledge will be generated. Only then will the diagnosis and treatment of swallowing disorders have a sound scientific basis.

SUMMARY

Numerous methods have been used to evaluate the pharyngeal stage of swallowing. This is a brief review and critique of three dynamic methods: videoradiography, manometry, and electromyography. The clinical utility and limitations of each method are discussed, with special attention to EMG. The physiology of normal and abnormal pharyngeal swallowing is an area of active clinical research.

Supported in part by a Clinical Investigator Development Award (1K08NS01211-01) from the NINCDS, a Clinician-Scientist Award from the Johns Hopkins University, and a Young Investigator Award from the Physical Medicine and Rehabilitation Education and Research Foundation.

References

1. Miller AJ. Deglutition. Physiol Rev 1982; 62:129–184.
2. Donner MW, Silbiger ML. Cinefluorographic analysis of pharyngeal swallowing in neuromuscular disorders. Am J Med Sci 1966; 251:600–616.
3. Miller RM. Evaluation of swallowing disorders. In: Groher ME, ed. Dysphagia: diagnosis and management. Boston: Butterworths, 1984:85.
4. Jones B, Krammer SS, Donner MW. Dynamic imaging of the pharynx. Gastrointest Radiol 1985; 10:213–224.
5. Logemann J. Evaluation and treatment of swallowing disorders. San Diego: College-Hill Press, 1983.
6. Siebens AA, Linden P. Dynamic imaging for swallowing reeducation. Gastrointest Radiol 1985; 10:251–253.
7. Palmer JB, Tanaka E, Siebens AA. Motions of the posterior pharyngeal wall in swallowing. Laryngoscope 1988; 98:414–417.
8. Code CF, Creamer B, Schlegel JF, Olsen AM, Donoghue FE, Anderson HA. An atlas of esophageal motility in health and disease. Springfield, IL: Charles C. Thomas, 1958.
9. Dodds WJ, Kahrilas PJ, Dent J, Hogan WJ. Considerations about pharyngeal manometry. Dysphagia 1987; 1:209–214.
10. Brasseur JG. A fluid mechanical perspective on esophageal bolus transport. Dysphagia 1987; 2:32–39.
11. Kimura J. Electrodiagnosis in diseases of nerve and muscle. Philadelphia: F.A. Davis, 1983.
12. Basmajian JV. Muscles alive. 4th ed. Baltimore: Williams and Wilkens, 1978.
13. Tanaka E, Palmer JB, Siebens AA. Bipolar suction electrodes for pharyngeal electromyography. Dysphagia 1986; 1:39–40.
14. Palmer JB, Tanaka E, Siebens AA. Electromyography of the pharyngeal musculature: technical considerations. Arch Phys Med Rehabil, in press.

Chapter Twenty-One

AGING-RELATED CHANGES IN PERIPHERAL NERVES IN THE HEAD AND NECK

LESLIE T. MALMGREN, Ph.D.

The elderly experience disorders of swallowing and of mechanisms preventing aspiration[1-6] as well as of the quality of vocalization.[7-11] In view of the complexity of these physiologic systems and of the requirement for precise interaction of the component sensory and motor systems for the achievement of normal performance,[12,13] it is perhaps not surprising that age-related dysfunctions are observed in the head and neck. Since a number of studies have reported age-related morphologic and physiologic changes in a variety of peripheral nerves,[14-24] it is likely that nerves in the head and neck are also affected by age, although there is little specific information available. However, the degree and nature of age-related changes in peripheral nerves vary between different nerves and are influenced by such variables as the pattern of nerve activity, the physiologic function of the nerve, the length of the axon, and the degree of age-related exposure to trauma,[25-31] and it is essential to determine the extent and characteristics of age-related changes in peripheral nerves in the head and neck. These data, in combination with information concerning parallel changes in the central nervous system and in the end-organs, should ultimately permit the elucidation of the pathogenetic mechanisms responsible for these disorders. This review summarizes the age-related changes that have been reported for peripheral nerves in general, with an emphasis on the data available for aging nerves in the head and neck.

PHYSIOLOGIC CHANGES IN AGING PERIPHERAL NERVE

It has been reported that the elderly display various clinical manifestations of an aging peripheral nervous system, including decreased vibratory sensitivity,[32-34] loss of touch sensation,[35-37] loss of the sensitivity of the cornea to air puffs,[36] and diminished tendon reflexes with evidence of peripheral causes.[38] The number of studies on head and neck systems is more limited. However, it has been reported that there is a six-fold increase in reflex glottic closure threshold from the second to the eighth and ninth decade.[1] Human electrophysiologic studies have indicated an age-related reduction of the maximum conduction velocity in sensory fibers, as well as an age-related drop in the amplitude of sensory potentials.[14,23] The conduction velocity in human motor fibers also shows a decrease with age.[17,18] Studies of conduction velocity in motor and sensory nerves of animal models do not show a decrease in conduction velocity with increasing age.[39,40]

MORPHOLOGIC CHANGES IN AGING PERIPHERAL NERVE

Nerve Fiber Loss

In human nerves, there is a general tendency for the loss of myelinated nerve fibers with increasing age (Fig. 21–1).[15,19,22,24] However, it should be stressed that there is typically a great deal of overlap in the individual values observed for young adult versus old individuals.[15,22,24] Furthermore, the most extensive losses of myelinated fibers have been reported for the anterior tibial nerve of the foot,[19] where it is likely that long-term trauma from badly fitting shoes accounts for an additional loss of myelinated fibers.[19,41] Reports of an age-related loss of myelinated fibers in animal models are less consistent (Fig. 21–2). Quantitative studies on myelinated fiber count in the rat soleus,[42] tibial and medial plantar,[43] and phrenic nerves[40] have not indicated an age-related change. Differing results have been obtained for the rat sciatic nerve: a quantitative study indicates the lack of an age-related change in the myelinated fiber count with age;[39] a qualitative study indicates a decreased fiber count; electrophysiologic data indicate an age-related reduction in the number of motor units.[44] In addition, a qualitative study reported extensive degeneration of fibers in the dorsal and ventral roots of aging rats,[25] and a quantitative study on the mouse posterior tibial nerve has indicated an age-related decrease in myelinated fibers.[45] The results of quantitative studies on the rat recurrent laryngeal[46] and superior laryngeal nerves[47] indicate no statistically significant age-

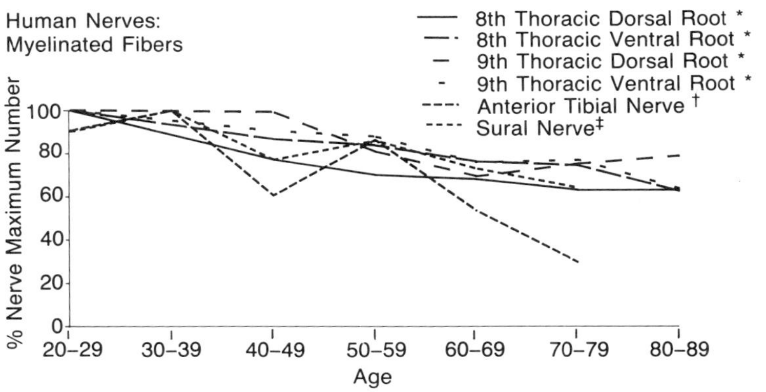

Figure 21-1 Graph shows general tendency for loss of myelinated nerve fibers with increasing age.
* Data from Corbin KB, Gardner ED. Decrease in number of myelinated fibers in human spinal roots with age. Anat Rec 1937; 68:63-74.
† Data from Swallow M. Fibre size and content of the anterior tibial nerve of the foot. J Neurol Neurosurg Psychiatry 1966; 29:205-213.
‡ Data from Jacobs JM, Love S. Qualitative and quantitative morphology of human sural nerve at different ages. Brain 1985; 108:897-924.

related changes in the numbers of either myelinated or unmyelinated nerve fibers.

Schwann Cell Changes

Schwann cells in aging human nerves display a wide variety of pathologic changes. These include an increase in Reich granules, demyelination, remyelination, reduction of mean internodal length, abnormally thin myelin, and disproportionately thick myelin.[20,21,24,48,49] Aging peripheral nerves of animal models also show extensive Schwann cell changes, including extremely disordered myelin ("myelin bubbling"), paranodal and segmental demyelination, remyelination, and an increase in Hirano bodies.[25,26,50-54] Similar changes have been reported to occur in the rat recurrent[46] and superior laryngeal nerves.[47]

An increase in the amount of adaxonal Schwann cell cytoplasm (Schwann cell cytoplasm adjacent to axon) is characteristic of axons undergoing degeneration during toxic neuropathies or nerve trauma,[55] and it is thought that these "fingers" of Schwann cell cytoplasm sequester and remove organelles from the axoplasm.[55] Qualitative studies have noted an age-related increase in adaxonal Schwann cell cytoplasm in rat plantar and tibial nerves[52,53] and in human sural nerves.[20] Recently, stereologic techniques have revealed a statistically significant and substantial increase in the volume fraction of adaxonal Schwann cell cytoplasm in the rat superior laryngeal nerve.[47]

Changes in the Size of the Nerve and Endoneurial Extracellular Space

One of the most consistent changes reported for aging human peripheral nerves is an increase in the percentage of the cross-sectional area of the nerve occupied by the endoneurial extracellular space.[16,19,24] This leads to a large increase in the total cross-sectional area of the nerve.[19] An increase in the size of the endoneurial space has also been reported to occur in animal models.[53] In stereologic studies on the rat recurrent laryngeal nerve[46] as well as in those on the superior laryngeal nerve,[47] there was not a statistically significant increase in the volume fraction of the endoneurial space in 25-month-old rats (mean survival for these rats is 24.6 months).[56] However, both of these nerves showed a statistically significant increase in this variable in 29- to 31-month-old rats.

Changes in Blood Vessels

Age-related changes in blood vessels are commonly reported for human peripheral nerves. Cottrell[16] described vascular changes in several aging human nerves that included endothelial proliferation, medial fibrosis and hyalinization, and, in the later decades, vascular occlusion. Ultrastructural studies on human nerves have revealed an age-related increased reduplication of the endothelial and pericytic basement membranes with an absence of membrane thickening.[24] It is indicated that there is

	Recurrent Laryngeal Nerve *		Superior Laryngeal Nerve (Int. Brn.) †	
	Old	Very Old	Old	Very Old
Number of Myelinated Fibers	No Change	No Change	No Change	No Change
Number of Unmyelinated Fibers	No Change	No Change	No Change	No Change
Mean Myelinated Fiber Size	No Change	No Change	No Change	No Change
Mean Unmyelinated Fiber Size	No Change	No Change	No Change	No Change
Fibers with Thin Myelin	↑	↑	No Change	No Change
Fibers with Pathology	↑	↑	↑	↑
Mitochondrial Volume Fraction in Axon	No Change	No Change	No Change	No Change
Microtubule Numerical Density in Axon	No Change	No Change	No Change	No Change
Neurofilament Numerical Density in Axon	No Change	No Change	↓	↓
Endoneurial Extracellular Space Volume Fraction	No Change	↑	No Change	↑
Adaxonal Schwann Cell Cytoplasm Volume Fraction			↑	↑

Figure 21–2 Summary of aging-related changes in recurrent laryngeal nerve and superior laryngeal nerve in animal model.
* Data from Malmgren LT, Ringwood MA. Aging of the recurrent laryngeal nerve: an ultrastructural morphometric study. In: Fujimura O, ed. Vocal physiology: voice production, mechanisms and functions. New York: Raven Press, in press.
† Data from Rosenberg SI, Malmgren LT, Woo P. Aging-related ultrastructural changes in the internal branch of the rat superior laryngeal nerve. Eleventh midwinter meeting of the Association for Research in Otolaryngology. Abstracts 1988; 189.

no change in the blood vessels in aging mouse posterior tibial nerves.[45] However, it is reported that in aging rat peripheral nerves, the adventitia of small blood vessels often appeared thickened in nerves showing other pathologic changes.[26]

Perineurium

In human peripheral nerves, light microscopic studies have reported an age-related increase in the overall thickness of the perineurium,[16] and ultrastructural studies have indicated an age-related thickening of the basement membrane of the perineurium.[24] This differs from the thickening in the perineurial basement membrane seen in diabetics where this change is observed in the inner layers of the perineurium,[57] since this occurs in the outermost layers of the perineurium in aging nerves.[24] The perineurium is a component of the blood-nerve barrier, and it acts both as a passive diffusion barrier[58,59] and also probably as a metabolically active barrier. It has a high sodium-potassium adenosine triphosphatase (ATPase) activity and is thought to regulate the ionic composition of the endoneurium.[60,61] It has been suggested that a dysfunction in the capacity of the perineurium to regulate the ionic composition of the endoneurium may be involved in the pathogenesis of the endoneurial edema seen in diabetics.[61,62] Further studies are necessary to determine if age-related changes in the perineurium contribute in this way to the changes characteristic of aging peripheral nerves.

Oxidative Metabolism and Mitochondrial Content

Oxidative metabolism provides the primary support for energy expenditures in peripheral nerves under resting conditions.[63] Since the mitochondrion is the organelle primarily responsible for this process, a number of studies have examined the mitochondrial content of axons in aging peripheral nerves. Samorajski[45] reported a decrease in the number of mitochondria per unit micrograph area in the aging mouse posterior tibial nerve. On the other hand, stereologic studies carried out on the rat recurrent laryngeal nerve[46] and the rat superior laryngeal nerve[47] have indicated that there is not a statistically significant age-related change in the percentage of the volume of the axon occupied by mitochondria. In considering these differing results, it is important to note that estimations of mitochondrial content on the basis of the number of mitochondria per unit micrograph area may also reflect age-related changes in mitochondrial size, shape, or orientation, rather than the actual numerical density or volume density of mitochondria in the tissue.[64] Stereologic determinations of the mitochondrial volume fraction are easier to interpret since they are not compromised by these potential artifacts. Nevertheless, it is also possible that age affects the mitochondrial contents of the mouse posterior tibial nerve differently than that of the rat recurrent and superior laryngeal nerves. Age-related changes in the activity patterns of each of these nerves may not be equivalent, in view of their extremely different functions, and the degree of aging can be influenced by system-specific variables such as activity.[28,30]

Microtubules and Neurofilaments

Microtubules and neurofilaments play important roles in axonal transport and intracellular support.[65,66] It has been reported that slow axonal transport decreases with age,[67,68] while the rate of fast axonal transport remains constant with increasing age, although the variance between animals increases with age.[69] Neither the rat recurrent laryngeal nerve[46] nor the rat superior laryngeal nerve[47] shows significant age-related changes in the numerical density of microtubules. However, a significant age-related reduction in the numerical density of neurofilaments is seen in the rat superior laryngeal nerve,[47] but not in the rat recurrent laryngeal nerve.[46] Studies on other systems have also reported age-specific microtubule and neurofilament contents that differ between systems. In the mouse, the neurofilament content in the pyramidal tract decreases with age,[70] but it shows no age-related change in the posterior tibial nerve,[45] and the microtubule content shows an age-related increase in the pyramidal tract,[70] but not in the posterior tibial nerve.[45] These differential changes may result in corresponding system-specific changes in axonal transport and intracellular support, but further studies in a variety of different peripheral nerves are necessary to examine this possibility.

CONCLUSION

With the exception of the recent studies reviewed concerning the morphologic changes observed in the aging recurrent laryngeal and superior laryngeal nerves of the rat animal model,[46,47] it appears that little is known about the system-specific characteristics of aging of peripheral nerves in the head and neck. These systems play complex and crucial roles in deglutition, respiration, and vocalization,[12,13] and although more data is needed with respect to the clinical characteristics of aging in these systems, the available data suggest that a variety of substantial dysfunctions in these systems are common in the elderly.[1-11] Some types of morphologic studies can be carried out on aging peripheral nerves in the human head and neck, and studies of this type are absolutely essential since it is unlikely that any animal model precisely reflects the exact changes seen in the corresponding human nerves. However, the range of morphologic techniques applicable to the study of aging human nerves in the head and neck is severely compromised by postmortem, paraneoplastic, and other pathologic changes in the available sources of human tissue. This review has pointed out a variety of age-related changes in the peripheral nerves in the head and neck of animal models that appear to parallel those reported for human nerves, and experimental studies concerning the pathogenetic basis for these changes should be productive. In addition to the need for reliable, quantitative morphologic data concerning the aging of peripheral nerves in the head and neck, comparable quantitative basic physiologic data is also essential. Finally, it should be emphasized that age-related disabilities in head and neck functions almost certainly also involve changes in sensory receptors and muscles, as well as changes in the central nervous system, and these research areas must also be the focus of future attention.

References

1. Pontoppidan H, Beecher HK. Progressive loss of protective reflexes in the airway with advance of age. JAMA 1960; 174:2209-2213.
2. Gelperin A. Sudden death in an elderly population from aspiration of food. J Am Geriatr Soc 1974; 22:135-136.
3. Zavala DC. The threat of aspiration pneumonia in the aged. Geriatrics 1977; 32:46-51.
4. Wolkove N, Kreisman H, Cohen C, Frank H. Occult foreign-body aspiration in adults. JAMA 1982; 248:1350-1352.
5. Ekberg O, Wahlgren L. Dysfunction of pharyngeal swallowing: a cineradiographic investigation in 854 dysphagial patients. Acta Radiol Diagn 1985; 26:389-395.
6. Braman SS, Davis SM. Wheezing in the elderly. Geriat Clin North Am 1986; 2:269-283.
7. Mysak ED. Pitch and duration characteristics of older males. J Speech Hear Res 1959; 2:46-54.
8. McGlone RE, Hollien H. Vocal pitch characteristics of aged women. J Speech Hear Res 1963; 6:164-170.
9. Hollien H, Shipp T. Speaking fundamental frequency and chronological age in males. J Speech Hear Res 1972; 15:155-159.
10. Honjo I, Isshiki N. Laryngoscopic and voice characteristics of aged persons. Arch Otolaryngol 1980; 106:149-150.
11. Mueller PB, Sweeney RJ, Baribeau LJ. Acoustic and morphological study of the senescent voice. Ear Nose Throat J 1984; 63:71-75.
12. Wyke BD, Kirchner JA. Neurology of the larynx. In: Hinchcliffe R, Harrison D, eds. Scientific foundations of otolaryngology. London: W. Heinemann, 1976:546.
13. Miller AJ. Deglutition. Physiol Rev 1982; 62:129-184.
14. Buchthal F, Rosenfalck A. Evoked action potentials and conduction velocity in human sensory nerves. Brain Res 1966; 3:1-402.
15. Corbin KB, Gardner ED. Decrease in number of myelinated fibers in human spinal roots with age. Anat Rec 1937; 68:63-74.
16. Cottrell L. Histologic variations with age in apparently normal peripheral nerve trunks. Arch Neurol Psychiat 1940; 43:1138-1150.
17. Wagman IH, Lesse H. Maximum conduction velocities of motor fibers of ulnar nerve in human subjects of various ages and sizes. J Neurophysiol 1952; 15:235-244.
18. Norris AH, Shock NW, Wagman IH. Age changes in the maximum conduction velocity of motor fibers of human ulnar nerves. J Appl Physiol 1953; 5:589-593.
19. Swallow M. Fibre size and content of the anterior tibial nerve of the foot. J Neurol Neurosurg Psychiatry 1966; 29:205-213.
20. Ochoa J, Mair WG. The normal sural nerve in man. II. Changes in the axons and Schwann cells due to aging. Acta Neuropathol (Berl) 1969; 13:217-239.
21. Stevens JC, Lofgren EP, Dyck PJ. Histometric evaluation of branches of peroneal nerve: technique for combined biopsy of muscle nerve and cutaneous nerve. Brain Res 1973; 52:37-59.
22. Kawamura Y, Okazaki H, O'Brien PC, Dyck PC. Lumbar motoneurons of man. I. Number and diameter histogram of alpha and gamma axons of ventral root. J Neuropathol Exp Neurol 1977; 36:853-860.
23. Buchthal F, Rosenfalck A, Behse F. Sensory potentials of normal and diseased nerves. In: Dyck PJ, Thomas PK, Lambert EH, Bunge R, eds. Peripheral neuropathy. Vol. 1. Philadelphia: WB Saunders, 1984:981.
24. Jacobs JM, Love S. Qualitative and quantitative morphology of human sural nerve at different ages. Brain 1985; 108:897-924.
25. Gilmore SA. Spinal nerve root degeneration in aging laboratory rats: a light microscope study. Anat Rec 1972; 174:251-258.
26. Steenis G, Kroes R. Changes in the nervous system and musculature of old rats. Vet Pathol 1971; 8:320-332.
27. Tucek S, Gutman E. Choline acetyltransferase activity in muscles of old rats. Exp Neurol 1973; 38:349-360.
28. Samorajski T, Rolsten C. Nerve fiber hypertrophy in posterior tibial nerves of mice in response to voluntary running activity during aging. J Comp Neurol 1975; 159:553-558.
29. Rosenheimer JL, Smith DO. Differential changes in the endplate architecture of functionally diverse muscles during aging. J Neurophysiol 1985; 53:1567-1581.
30. Rosenheimer JL. Effects of chronic stress and exercise on age-related changes in endplate architecture. J Neurophysiol 1985; 53:1582-1589.
31. Spencer PS, Schaumburg HH. Experimental models of primary axonal disease induced by toxic chemicals. In: Dyck PJ, Thomas PK, Lambert EH, Bunge R, eds. Peripheral neuropathy. Vol. 1. Philadelphia: WB Saunders, 1984:636.
32. Skre H. Neurological signs in a normal population. Acta Neurol Scand 1972; 48:575-606.

33. Steiness I. Vibratory perception in normal subjects. Acta Med Scand 1957; 158:315–325.
34. Goff GB, Rosner BS, Detre T, Kennard D. Vibration perception in normal man and medical patients. J Neurol Neurosurg Psychiatry 1965; 28:503–509.
35. Dyck PJ, Schultz PW, O'Brien PC. Quantitation of touch-pressure sensation. Arch Neurol 1972; 26:465–473.
36. Millodot M. The influence of age on the sensation of the cornea. Invest Ophthalmol Vis Sci 1977; 16:240–243.
37. Bruce MF. The relation of tactile thresholds to histology in the fingers of elderly people. J Neurol Neurosurg Psychiatry 1980; 43:730–734.
38. Larsson L. Morphological and functional characteristics of the aging skeletal muscle in man. Acta Physiol Scand 1978; Suppl 457:1–36.
39. Birren JE, Wall PD. Age changes in conduction velocity, refractory period, number of fibers, connective tissue space and blood vessels in sciatic nerve of rats. J Comp Neurol 1956; 104:1–16.
40. Smith DO, Rosenheimer JL. Factors governing speed of action potential conduction and neuromuscular transmission in aged rats. Exp Neurol 1984; 83:358–366.
41. Gairns FW, Garven HSD, Smith G. The digital nerves and the nerve endings in progressive obliterative vascular disease of the leg. Scott Med J 1960; 5:382–391.
42. Gutmann E, Hanzlikova V. Motor unit in old age. Nature 1966; 209:921–922.
43. Sharma AK, Bajada S, Thomas PK. Age changes in the tibial and plantar nerves of the rat. J Anat 1980; 130:417–428.
44. Caccia MR, Harris JB, Johnson MA. Morphology and physiology of skeletal muscle in aging rodents. Muscle Nerve 1979; 2:202–212.
45. Samorajski T. Age differences in the morphology of posterior tibial nerves of mice. J Comp Neurol 1974; 157:439–452.
46. Malmgren LT, Ringwood MA. Aging of the recurrent laryngeal nerve: an ultrastructural morphometric study. In: Fujimura O, ed. Vocal physiology: voice production, mechanisms and functions. New York: Raven Press, in press.
47. Rosenberg SI, Malmgren LT, Woo P. Aging-related ultrastructural changes in the internal branch of the rat superior laryngeal nerve. Eleventh midwinter meeting of the Association for Research in Otolaryngology. Abstracts 1988; 189.
48. Vizoso AD. The relationship between internodal length and growth in human nerves. J Anat 1950; 84:342–353.
49. Lascelles RG, Thomas PK. Changes due to age in internodal length in the sural nerve of man. J Neurol Neurosurg Psychiatry 1966; 29:40–44.
50. Berg BN, Wolf A, Simms HS. Degenerative lesions of spinal roots and peripheral nerves in aging rats. Gerontology 1962; 6:72–80.
51. Griffiths IR, Duncan ID. Age changes in the dorsal and ventral lumbar nerve roots of dogs. Acta Neuropathol 1975; 32:75–85.
52. Thomas PK, King HM, Sharma AK. Changes with age in the peripheral nerves of the rat. Acta Neuropathol 1980; 52:1–6.
53. Grover-Johnson N, Spencer PS. Peripheral nerve abnormalities in aging rats. J Neuropathol Exp Neurol 1981; 40:155–165.
54. Krinke G. Spinal radiculoneuropathy in aging rats. Demyelination secondary to neuronal dwindling? Acta Neuropathol 1977; 59:63–69.
55. Spencer PS, Thomas PK. Ultrastructural studies with the dying back process. II. The sequestration and removal by Schwann cells and oligodendrocytes of organelles from normal and diseased axons. J Neurocytol 1974; 2:763–783.
56. Festing MFW, Blackmore DK. Life span of specific-pathogen-free (MRC category 4) mice and rats. Lab Anim 1971; 5:179–192.
57. Johnson PC, Brendel K, Meezan E. Human diabetic perineurial cell basement membrane thickening. Lab Invest 1981; 44:265–270.
58. Olsson Y, Reese TS. Permeability of vasa nervorum and perineurium in mouse sciatic nerve studied by fluorescence and electron microscopy. J Neuropathol Exp Neurol 1971; 30:105–119.
59. Malmgren LT, Olsson Y. Differences between the peripheral and the central nervous system in permeability to sodium fluorescein. J Comp Neurol 1980; 191:103–117.
60. Shanthaveerappa TR, Bourne GH. The "perineurial epithelium": a metabolically active, continuous, protoplasmic cell barrier surrounding peripheral nerve fasciculi. J Anat 1962; 196:527–537.
61. Llewelyn JG, Thomas PK. Perineurial sodium-potassium-ATPase activity in streptozotocin-diabetic rats. Exp Neurol 1987; 97:375–382.
62. Jakobsen J. Peripheral nerves in early experimental diabetes. Expansion of the endoneurial space as a cause of increased water content. Diabetologia 1978; 14:113–119.
63. Greene DA, Winegrad AI. Effects of acute experimental diabetes on composite energy metabolism in peripheral nerve axons and Schwann cells. Diabetes 1981; 30:967–974.
64. Gundersen HJG. Stereology of arbitrary particles. J Microsc 1986; 143:3–45.
65. Ochs S. Basic properties of axoplasmic transport. In: Dyck PJ, Thomas PK, Lambert EH, Bunge R, eds. Peripheral neuropathy. Vol. 1. Philadelphia: WB Saunders, 1984:453.
66. Pleasure D. The structural proteins of peripheral nerve. In: Dyck PJ, Thomas PK, Lambert EH, Bunge R, eds. Peripheral neuropathy. Vol. 1. Philadelphia: WB Saunders, 1984:441.
67. Komiya Y. Slowing with age of the rat of slow axonal flow in bifurcating axons or rat dorsal root ganglion. Brain Res 1980; 183:477–480.
68. Jablecki C, Brimijoin S. Axoplasmic transport of choline acetyltransferase activity in mice: effect of age and neurotomy. J Neurochem 1975; 25:583–593.
69. Ochs S. Effect of maturation and aging on the rate of fast axoplasmic transport in mammalian nerve. Prog Brain Res 1973; 40:349–362.
70. Samorajski T, Friede RL, Ordy JM. Age differences in the ultrastructure of axons in the pyramidal tract of the mouse. J Gerontol 1971; 26:542–551.

ONCOLOGY AND AGING

INTRODUCTION

JOHN CONLEY, M.D.

First of all, I would like to state how pleased I am to be a member of this meeting and to be able to experience the new thrusts and the new developments and participate in the excitement of what is really going on. I was delighted with the introduction on the biology of aging, which is really the biology of life itself. Then the presentation moved from that subtly into the effect that this process has on people and the humanistic approach to it, the recognition of individual autonomy. It just kept escalating and building in an exciting way. The presentation had a beautiful rhythm to it, up into the consequences of the aging process. I am a bit overwhelmed by data and statistics and by some charts and utility of the information that is coming in, planning a force and energy of the forward movement that you can feel. Then, of course, there is always a certain amount of manipulation. This manipulation casts light into the future and helps us to understand the meaning of this experience in geriatrics, which is a new, highly recognized situation that is becoming well-organized, and also to understand the direction it is taking. Most of the things of the past 2 days have concerned themselves with our special senses. The only sense that was left out, and I must say common sense was not left out, was the sense of the eye. The others of balance, hearing, taste, smell, swallowing, speaking, and touching are what we are concentrating on at this particular meeting. There is a lot more, of course, to the aging process than that, but this is a focal point. Some other things were mentioned such as locomotion, dizziness, falling down, and eating. Nobody has mentioned sex; I'm surprised! A large part of this has been associated with tests and analysis, and there isn't any question about it: modern man is moving toward a technical type of analytical definition of his existence. I can't tell you whether that is good or bad, but these tests have two fascinations for me. One is the mystical fascination as to whether they mean anything (and, you know, about 80 percent of the tests that are proposed are eventually relegated to the realm of oblivion), but no matter how many tests are done, or how much they cost, one test seems to lead to another test. Indeed, the results of one test might lead to 10 additional tests, and this is occurrent again in a rhythm, the movement of investigation; this is absolutely essential. These tests relate to perceptions; you can't eliminate that. They relate to function; that's all part of the living process. Then you come down to the more realistic matter of equipment. What is equipment? What is the gadget? What is the thing? Then there is the pharmacology. How many pills are you going to take? What kinds of chemicals are you going to take? Then, of course, in the end, there is always the technical thing because in all of these enterprises you need technical experience. You have to have high class carpenters and high class plumbers and high class doctors working in laboratories on animals and with pharmaceutical agents and ultimately with people. Now, this brings me to another focus that I'm experiencing during this geriatric ordeal, and that is cancer because my assignment here was on oncology in the older age group. I would like to put in something we have been missing a little bit, and righteously so up to this time. That is that cancer brings a heavy shadow with it. It brings a silence and some moans and groans, but cancer is life-threatening and, in many instances, it is the beginning of the dying process for that human being. I would like to now come down the funnel into the cancer part of this experience. I will make just a few more introductory remarks, and Dr. Cantrell and Dr. Wolfe will amplify the meaning of this as far as the geriatric situation is concerned.

The need for oncologic services in the geriatric group is broad and multifocal. It is real because we are dealing with a potential life-threatening disease that has its highest incidence in the geriatric group. The human dimensions of this condition are that it afflicts an area of the body that is associated with basic function and aesthetics, thus inserting itself poignantly into the quality of life. The societal aspects of this condition are its needs for resources and human attention.

There are approximately 70,000 cases of cancer in the area of the head and neck every year in the United States, and the average mean age of those suffering from these problems is 59 years. Eighty percent of these cancers are of the squamous cell type, and they occur primarily in the aerodigestive system. The remaining 20 percent are adenocarcinomas and sarcomas, and they occur in glandular tissue or mesodermal elements in the area of the head and neck. The average age of the squamous cell group is slightly over the 59-year mean, and the glandular mesodermal group slightly less than the 59-year mean. The overall 5-year survival rate is approximately 67 percent in the management of localized disease (Stage 1) and 30 percent in those with regional metastasis (Stage 2). The cure rate for Stage 3 in patients with distant hemogenous metastasis is miniscule.

One cannot escape the impact of societal forces in the etiology of many of these conditions. When the still enigmatic genetic factors are eliminated, we come into the etiologic aspects of the living condition, namely, noxious pollutants in air, water, and food; harmful social habits of smoking and drinking; and undesirable exposure in the working place relative to mining, coke ovens, woodworking, the preparation of leather products, work associated with phosphorus, and exposure to radioactive substances, to mention only a few. The hazards of exposure to sun and the deprivations of malnutrition are so ubiquitous that we have begun to consider these factors as almost normative.

The specific implications to the patient are an alteration in some of the basic physiologic functions of swallowing, breathing, eating, and speaking. Many of these alterations are crippling to various degrees and are concentrated in certain essential anatomical structures, and the attack on these structures affects aesthetics, basic physiologic activity, the autonomy of the person, and the quality of life to varying degrees. When this is integrated into a functional therapeutic process that includes surgery, irradiation, and chemotherapy as a specific attack on certain aspects of the body, with its response, and the concomitant involvement of the medical and paramedical personnel along with the necessary administrative factors, there begins to develop some identification of the magnitude of the problem. When this is combined with the significant increase in longevity that is happening today, the rising volume of older people, and its effect on society, it places a special emphasis on otolaryngology and cancer of the head and neck in the geriatric group.

Chapter Twenty-Two

ETIOLOGIC FACTORS IN THE DEVELOPMENT OF CANCER

ROBERT W. CANTRELL, M.D., F.A.C.S.

INTRODUCTION

It is not known when man first thought cancer was caused by contact with elements of the environment, but one of the earliest scientific reports of this relationship was by Sir Percivall Pott,[1] who noted the high incidence of scrotal cancer in chimney sweeps in his treatise, *Chirurgical Observations Relative to the Cataract, Polypus of the Nose, The Cancer of the Scrotum, The Different Kinds of Ruptures and Mortification of the Toes and Feet,* published in London in 1775. Pott discussed the occupationally-induced cancers epidemic at that time in English chimney sweeps, and he rightly pinpointed soot as the cause. During that period in England, small boys, 4 to 7 years of age, were required to crawl naked up the narrow, tortuous chimneys to scrape loose the soot. A high percentage of these unfortunate lads, who bathed as rarely as annually, developed scrotal cancers around age 30. Pott's description is:

> "... there is a disease peculiar to a certain set of people, which has not, at least to my knowledge, been publickly noticed; I mean the chimney sweepers' cancer.
>
> "The first attack occurs on the inferior part of the scrotum where it produces a superficial, painful, ragged, ill-looking sore with hard and rising edges. The trade calls it the soot-wart. I never saw it under the age of puberty...in no great length of time, it pervades the skin, dartos, and membranes of the scrotum, and seizes the testicle, which it enlarges, hardens, and renders truly and thoroughly distempered, from whence it makes its way up the spermatic process into the abdomen, most frequently indurating and spoiling the inguinal glands. When arrived within the abdomen, it affects some of the viscera, and then very soon becomes painfully destructive.
>
> "The fate of these people seems singularly hard; in their early infancy, they are most frequently treated with great brutality and almost starved with cold and hunger; they are thrust up narrow and sometimes hot chimnies where they are bruised, burned and almost suffocated and when they get to puberty, become peculiarly liable to a most noisome, painful and fatal disease."

Some physicians had difficulty in accepting the relationship between environmental factors and cancer development owing to the long lag time of approximately 25 years between exposure and the manifestation of the cancer. Additionally, this cancer was much less common among chimney sweeps on the continent and in America. The problems of latent periods and geographic variations in cancer incidence continue to plague epidemiologists to the present day.

In time it was determined that the lack of protective clothing, which exposed the scrotum to abrasion with imbedding of soot particles, the poor personal hygiene, and the high concentration of carcinogens in English soot as opposed to soot from other countries accounted for the increased incidence of scrotal cancer in England.

One hundred and forty years elapsed before Yamagiwa and Ichikawa,[2] in 1914, reported inducing cancer on the ears of rabbits by repeated applications of coal tar, an ingredient of soot. Their work closely followed the experiment of Fibiger[2] who, in 1913, reported inducing carcinoma in the stomach and esophagus of rats by infecting them with spiroptera. This was probably the first report of experimentally-induced cancer. Presumably these parasites caused chronic irritation of the mucous membrane, thereby leading to the development of carcinoma and proving Virchow's hypothesis that chronic irritation can cause cancer.

Cook, Hewett, and Hieger[3] in 1933 isolated 3, 4-benzpyrene from coal tar as the chemical carcinogen. It had taken 158 years from the time the epidemiologic relationship between chimney sweeping and scrotal cancer was first suspected until the exact carcinogenic agent was identified.

Even though the specific etiologic agent was not known in England in Pott's time, the public outcry, particularly from the clergy and physicians, prompted Parliament to pass laws in 1788, the year of Pott's death, that raised the minimum age for chimney sweeps and mandated protective clothing and hygiene. This was one of the earliest examples of legislation designed to prevent occupational illnesses.

The major contributions of Fibiger, Yamagiwa, and Ichikawa,[2] largely unheralded, had this significance: if man could induce cancer experimentally and could identify carcinogens in the environment, man might also be able to control cancer, either through avoidance or modification of the carcinogens or by altering man's response to them.

MECHANISM OF EXPOSURE TO CARCINOGENS

Table 22-1 lists ways humans can become exposed to carcinogens. By far the largest number of people are exposed to irradiation in the form of ultraviolet rays from the sun. Not surprisingly, a large number of cancers are skin cancers: basal cell carcinomas, squamous cell carcinomas, and melanomas, in decreasing order of frequency. People with light skin are more susceptible than dark-skinned people, and the danger of developing skin cancer increases when light-skinned individuals move closer to the equator.[4]

Skin cancers are increasing in frequency,[4] and whether attributable to a decrease in the ultraviolet (UV) filtering ozone layer of the atmosphere caused by air pollution, owing to the migration from colder northern climates to the sun belt, or both, is problematic. Broad-brimmed hats, sun screen lotions, and protective clothing can diminish this incidence.

Other methods of exposure are through contact of the skin or mucous membrane with carcinogens, either by direct contact as in snuff dipping, by breathing contaminated air, or by ingesting contaminated food or water. In some cases, the inspired air contains a carcinogen, such as tobacco tar, which is deposited in the lungs where the contact occurs, or in the case of breathing radon gas, the inspired contaminant is carcinogenic through irradiation of lung tissue.

Epidemiologists attempt to identify agents in the environment that are carcinogenic. Higginson,[5] in reviewing epidemiologic trends in cancer development in 1968, estimated that approximately 90 percent of all human cancers are influenced by exogenous factors. Others[6] have put the percentage even higher, feeling that perhaps all cancers are caused by environmental factors.

A single exposure to some carcinogens is sufficient to induce a cancer under laboratory conditions. Examples of this are dimethylnitrosamine,[7] aflatoxin,[8] and ionizing radiation.[9] The lag time between exposure and the appearance of the cancer applies in these cases, and if single exposure causes cancer in humans, identification of the carcinogen is difficult, if not impossible, since the exposure may not be recognized or the incident forgotten. Fortunately, it is felt that relatively few cancers in humans occur after a single exposure.

Generally, repeated exposure to a carcinogen over many years is required before a cancer develops. This is fortunate since it allows us to avoid the carcinogen once it is identified and markedly decreases the chance of allowing a cancer to develop.

Repeated exposures over time are the primary reason cancer is an affliction of older people. Another reason given for the cancer incidence being higher in the elderly is deterioration of the immune system with age. Regardless of the mechanism, there is a direct relationship with age and cancer incidence. Cairns[6] points out that, as we eradicate infections and other diseases that kill younger members of society, thus allowing the population to live longer, we see a relative increase in

TABLE 22-1 Mechanism of Exposure to Carcinogens

Irradiation
   Natural
     Ultraviolet (sun)
     Radon gas
     Uranium ore
   Man-made
     Alpha-rays
     Beta-rays
     Gamma-rays
     X-rays

Direct Contact
   Coal tar
   Snuff
   Chewing tobacco
   Betel nut
   Pan

Respiration
   Tobacco smoke
   Industrial air pollution
   Radon gas
   Asbestos
   Wood dust

Alimentation
   Polluted water
   Food contaminated with natural or artificial carcinogens (nitrosamines, red dye#2).

Iatrogenic
   Agents administered through invasive techniques
   Pharmacologic agents

the degenerative diseases that accompany aging, e.g., heart disease and stroke. Cancer is included in this category.

The largest single causative factor in the development of cancer today is tobacco use, primarily cigarette smoking. Socioeconomic and political arguments to the contrary, the epidemiologic relationship between tobacco use and cancer development is irrefutable. When this is combined with the heart and lung diseases also linked to tobacco use, one sees that this unnecessary human social habit is responsible for more than 360,000 premature deaths annually. This is more than the deaths caused by motor vehicle accidents, homicides, suicides, alcoholism, drug abuse, AIDS, and fires combined.[10]

This discussion will focus on specific etiologic factors implicated in cancers of the respiratory tract and the upper digestive tract.

GENETIC FACTORS

Some investigators have attempted to implicate genetic factors in the development of cancer. This presumably grew from the knowledge that certain inbred strains of rodents develop cancer spontaneously or on exposure to any one of several stimuli. Further, the degree of skin pigmentation in humans is inversely related to the development of skin cancers, and certain rare familial conditions (xeroderma pigmentosum, basal cell nevus syndrome) show genetic susceptibility in cancer development. Nasopharyngeal carcinoma (NPC), a disease in which the Epstein-Barr virus is implicated, has a higher incidence in Chinese living in southern China, Hong Kong, and Singapore, as well as in Eskimos, North Africans, and East Africans. Whether this represents environmental factors, genetic susceptibility, or both is uncertain at this time. In Singapore, the incidence of NPC in Chinese is 18.6 per 100,000 per year, 4.8 per 100,000 per year in Malays, and only 0.9 per 100,000 per year in Indians.[11] This suggests a genetic susceptibility.

Gastric cancer, on the contrary, has a relatively high incidence in Japan, but assumes a lesser incidence when Japanese immigrate to California. Japanese born in California have an incidence of gastric carcinoma similar to Caucasians living in California.[6] Presumably, this is attributable to environmental factors, such as diet, and not genetic factors. Furthermore, known carcinogens such as tobacco or nitrosamines are capable of inducing cancer in all humans exposed, regardless of race, sex, or other genetic factors.

This is not to say that individual resistance or susceptibility plays no role. Every person exposed to a given carcinogen does not develop cancer. Obviously, more than one factor is involved.

MULTIPLE FACTORS

Many investigators have noted that a specific type of cancer can be induced by several different stimuli. Squamous cell carcinoma of the oral cavity has been related to cigarette smoking, snuff dipping, chewing tobacco, chewing betel nuts, using Pan (pan leaf, betel nuts, tobacco, and slaked lime), heat, syphilis, and ill-fitting dentures. Oral cavity cancer in the United States accounts for approximately 1.6 percent of all cancers, but in India where Pan use is widespread, oral cavity cancer, primarily squamous cell carcinoma of the buccal mucosa, accounts for 45 percent of all cancer.

Several factors can combine to induce a cancer. For example, esophageal cancer is more common in alcoholics. This may be attributable to a direct irritating effect of the alcohol, diminution in the immune mechanism through liver damage, or the action of the alcohol as a solvent for other carcinogens, such as tobacco tars. Malnutrition, which is frequently present in alcoholics, and viruses may also contribute to cancer development in alcoholics.

INFECTIOUS AGENTS

The development of gastric cancer in rats infected with the parasite spiroptera was mentioned. Recent efforts to link cancer to infectious agents has concentrated mainly on viruses as the etiologic agent, particularly in leukemias and lymphomas. Burkitt,[12] in 1958, noted that African children in Uganda developed tumors of the jaw that he initially thought were sarcomas, but that later proved to be malignant lymphoma. Subsequent investigation[13] showed this tumor to afflict mainly children between 2 and 14 years of age with a peak incidence at 5 years of age. This accounted for 50 percent of all childhood cancers seen in Uganda. Of 200 cases occurring in 8 years, 140 involved the jaws. This tumor was subsequently found to occur across tropical Africa, but never at elevations above 5,000 feet, in areas where the temperature dropped below 60° F annually, or where the rainfall was below 20 inches per year. This led Burkitt to conclude that an infectious agent, probably a virus transmitted by a mosquito, was responsible.[13]

We now know that the Epstein-Barr virus is implicated in malignant (Burkitt's) lymphoma and also in infectious mononucleosis and in nasopharyngeal carcinoma.[11,14] As mentioned earlier, genetic factors may play a role in the development of NPC as well as environmental factors, such as cigarette smoking and eating Cantonese salted fish. Traces of dimethylnitrosamine have been found in the salted fish. Environmental factors are implicated further since Chinese living in the United States have a lower incidence of NPC.

Slow viruses, or human retroviruses, which have been identified only recently and of which the human immunodeficiency virus (HIV) responsible for AIDS is one, may be implicated in carcinogenesis. The Kaposi's sarcoma found in many of those afflicted with AIDS may be viral-induced.

Human papillomavirus (HPV) is known to induce verruca vulgaris (common warts), condyloma acuminatum (venereal warts), epidermodysplasia verruciformis, and laryngeal papillomatosis. This virus has been postulated to induce bowenoid papulosis, florid oral papillomatosis, and oral focal epithelial hyperplasia (Heck's disease), as well as squamous carcinoma of the cervix and of the esophagus. Hille and co-workers[15] in 1986 reported finding morphologic manifestations of HPV infection in 23 cases (33 percent) of 70 patients with invasive squamous cell carcinoma of the esophagus. HPV antigens were demonstrated by immunohistochemical staining in seven of the 23 cases. Kashima and co-workers[16] identified human papillomavirus capsid antigens in tissue taken by biopsy from 14 of 20 patients with carcinoma in situ of the larynx.

Problems related to establishing epidemiologic relationships in infectious agents as a cause of cancer lie in individual resistance or susceptibility to infection by viruses plus synergism with other carcinogens. If viruses cause cancer, we would expect to see epidemics of cancer, and except for some villages in Uganda where Burkitt noted an increased incidence of lymphoma, these cancer epidemics have not materialized. Children, who contract more viral diseases than do adults, would have more cancers than adults. Burkitt's lymphoma does occur primarily in children, and childhood leukemias may represent cancers in which viruses play a role. The increased incidence of cancer with age indicates factors other than viruses as the major etiologic agents. Carcinogenic chemicals, other environmental carcinogens, or diminution in the immune system remain the major suspected contributors to cancer development.

EPIDEMIOLOGIC LIMITATIONS

Deriving conclusions based on epidemiologic studies can be misleading. Higginson[5] showed a correlation between the degree of industrialization and the incidence of carcinoma of the colon in males. Nigeria, with the lowest industrialization, had the lowest incidence of colon carcinoma. The United States, with the greatest degree of industrialization, had the highest incidence of colon carcinoma. Cairns[6] presented a similar graph (Fig. 22-1) that included New Zealand and that related colon carcinoma to per capita consumption of beef. In this case New Zealand had the highest per capita beef consumption and the highest incidence of colon carcinoma. The United States was second in both categories with Nigeria being the lowest in both categories. Seen another way, the incidence of colon carcinoma is also correlated with the cereal content of the diet, which is highest in Nigeria and lowest in New Zealand. These seemingly contradictory observations might be explained by a logical hypothesis: a carcinogen in beef (nitrosamine?) or other carcinogens produced by industrialization and ingested orally may have a lower fecal transit time in those societies with low fiber diets, thus resulting in a longer colonic mucosal exposure to the carcinogen(s).

SPECIFIC ETIOLOGIC AGENTS

Throughout the many reports reviewed for this communication, cigarette smoking and other forms of tobacco use are always associated with an increased incidence of cancer of the upper aerodigestive tract. Closely associated with increased cancer incidence was heavy alcohol consumption, and when these two factors were combined there appears to be synergism.

Cigarette smoking accounts for approximately 360,000 premature deaths annually, and merely eliminating this unnecessary social habit would result in these 360,000 victims living an additional 15 years.[10] Not all of these patients die of cancer, but more than half of them do, and the largest number die from lung cancer, which makes up 25 percent of all cancers.

Lung cancer was not a prevalent disease around 1900 when cigarette smoking began to grow in popularity. Since smoking one cigarette does not produce a cancer, but rather heavy smoking, usually greater than one pack per day for 15 to 20 years, one would expect an increase in lung cancer to parallel the increase in cigarette smoking, but 15 or 20 years later. That is what we see. Cairns[6] shows this in Figure 22-2. Evidence that this is not attributable to other factors is seen in lung cancer rates in women. Prior to World War II, lung cancer was

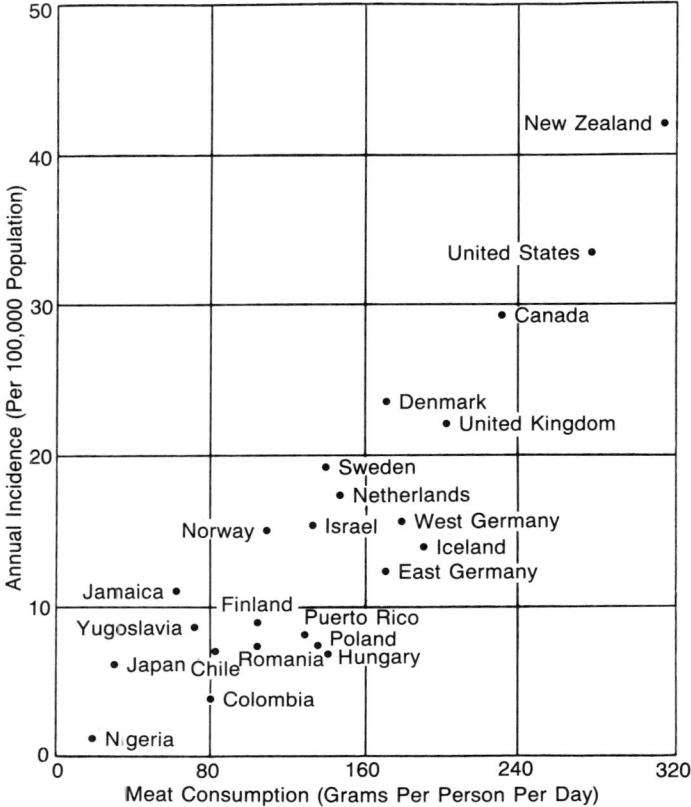

Figure 22-1 Incidence of colon carcinoma related to per capita consumption of beef. There is also a relationship to the low consumption of cereals. With permission from Cairns J. The cancer problem. Sci Am 1975; 233(5):64–78.

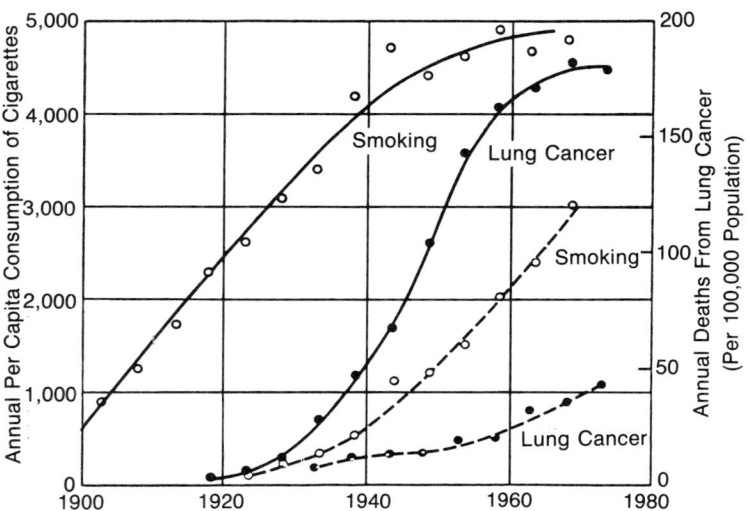

Figure 22-2 The incidence of carcinoma of the lung paralleling the incidence of cigarette smoking by men and women. The lung cancer occurs only after many years of heavy smoking. Solid line is men; broken line is women. With permission from Cairns J. The cancer problem. Sci Am 1975; 233(5):64–78.

rare in women. Few women smoked cigarettes. With the upheaval attending World War II, many women were required to enter the work force to replace men called into military service. As these women assumed men's work habits, they also assumed some of men's bad social habits, particularly cigarette smoking. Once addicted to smoking cigarettes, it is difficult to overcome. Again, one would expect to see the lung cancer incidence in women begin to increase approximately 20 years after World War II, and that is exactly what happened. As more and more women began smoking, the lung cancer incidence in women began to rise, and by the early 1980s, the American Cancer Society predicted that, based on cigarette smoking patterns in women and on cancer trends, lung cancer would be the leading cause of cancer deaths in women by 1985. This prediction proved correct and lung cancer has remained the leading cause of cancer deaths in women since 1985.

ALCOHOL CARCINOGENESIS

The role of alcohol in carcinogenesis is less clear, but nevertheless directly correlated. Warren,[17] in 1836, observed that lingual cancer in a tobacco chewer was "generated by the long use of ardent spirits." Multiple studies since have shown the correlation between chronic alcohol consumption and an increased incidence of cancer of the oral cavity, esophagus, and supraglottic and glottic larynx.[18] These studies show that, although there is marked synergism when chronic alcohol consumption is combined with heavy tobacco use, an increased incidence of esophageal and liver cancers occurs with heavy alcohol consumption in the absence of tobacco use. This incidence is related directly to the total amount of alcohol consumed and is independent of the type of alcoholic beverage.

Various theories have been proposed for the carcinogenic effects of alcohol. Carcinogens other than ethanol may be present in alcoholic beverages. Higher alcohols present, such as isoamyl, isobutyl, and n-propyl alcohol, can cause liver cancer in rats, and traces of nitrosamines are present in alcoholic beverages. The nutritional deficiencies commonly associated with alcoholics may play a role, and alcohol can lead to impaired absorption of nutrients and vitamins. Ethanol is capable of decreasing vitamin A levels, and this vitamin participates in the regulation of epithelial cell differentiation.[18] Epithelium is also adversely affected by deficiencies in riboflavin and zinc. These elements are known to be decreased in chronic alcoholics. Chronic ethanol consumption alters intracellular metabolism of epithelial cells at target sites, thus resulting in enhanced metabolic activation of tobacco-associated carcinogens.

Alcohol may serve as a solvent for tobacco-related or other carcinogens, thus permitting easier passage through the cellular membrane. This could apply to oral cavity or esophageal cancer, but would not explain the increased incidence of glottic or liver cancer in alcoholics.

It has been known for some time that chronic ethanol consumption leads to enhancement of the liver microsomal drug-metabolizing capability. It has been shown[18] that the metabolism of the hepatocarcinogen N-nitrosopyrrolidine is increased in ethanol-consuming animals.

Decreased liver metabolism in a severely cirrhotic patient may result in a decreased hepatic ability to detoxify carcinogens, thereby resulting in an increased circulating systemic concentration of carcinogens. Other possibilities are diminution of the hepatic contribution to the immune system or the development in the damaged liver of an immune globulin protective of cancer cells.

OTHER CARCINOGENS

Table 22-2, modified from Higginson,[5] lists some known human carcinogens. Obviously, to decrease cancer incidence, exposure to these agents should be minimized or avoided. Table 22-3, also from Higginson, lists agents known to be carcinogenic in animals and potentially carcinogenic in humans.

The Food and Drug Administration (FDA) has tested approximately 6,000 chemicals and found about 500 to be carcinogenic. This work was done in animals and extrapolated to humans. Owing to individual susceptibility and to the fact that no one knows what is a minimally permissible dose of car-

TABLE 22-2 Known Human Carcinogens

Coal tar and soot[19]	Aromatic amines[24]
Creosote[19]	Tobacco[25]
Mineral oils[19,20]	Betel quid[26]
Residues of petroleum	Ionizing radiation[9]
Cracked[19]	Ultraviolet radiation[27]
Waxes[21]	Burns[28]
Isopropyl oil[19]	Nickel, Chromium, Arsenic[19]
Benzol[19]	Asbestos[29]
Alcoholic drinks[22]	Parasites
Alkylating drugs[22]	Conorchiasis[30]
	Schistosomiasis[31]

With permission from Higginson J. Present trends in cancer epidemiology. In: Organ JF, ed. Proceedings of the Eighth Canadian Cancer Research Conference. Oxford: Pergamon Press, 1968; 8:40.

TABLE 22-3 Experimental Carcinogens to Which Man Has Been Exposed, but for Which Evidence of a Significant Role Remains to be Demonstrated

Agent	Susceptible Species	Major Organ Affected	Source of Human Exposure
Dimethyl amino azo-benzene(DAB)	M, R, D	Liver	Coloring agent[32]
Isoniazid	M	Lung	Chemotherapy[33]
Iron dextran	M, R	Soft tissue	Therapy[34]
Luteoskyrin	R	Liver	Rice (moldy)[35]
Penicillin G	R	Soft tissue	Chemotherapy[36]
Senecio alkaloids (i.e., retrorsine)	R	Liver	Food[37]
Tannic acid	M, R	Liver	Beverages[30,38]
SV 40 virus	H	Soft tissue, brain	Vaccine[39]

M=Mouse; D=Dog; R=Rat; H=Hampster
With permission from Higginson J. Present trends in cancer epidemiology. In: Organ JF, ed. Proceedings of the Eighth Canadian Cancer Research Conference. Oxford: Pergamon Press, 1968; 8:40.

cinogen, the FDA states a given agent is, or is not, carcinogenic without any effort to quantify dosage.

It is at this point that socioeconomic considerations and the weighing of risk versus benefits begin to intrude into purely scientific considerations. Should a known carcinogen in animals that is potentially carcinogenic in humans, but that offers some benefits to humans, be avoided in all cases? Isoniazid is an example. It is known to cause lung cancer in rats. It has also saved hundreds of human lives through its use in the treatment of tuberculosis. Fortunately, it was in widespread use prior to the discovery of its carcinogenic potential in mice, and no increased incidence of cancer had been noted in humans treated with isoniazid.

Saccharin is another example. It is known to cause cancer in laboratory animals, but when the FDA attempted to remove it from the market as they had cyclamates previously, diabetics (and saccharin producers) raised enough objections that saccharin was allowed to remain on the market. A warning, nearly too small to read, has been affixed to each packet stating, "Use of this product may be hazardous to your health. This product contains saccharin, which has been determined to cause cancer in laboratory animals." Apparently, at least in the eyes of the Congress, the benefits of saccharin outweighed its risks.

This also raises the argument between those who hold that animal results are not always transferrable to humans and those who state that a carcinogen in any mammalian species is potentially dangerous for humans.

The number of work-related cancers is relatively small when compared to the large numbers of tobacco and alcohol-related cancers. Yet the current system not only permits, but insists, on identifying cancers caused by industrial exposures and on compensation for the victim by the industry involved.

United States Surgeon General Koop released the seventeenth *Smoking and Health* report in December, 1985, 22 years after the first was released by Surgeon General Terry in 1964 that linked cigarette smoking and cancer. In his report, Koop declared that cigarettes represent a greater cause of death and disability than any other hazard in the working environment. This report was not greeted with enthusiasm by the unions, who were worried that employers might use this information to shield themselves from legal liability for workers suffering from occupational illness aggravated by smoking.[40]

Work-related carcinogens receive a disproportionately higher level of investigation and attention. Moreover, in many cases in which industrial agents are suspected of being carcinogenic or are actually proven to be so, many epidemiologic studies have not taken into account the synergistic effect of tobacco smoking.

Koop,[40] in reference to Selikoff's work,[41] pointed out that workers exposed to asbestos for 20 years increase their risk for lung cancer five-fold, while male smokers not exposed to asbestos increase their risk for lung cancer 10-fold. If the asbestos worker smokes, his risk of lung cancer is increased 50-fold; if he smokes more than one pack of cigarettes a day, his risks are increased 90-fold.

All monetary awards for damage to those developing asbestos-related cancers have come from the asbestos producers, and no monetary awards have come from tobacco companies.

This should not be interpreted as an apology for industrial pollution. Any industrial carcinogen identified and clearly shown to cause diseases in humans must be eliminated from the environment. Industries that produce pollutants must be required to clear the pollution they produce and to dispose of it properly. This is a plea to consider *all* sources of carcinogens and to allocate damages proportionately. All other industries except tobacco companies and alcohol producers have the standards of product liability applied. It is time that the vast health care costs arising from these two latter industries be allocated back to those who profit from producing these carcinogens.

Do not expect much help in this from the government. It is unlikely that it will ever be politically feasible to curb an industry (tobacco) that employs 500,000 farm families and that brings 6 billion dollars of tax money into the government annually. Or, as Cairns[6] states,

> "There is every reason to believe that the abolition of cigarette smoking would largely eliminate lung cancer, the commonest of all forms of death from cancer. So far, however, there is no sign that smoking will be abolished. The professional classes smoke less than they once did, but the poor smoke more. It could even be argued that few Western societies could afford to abolish a habit that creates a large secondary industry, generates considerable revenue and kills mostly the older members of the population, who otherwise would draw on government welfare and social security benefits."

FUTURE TRENDS

It has been stated that the billions of dollars allocated for research into a cure for cancer have not been well-spent. If one were to consider only the age-adjusted mortality rates, where a death occurring at age 75 is considered the same as a death at age 5, this might seem to be the case. In 1950 cancer caused 15 percent of all deaths in the United States; in 1985 cancer was responsible for 24 percent of all deaths.[42] Looking back further, in 1900 cancer was the ninth leading cause of death, with stomach cancer leading and lung cancer rare. Today, cancer is the second leading cause of death, with lung cancer being most common and stomach cancer rare.

Early diagnosis through Papanicolaou cervical smears and mammography results in slightly improved cure rates, and improved surgery, irradiation, and chemotherapy have resulted in lowering cancer mortality rates slightly. Etiologic factors, particularly cigarette smoking, which causes more than 30 percent of all cancers, have been identified, and attempts at reducing or controlling exposures to these carcinogens have been undertaken with some success.

If years of potential life lost (YPLL) is used as an indicator of cancer mortality, rather than age-adjusted mortality, different trends are noted. In 1980 cancer accounted for 1.824 million YPLL to age 65. If the cancer rates of 1950 had persisted, 2.093 million YPL would have been lost. This means that 269,000 years of potential life to age 65 were saved, and if this is carried through to 1986, more that 1 million years of potential life to age 65 have been saved, indicating that considerable progress against cancer has been made.[42] Even when applying age-adjusted mortality rates, cancer mortality has declined 25 percent to 65 percent in various age groups through age 44. Unfortunately, above age 54 the age-adjusted mortality rates have risen, in some age groups significantly. This is attributable to increasing lung cancer death rates in the age groups above 54. Mortality from malignant neoplasms not of the respiratory system have either leveled off or declined in those over age 54.[42]

The National Cancer Program has begun to concentrate on prevention and screening in addition to improving treatment in order to reduce mortality from cancer up to 50 percent by the year 2000. The Surgeon General, along with the American Cancer Society, has adopted a goal of a tobacco-free society by 2000. This is a laudable, but perhaps a somewhat unrealistic, goal. Even a slight decrease, reducing the number of adults who smoke from 34 percent to 15 percent, would result in an 8 to 15 percent reduction in mortality. By reducing fat consumption from 38 percent to 25 percent of total energy intake and increasing consumption of fiber from 8 to 12 to 20 to 30 g per day, another mortality reduction of 8 percent could be achieved. Increased screening offers an additional 3 percent decrease in mortality, and adoption of state-of-the-art treatment can lower the mortality an additional

10 to 26 percent. This would be a total reduction in cancer mortality of 25 to 50 percent by the year 2000. This goal is attainable, and up to a third of the reduction can be achieved by decreasing or ceasing cigarette smoking and heavy alcohol consumption and by adjusting dietary habits, actions that can be initiated by the individual at little or no cost. This information must be communicated to the public.

CONCLUSION

This review has dealt with factors in the environment that are capable of inducing cancer. It is conservatively estimated that more than 90 percent of all cancers are caused by environmental factors that can be avoided, minimized, or our response to them modified. Assuming this is true, it behooves clinicians to support efforts by epidemiologists to identify carcinogens and then to prevail on our patients and on the public to avoid these lethal agents.

The one exposure most prevalent and the carcinogen responsible for inducing the majority of cancers of the head, neck, and lungs (approximately 30 percent of all cancers) is cigarette smoking, followed closely by chronic alcohol consumption. Not only should physicians prevail on patients under our care who have cancer to avoid these carcinogens and thus avoid inciting a new lesion once the primary tumor is controlled, we should take the lead in urging *all* patients and the public to decrease or cease smoking cigarettes and to avoid chronic alcohol abuse.

References

1. Pott P. Chirurgical observations relative to the cataract, polypus of the nose, the cancer of the scrotum, the different kinds of ruptures and mortification of the toes and feet. London, L. Hawes, W. Clarke, and R. Collins, 1775. In: Melicow MM. Percivall Pott (1713–1788): 200th anniversary of first report of occupation-induced cancer of scrotum in chimney sweepers (1775). Urology 1975; 6(6):745–749.
2. Yamagiwa K, Ichikawa K. Experimental study of the pathogenesis of carcinoma. J Cancer Res 1918; 3(1):1–19.
3. Heuper WC. Occupational tumors and allied diseases. Springfield: Charles C Thomas, 1942:196.
4. Cantrell RW. Malignant neoplasms of the skin of the head. In: English GM. Otolaryngology. Vol 5. Philadelphia: Harper & Row, 1982:Ch. 59.1.
5. Higginson J. Present trends in cancer epidemiology. In: Organ JF, ed. Proceedings of the Eighth Canadian Cancer Research Conference. Oxford: Pergamon Press, 1969; 8:40.
6. Cairns J. The cancer problem. Sci Am 1975; 233(5):64–78.
7. Magee PN, Barnes JM. The production of malignant primary hepatic tumours in the rat by feeding dimethylnitrosamine. Br J Cancer 1956; 10:114–122.
8. Carnaghan RBA. Hepatic tumours and other chronic liver changes in rats following a single oral administration of aflatoxin. Br J Cancer 1967; 21:811–814.
9. Upton AC. Comparative observations on radiation carcinogenesis in man and animals. In: Carcinogenesis, a broad critique. Baltimore: Williams & Wilkins, 1967:631.
10. Warner KE. Health and economic implications of a tobacco-free society. JAMA 1987; 258(15):2080–2086.
11. de The G. Role of Epstein-Barr virus in human diseases: infectious mono-nucleosis, Burkitt's lymphoma, and nasopharyngeal carcinoma. In: Klein G, ed. Viral oncology. New York: Raven Press, 1980:769.
12. Burkitt D. A sarcoma involving the jaws in African children. Br J Surg 1958; 46:218–223.
13. Burkitt D. A children's cancer dependent on climactic factors. Nature 1962; 194(4825):232–234.
14. Halpin J, Scott AL, Jacobson L, et al. Enzyme-linked immunosorbent assay of antibodies to Epstein-Barr virus nuclear and early antigens in patients with infectious mono-nucleosis and nasopharyngeal carcinoma. Ann Intern Med 1986; 104(3):331–337.
15. Hille JJ, Margolius RA, Markowitz S, et al. Human papillomavirus infection related to oesophagela carcinoma in black South Africans. S Afr Med J 1986; 69:417–420.
16. Kashima H, Mounts P, Kuhajda F, et al. Demonstration of human papillomavirus capsid antigen in carcinoma in situ of the larynx. Ann Otol Rhinol Laryngol 1986; 95(6):603–607.
17. Warren JC. Surgical observations on tumours with cases and observations. In: Wynder EL. A corner of history. Prev Med 1976; 5:317–319.
18. McCoy GD, Wynder EL. Etiological and preventive implication in alcohol carcinogenesis. Cancer Res 1979; 39:2844–2850.
19. Heuper WC, Conway WD. Chemical carcinogenesis and cancers. Springfield, IL: Charles C Thomas, 1964.
20. Boyd JT, Doll R. Gastro-intestinal cancer and the use of liquid paraffin. Br J Cancer 1954; 8:231–237.
21. Shubik P, Saffiotti U, Lijinsky W, Pietra G, Rappaport H, Toth B, Raha CR, Tomatis L, Feldman R, Ramahi H. Studies on the toxicity of petroleum waxes. Toxicol Appl Pharmacol 1962; 4(Suppl):1–62.
22. Wynder EL, Bross IJ. A study of etiological factors in cancer of the esophagus. Cancer 1961; 14:389–413.
23. Roe FJ. The relevance of preclinical assessment of carcinogenesis. Clin Pharmacol Ther 1966; 7:77–111.
24. Bonser GM. Factors concerned in the location of human and experimental tumours. Br Med J 1967; 2:655–660.
25. Wynder EL, Hoffman D. Experimental tobacco carcinogenesis. In: Haddow A, Weinhouse S, eds. Advances in cancer research. New York: Academic Press, 1964:249.
26. Hirayama T. An epidemiological study of oral and pharyngeal cancer in Central and South-East Asia. Bull WHO 1966; 34:41–69.
27. Blum HF. Carcinogenesis by ultraviolet light. Princeton: Princeton University Press, 1959.
28. Treves N, Pack GT. The development of cancer in burn scars. Surg Gynecol Obstet 1030; 51:749.
29. Gilson JC. Wyers Memorial Lecture 1965: Health hazards of asbestos—recent studies on its biological effects. Trans Soc Occup Med 1966; 16:62–74.
30. Higginson J. The geographical pathology of primary liver cancer. Cancer Res 1963; 23:1624–1633.
31. Higginson J. Cancer: statistical aspects and epidemiology. In: Raven RW, ed. Cancer progress. London: Butterworths, 1963:73.
32. Peacock PR. Problems arising from the use of chemicals in food—colouring matter in food. Chem Indust 1952; 10:238–241.

33. Hammond EC, Selikoff IJ, Robitzek EH. Isoniazid therapy in relation to later occurrence of cancer in adults and in infants. Br J Med 1967; 2:792-795.
34. Haddow A, Roe FJC, Mitchley BC. Induction of sarcomata in rabbits by intramuscular injection of iron-dextran ("Imferon"). Br J Med 1964; 2:1593-1594.
35. Kobayashi Y, Uraguchi K, Sakai F, Tatsuno T, Tsu kioke M, et al. Toxicological studies on the yellowed rice by P. Islandicum. Suppl. III. Proc Japan Acad 1959; 35:501-506.
36. Dickens F. Mold products including antibiotics as carcinogens. In: Carcinogenesis—a broad critique. Baltimore: Williams & Wilkins, 1967:447.
37. Bras G. Nutritional aspects of cirrhosis and carcinoma of the liver. Fed Proc 1961; 20:353-360.
38. Korpassy B, Mosonyl M. The carcinogenic activity of tannic acid—liver tumours induced in rats by prolonged subcutaneous administration of tannic acid solutions. Br J Cancer 1950; 4:411-420.
39. Fraumeni JF Jr, Ederer F, Miller RW. An evaluation of the carcinogenicity of Simian virus 40 in man. JAMA 1963; 185:713-718.
40. Korcok M. US surgeon general ignites furor with findings on smoking in the workplace. Can Med Assoc J 1986; 134:801-804.
41. Selikoff IJ, Hammond EC, Churg J. Asbestos exposure, smoking and neoplasia. JAMA 1968; 204:106-112.
42. Breslow L, Cumberland WG. Progress and objectives in cancer control. JAMA 1988; 259:1690-1694.

Chapter Twenty-Three

AGING, THE IMMUNE SYSTEM, AND HEAD AND NECK CANCER

GREGORY T. WOLF, M.D., F.A.C.S.

INTRODUCTION

Head and neck squamous carcinoma is a malignancy that occurs predominantly in adult individuals who have been long-term users of tobacco and alcohol. The stage of disease at time of diagnosis is usually advanced, and at least half of affected patients are older that 60 years when first diagnosed. The increasing incidence of these cancers with age is probably attributable to two interrelated effects of age. The first is a permissive effect in which time is allowed for the expression of previous carcinogenic stimuli, and the second is an enhancement effect related to specific changes in cellular metabolism or biochemistry that are results of the aging process. Of prime importance in the enhancement effect may be age-related changes in the immune system. Profound deficits in cellular immune reactivity are commonly detected in patients with head and neck cancer,[1] however, the relationship of these deficits to age, nutritional status, genetic factors, social habits, tumor extent, or prognosis remains unclear. What is clear is that the induction and progression of head and neck cancer is probably a multistep process that takes place after long-term exposure to carcinogens and promoters and that is associated with a concomitant failure of natural immunologic homeostasis.

A major component of the aging process is a gradual senescence of the immune system that has been associated with an increased incidence of neoplasia, autoimmune disorders, and infectious diseases.[2,3] Research interest in the effects of age on immune function and cancer has been stimulated by the longstanding assumption that a failure in immune competence is closely related to the development of neoplasia and that the progression of a neoplastic process can be altered by immunologic mechanisms. Unfortunately, the effects of age itself on cancer growth are not clearly understood, and our knowledge of mechanisms responsible for the effects of aging on immune reactivity is incomplete. The incidence of malignancy increases with age; 50 percent of all cancers occur in those over 65 years of age.[4,5] In fact, age has been cited as the most significant risk factor for the development of cancer.[6] Despite these facts, cancer growth and the development of metastases have been reported to be slower in older individuals compared with younger ones.[7-9] Further, some studies in patients with head and neck cancer have suggested that tumors occurring in younger patients have a more aggressive biologic behavior and a poorer prognosis; however, the numbers of young patients with these cancers are few and reliable data are lacking. Many of the conclusions regarding aging and cancer have been extrapolated from the results of animal studies using aged mice and as such may not be pertinent to the human setting.

The effects of immunologic senescence on cancer growth are also unclear. A uniform decline in immune competence as a result of thymic and splenic involution is well documented.[10-12] However, specific alterations in cellular and humoral immune function that are associated with aging are highly variable and probably influenced by a number of factors besides thymic degeneration. Using different model systems, both suppression and facilitation of tumor growth can be demonstrated with age-related immune depression.[13-16] Until the effects of specific immune abnormalities on neoplasia are better understood, the association of age-induced immune suppression on cancer growth in man will remain speculative.

Despite these limitations, considerable new knowledge about immune mechanisms has been achieved through advances in biochemistry, molecular biology, and hybridoma technology. Recently emphasized in tumor immunology have been the functions of T lymphocytes as mediators of tumor rejection and the role of regulatory lymphokines, such as the interleukins, as critical cofactors in the maintenance and amplification of the immune response.[17] Although this chapter will discuss general effects of aging on immune competence, the major emphasis will be on T cell mechanisms felt to be most important in the clinical course of patients with head and neck cancer.

THE IMMUNE NETWORK

A prerequisite to discussion of specific features of the effects of aging on immune reactivity is an understanding of the cellular components involved in the immune response. Classically, the immune system has been divided into "humoral" and "cellular" divisions. The humoral component represents bone marrow stem cell development that leads to the production of immunocompetent, antibody-producing plasma cells and B lymphocytes. The cellular component represents stem cell development that leads to the production of thymic-derived, antigen reactive T lymphocytes that are multifunctional. Traditionally, in tumor immunology the greatest importance has been placed on the role of the cellular system. Furthermore, aging appears to have its major effects on the cellular immune system and to have only modest effects on humoral immunity.[2,3] Distinct separation of these two components of immune response is becoming increasingly difficult, however, since humoral immunity is under the regulatory influence of subsets of T lymphocytes. Also, humoral mechanisms such as antibody-mediated tumor cell destruction, immune complex formation, and cytophilic antibody arming of macrophages are important ancillary mechanisms in tumor cell recognition and immune rejection.

The major mechanisms of cytotoxicity against tumor cells are mediated by thymus-dependent lymphocytes (T cells). Under the influence of the thymic microenvironment, precursor T lymphocytes differentiate into mature T cells that can react directly with antigens via specific membrane receptors to become, functionally, "helper" cells, effector cells, or immune regulatory cells. Monoclonal antibodies have been developed that recognize specific surface receptors and differentiation antigens on T lymphocytes. These antibodies have been used to subgroup these morphologically similar cells into subsets according to function. Some of the common designations[18] used for lymphocyte subpopulations are listed in Table 23–1. Various subsets of T cells are responsible for mediating tumor cell destruction, amplifying the response of other T and B cells through lymphokine production, suppressing the immune response, and influencing the recruitment and retention of other inflammatory cells to a tissue site of reaction. In response to antigen stimulation and monocyte-derived soluble factors, helper-inducer T lymphocytes produce lymphokines that are critical for the proliferation of other T lymphocyte-effector cell populations. Activities of these effector cells include cytotoxicity and feedback suppression of responses. Initiation of proliferation also requires activation of the precursor cells by antigen and expression of appropriate lymphokine receptors on their cell membrane surface. Soluble mediators that play an important role in both initiating and regulating lymphocyte proliferation include the family of lymphokines termed the interleukins.[17] At least five different interleukin molecules have been described with differing activities and target cells. Interleukin 2 (IL2) in particular has been found to be the important second signal in the proliferation of a population of cytolytic "killer" cells that may be important in immunologically-mediated tumor regression.[19,20] A schematic representation of currently

TABLE 23–1 Human T Cell Differentiation Antigens

Antigen	Common Designation	% Positive Cells in Peripheral Blood	Specificity
T11	CD2	80	E-rosette receptor
T3, Leu 4	CD3	70	T cell antigen receptor
T4	CD4	45	Helper/inducer, Class II MHC reactive
T8	CD8	30	Cytotoxic-suppressor, Class I MHC reactive
T6	CD1	0.5	Thymocytes, Langerhans cells
T9	T9	—	Transferrin receptor, activated T cells
Leu 7	Leu 7	10	Large granular lymphocyte and T cells
Leu 11	CD16	4	Natural killer
Tac	CD25	—	IL2 receptor, activated T cells

understood interactions of IL2 and the IL2 membrane receptor leading to proliferation of cytotoxic cells is shown in Figure 23-1.

Failure of immunologically-mediated tumor eradication is most likely attributable to a combination of events that includes poor immune recognition of a tumor and impaired immune effector mechanisms. These functional deficits are caused in part by intrinsic abnormalities in cellular proliferation and tumor-derived immunosuppressive substances. A consistent observation in immunologic studies in aged individuals is the presence of a variety of cellular immune abnormalities that are similar to those seen in patients with cancer and that may be related to the senescence of the thymus gland. Considerable evidence exists that documents the importance of the thymus gland in maintaining immunocompetence in animal models.[21] A central role for the thymus gland in human immunodeficiency is less clear, but is supported by the profound defects associated with congenital thymic dysplasias that can be abrogated by administration of thymic extracts.[21,22] The active hormonal components of thymus gland extracts have been isolated and found to consist of a family of peptides that influence the maturation and differentiation of T lymphocytes. Extensive studies using both crude thymus extracts and purified, synthetic thymic peptides have demonstrated enhanced survival in tumor-bearing animals and improvements in immune parameters in immunosuppressed human cancer patients. In some studies, this improvement has correlated with improved survival.[23,24] Because aging is associated with a significant decrease in thymic mass and in circulating levels of thymic hormones,[10,12,25] and because of the central role of the thymus gland in T cell maturation, it is possible that treatment strategies of immune reconstitution with thymic hormones in elderly patients may be beneficial.

IMMUNE DEFICITS ASSOCIATED WITH AGING

Many of the changes in the cellular immune system that are associated with aging are attributable to a gradual loss of a cell's ability to proliferate.[26] However, the decline in immune function is complex and also involves changes in multiple lymphocyte subsets and in cellular interactions that regulate responses. The most consistently demonstrated alterations include decreased lymphocyte reactivity,[27-29] decreased lymphokine (interleukin 2) production,[30-33] and decreased levels of CD8 (cytotoxic-suppressor) cells,[34-36] CD4 (helper) cells,[34,37] and lymphocytes in general.[38] Both increases[35] and decreases[39] in levels of natural killer cells (Leu 7) have been reported. Since natural killer (NK) cells are believed to play an important role in immune surveillance, abnormalities in their number or function could be a factor in the increased incidence of cancer in the elderly. Abnormalities of NK cell levels[1,40,41] and function[42,43] are commonly seen in head and neck cancer and have been associated with an increased rate of distant metastases.[44] Probably of greater importance, however, are decreases in antigen specific T cell cytotoxic function associated with aging. Decreased levels of CD8 cells have been shown to be directly related to early tumor relapse in head and neck cancer.[45] The proliferation of these cells and of other less specific killer cells (e.g., LAK cells) appears to be mediated by interleukin 2. It is well-documented that production of IL2 declines with increasing age. This has been related to an inability of aged lymphocytes to express IL2 messenger ribonucleic acid (RNA).[46] Impaired activation of lymphocytes and expression of Ia antigens in response to mitogens have also been reported, and these deficits are similar among aged normal subjects and patients with

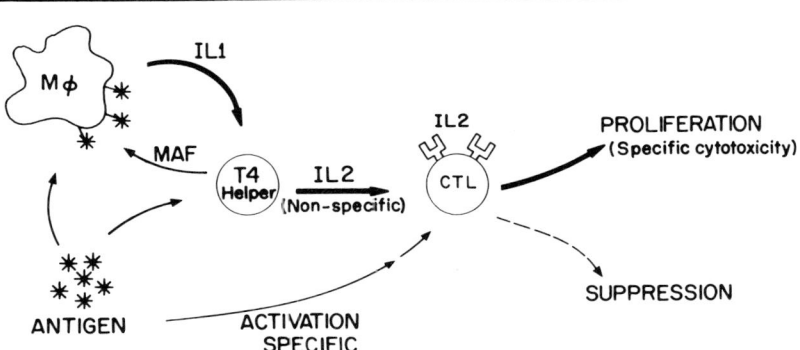

Figure 23-1 Schematic representation of cellular interactions involved in the generation and proliferation of cytotoxic lymphocytes. Production of interleukin 2 by helper T lymphocytes plays a central role in these interactions. Antigen recognition and processing by macrophages (MΦ) and helper cells result in elaboration of IL1 and IL2, respectively. Antigen stimulation of cytotoxic precursors (CTL) and helper cells results in expression of IL2 receptors, which in turn, together with IL2, leads to proliferation of cytotoxic effector cells. (MAF = macrophage activating factor.)

head and neck cancer.[47] These impairments may contribute to low levels of T cell cytotoxic function and impaired IL2 production. In addition, expression of IL2 receptors is also decreased in aging,[31] and levels of immunosuppressive serum glycoproteins are elevated.[48] Whether lymphocytes from aged individuals are normally responsive in vitro to exogenous IL2 is unclear since some investigators report normal responsiveness[39,49,50] and others report impaired responsiveness.[31,32] The ability of IL2 to reconstitute age-related T cell responses in vivo remains unknown. The defects in IL2 production and T cell responsiveness appear directly related to the aged T lymphocyte itself and not to impaired monocyte function, suppressor cell function, elevated prostaglandin levels, or depressed interleukin 1 levels.

A number of other integumentary changes affecting skin and mucosa occur with aging that may be important in the immunology of cancer. The skin is currently believed to be both a target organ for immune reactions and an organ that has its own unique immunomodulating properties in T cell differentiation. The latter role is supported by experimental evidence for thymic hormone binding to epithelial cells and the production of epidermal thymocyte-activating factors (ETAF) by normal epidermal cells.[51] External influences on the skin, particularly ultraviolet radiation, affect systemic immune responses by altering T cell reactivity, lymphokine production, keratinocyte production of ETAF, and the morphology of the resident immune cell of the skin, the Langerhans cell. Density of Langerhans cells in the skin decreases with age, as does the responsiveness to cytokines such as ETAF.[51] These changes in immune function may be important generally and at the local site of tumor development in the skin. Whether similar immunologic changes are associated with age-related atrophy of mucous membranes in the upper aerodigestive tract is unknown.

An interesting paradox in this catalog of immune derangements associated with aging is the increased incidence of autoimmune disorders that occurs at a time when immune function and thymic gland activity are declining. In both mice and man, production of monoclonal immunoglobulins and of autoantibodies is increased and suggests that aging is associated with altered immune homeostasis, not just immune impairment. Interestingly, some investigators have suggested an important role for autoimmunity in the facilitation of tumor growth,[13,16] and our own studies of lymphocyte subpopulations in head and neck cancer patients have suggested that patients who relapse have subpopulation profiles that are similar to those seen in autoimmune disorders.[45]

IMMUNE DEFICITS AND CANCER

Although a definite role for immune competence in cancer growth and treatment outcome has long been assumed, correlations of parameters of immune reactivity with prognosis have been limited. Animal models of regressing tumors document the critical role of tumor infiltration by T lymphocytes, and such models have been used to demonstrate successful immunotherapy by use of a variety of immune manipulations, including adoptive transfer of cultured "killer" lymphocytes. These exciting discoveries are now being investigated clinically.

Pertinent observations of potential importance in patients with head and neck cancer include correlations of disease-free survival with the degree of tumor infiltration by helper-inducer T4 lymphocytes and correlations of early disease relapse and distant metastases with peripheral blood levels of CD8 (cytotoxic) cells and NK activity, respectively.[44,45,52] Regulation of CD8 cell proliferation appears to be influenced by a subpopulation of helper- ($CD4^+$ $2H4^+$) inducer cells and by levels of helper cell production of IL2. NK activity also appears to be augmented directly by IL2.[53] Thus, the correction of peripheral blood immune deficits that are significantly associated with prognosis in head and neck cancer may be mediated by approaches directed at enhancing IL2 production and helper-inducer cell function. The mechanisms controlling the migration, retention, and activation of helper cells at a tumor site are unknown, but indirect evidence for impaired helper cell function in head and neck cancer is supported by impaired in vitro production of leukocyte migration inhibitory factor, IL2, and interferon in untreated patients,[40,54,55] and by the significant, longlasting decreases in both helper cell and cytotoxic cell levels associated with radiation therapy (Table 23–2).[56,57] Strategies of immunorestorative treatment that are used as an adjuvant to conventional treatment in such patients and that might benefit the elderly patient with cancer include adoptive replacement of affected cell populations and lymphokines or stimulation of appropriate lymphokine production and lymphocyte proliferation in vivo. Adoptive transfer of immune reactive cells and IL2 has not yet been studied in head and neck cancer, but has shown promising results in patients with advanced melanoma and renal cell carcinoma.[58,59] These studies have been associated with severe toxicity that would not be acceptable as adjuvant treatment in patients who are potentially curable by

TABLE 23-2 Serial Absolute Lymphocyte Subsets in Postoperative Radiation Therapy (RT) Patients

(n)	Preoperative (11)	Postoperative (11)	During RT (7)	Completion RT (7)	1 - 2 Months (11)	4 - 6 Months (8)
T11	1105 ± 164	1565 ± 340	337 ± 33	413 ± 112	362 ± 43	227 ± 59
T3	909 ± 141	1479 ± 337	308 ± 29	325 ± 96	304 ± 40	196 ± 50
T4	690 ± 83	944 ± 203	187 ± 22	209 ± 58	179 ± 27	116 ± 29
T8	362 ± 68	534 ± 149	111 ± 24	154 ± 47	138 ± 26	94 ± 29
T6	39 ± 22	60 ± 37	6 ± 3	14 ± 7	5 ± 1	11 ± 6
T9	38 ± 19	68 ± 23	8 ± 3	32 ± 20	6 ± 1	20 ± 11
T10	85 ± 20	186 ± 40	51 ± 20	65 ± 21	97 ± 23	48 ± 18
Leu 7	181 ± 59	322 ± 100	36 ± 13	103 ± 36	96 ± 17	61 ± 20
T4/T8	1.80 ± 0.21	1.98 ± 0.26	2.09 ± 0.42	1.55 ± 0.20	1.49 ± 0.18	1.51 ± 0.28

conventional means or as cancer prevention regimens in the elderly population. Other immunorestorative measures that use better tolerated natural products such as the thymic hormones, retinoids, or essential trace elements may be more practical for tumor-free patients.

IMMUNE RESTORATION, AGING, AND CANCER

Perhaps the most interesting relationship between cancer and aging involves the thymus gland. Decline in immune function with age has been correlated with a preceding decline in thymic function, involution of the thymus gland, and decrease in circulating thymic hormones.[12,60] The thymic hormones are peptides, produced by the thymus gland, that influence the maturation and function of T lymphocytes. A variety of biologically active peptides has been isolated and characterized.[25] One of the first to be fully sequenced and synthesized was thymosin alpha$_1$, which was found to stimulate the maturation and function of helper T cells and to be 100 times more active in biologic assays than the partially-purified parent preparation, thymosin fraction V.[61] Thymosin alpha$_1$ enhances impaired helper T cell function in both aged mice and man[25] and has been shown to restore impaired lymphokine production in vitro in patients with head and neck cancer and in vivo in animal models of radiation-induced immune suppression.[62,63] Of specific interest is the potential relationship of the lymphokine IL2 to both aging and immune function since production of IL2 is decreased in elderly subjects and IL2 is of central importance in the proliferation of cytotoxic cells. Levels of thymosin alpha$_1$ decrease with age[64] in parallel with thymic involution and with the decreasing ability of aged lymphocytes to produce IL2 in vitro. Most recently, production of IL2 by aged human peripheral blood lymphocytes has been shown to be markedly enhanced by a variety of thymic hormones, including thymosin alpha$_1$.[65-67] In addition to enhancing IL2 production, thymosin alpha$_1$ also enhances NK activity.[68] These potential restorative effects on helper cell activity and on the production of lymphokines that are important in the proliferation of cytotoxic cells suggest that thymic hormones could play a role as adjuvants in immunocompromised or elderly cancer patients.

In head and neck cancer therapy, radiation is the most immunosuppressive modality commonly used. In patients with advanced disease and preexisting immune abnormalities, the addition of postoperative radiation results in prolonged immune depression.[56,57] In particular, we have documented persistently decreased levels of CD8 cells after postoperative radiation (Fig. 23-2) that are poten-

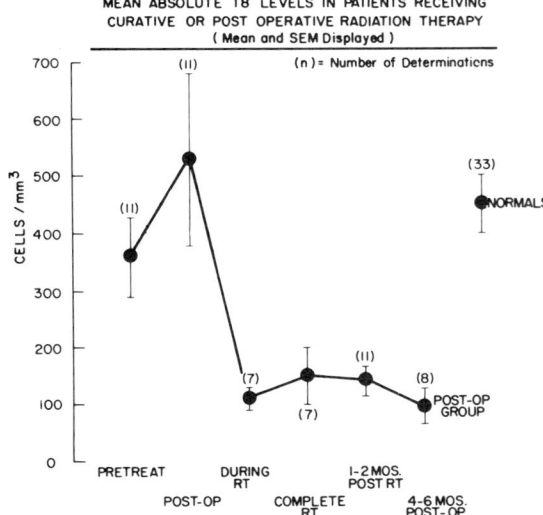

Figure 23-2 Serial absolute levels of CD8-positive lymphocytes prior to and following postoperative radiation therapy in patients with Stage III or IV head and neck squamous carcinoma. Mean levels at 6 months post-therapy remain significantly lower than pretreatment ($p < 0.05$).

TABLE 23-3 Serial Mean (±SE) Percent and Absolute (abs.) Lymphocyte Subpopulation Levels in Patients Receiving Thymosin Alpha$_1$* After Postoperative Radiation Therapy (RT)

	Pretreatment	End RT	1 Month	3 Month
% T11	80 ± 3	72 ± 4	81 ± 1†	78 ± 3
% T4	49 ± 2	37 ± 4	38 ± 2	37 ± 3
% T8	26 ± 2	26 ± 2	33 ± 2†	33 ± 4†
% Leu 7	21 ± 7	16 ± 2	23 ± 2†	22 ± 3
Abs T11	1314 ± 174	451 ± 86	703 ± 113	536 ± 114
Abs. T4	826 ± 118	239 ± 51	325 ± 55	234 ± 60
Abs. T8	408 ± 56	182 ± 43	281 ± 45†	248 ± 74
Abs. Leu 7	325 ± 91	121 ± 31	218 ± 43	162 ± 45

* 900 μg/m^2 twice a week × 4 weeks
† Differs from end RT value, p <0.05

tially detrimental, since levels of CD8 cells have been shown to be directly associated with prognosis in head and neck cancer.[45,56,69] Under normal circumstances, levels of CD8 cells appear to be regulated by helper cells and IL2. In pilot studies of the potential immune restorative effects of thymosin alpha$_1$ in head and neck cancer patients, twice weekly injections (900 μg/m^2) resulted in significant increases in absolute and percent CD8 cell levels, overall T cell levels, and percent NK cells by 1 month postradiation (Table 23-3). Similar significant increases in CD8 cell levels have also been reported with the use of thymic hormone after induction chemotherapy in head and neck cancer patients.[70]

These encouraging preliminary findings have led to an ongoing multi-institutional, placebo controlled, prospective trial using thymosin alpha$_1$ in patients with Stage III or IV head and neck squamous carcinoma who are treated with combined surgery and postoperative radiation (Fig. 23-3). It is hoped that thymic hormone immune reconstitution of helper cell function in this immunocompromised population will result in enhanced proliferation of cytotoxic effector cells and prevent the development of both distant metastases and second primary

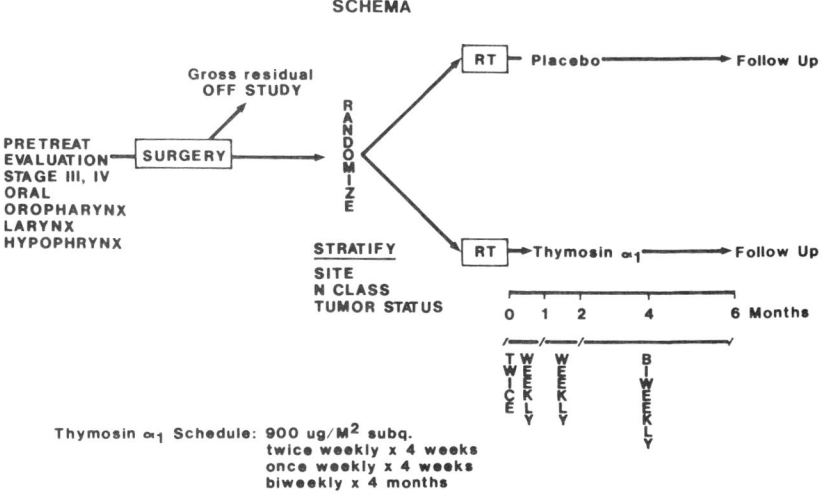

Figure 23-3 Schema of ongoing prospective placebo-controlled trial of thymosin alpha$_1$ as an immune restorative agent after postoperative radiation therapy in patients with head and neck squamous carcinoma. This study is being conducted at the University of Michigan and the University of South Florida.

tumors. Such studies should provide fundamental knowledge regarding the role of thymic hormones in the regulation of the immune response and should also provide insight into their efficacy in the correction of immune impairments associated with cancer and the aging process.

References

1. Wolf GT. Head and neck tumor immunology: an overview. In: Veldman JE, ed. Immunobiology, histophysiology and tumor immunology in otolaryngology. Amsterdam: Kugler, 1986:343.
2. Weksler ME. Senescence of the immune system. Med Clin North Am 1983; 67:263–272.
3. Ford PM. The immunology of ageing. Clin Rheum Dis 1986; 12:1–10.
4. Kelly JF. Clinical pharmacology of chemotherapeutic agents in old age. Front Radiat Ther Oncol 1986; 20:101–111.
5. Dix D, Cohen P, Flannery J. On the role of aging in cancer incidence. J Theor Biol 1980; 83:163–173.
6. Newel GR, Boutwell WB, Morris OL, Titley BC, Branyon ES. Epidemiology of cancer. In: DeVita VT, Hellman S, Rosenberg SA, eds. Cancer: principles and practice of oncology. Philadelphia: JB Lippincott, 1982.
7. Tsuda T, Kim YJ, Siskind GW, et al. Role of the thymus and T-cells in slow growth of B16 melanomas in old mice. Cancer Res 1987; 47:3097–3100.
8. Ershler WB. The change in aggressiveness of neoplasms with age. Geriatrics 1987; 42:99–103.
9. Poste G, Fidler IJ. The pathogenesis of cancer metastasis. Nature 1980; 283:139–146.
10. Singh J, Singh AK. Age-related changes in human thymus. Clin Exp Immunol 1979; 37:507–511.
11. Boyd E. The weight of the thymus gland in health and in disease. Am J Dis Child 1932; 43:1162–1214.
12. Lewis VM, Twomey JJ, Bealmear P, et al. Age, thymic involution and circulating thymic hormone activity. J Clin Endocrinol Metab 1978; 47:145–159.
13. Prehn RT. The immune reaction as a stimulator of tumor growth. Science 1972; 176:170–171.
14. Fidler IJ. Immune stimulation-inhibition of experimental cancer metastasis. Cancer Res 1974; 34:491–498.
15. Chee DO, Bodurtha AJ. Facilitation and inhibition of B16 melanoma by BCG in vivo and by lymphoid cells from BCG-treated mice in vitro. Int J Cancer 1974; 14:137–143.
16. Prehn RT, Prehn LM. The autoimmune nature of cancer. Cancer Res 1987; 47:927–932.
17. Gillis J. Interleukin-2: biology and biochemistry. J Clin Immunol 1983; 3:1–15.
18. Committee on Human Leukocyte Differentiation Antigens. Immunol Today 1984; 5:158.
19. Rosenberg SA, Mule JJ, Spriss PJ, et al. Regression of established pulmonary metastases and subcutaneous tumor mediated by the systemic administration of high-dose recombinant interleukin-2. J Exp Med 1985; 161:1169–1188.
20. Grimm EA, Maxumder A, Zhang UZ, Rosenberg SA. Lymphokine-activated killer cell phenomenon: lysis of natural killer-resistant fresh solid tumor cells by interleukin-2 activated autologous human peripheral blood lymphocytes. J Exp Med 1982; 155:1823–1841.
21. Schulof RS. Thymic peptide hormones: basic properties and clinical applications in cancer. CRC Crit Rev Oncol Hematol 1985; 3:309–368.
22. Wara DW, Barret DJ, Amman AF, Cowan MJ. In vitro and in vivo enhancement of mixed leukocyte culture reactivity by thymosin in patients with primary immunodeficiency disease. Ann NY Acad Sci 1979; 332:128–134.
23. Cohen MH, Chretient PB, Idhe DL, et al. Thymosin fraction 5 and intensive combination chemotherapy prolonging survival of patients with small cell lung cancer. JAMA 1979; 241:1813–1815.
24. Schulof RS, Lloyd MJ, Cleary PA, et al. A randomized trial to evaluate the immunorestorative properties of synthetic thymosin- alpha 1 in patients with lung cancer. J Biol Response Mod 1985; 4:147–158.
25. Zatz MM, Goldstein AL. Thymosin, lymphokines and the immunology of aging. Gerontology 1985; 31:263–277.
26. Makinodan T, Kay MM. Age influence on the immune system. Adv Immunol 1980; 29:287–330.
27. Brohee D, De Maertelaer V, Piro P, Kennes B, Neve P. Specific effect of age on lectin-induced mitogenesis of lymphocytes from diseased patients. Gerontology 1986; 32:74–80.
28. Deviere J, Kennes B, Closset J, DeMaertelaer V, Neve P. Immune senescence: effect of age, sex and health on human blood mononuclear subpopulations. Arch Gerontol Geriatr 1985; 4:285–293.
29. Mursko DM, Nelson BJ, Silver R, Matour D, Kaye D. Immunologic response in an elderly population with a mean age of 85. Am J Med 1986; 81:612–618.
30. Thoman ML. Role of interleukin-2 in the age-related impairment of immune function. J Am Geriatr Soc 1985; 33:781–787.
31. Negoro S, Hara H, Miyata S, et al. Mechanisms of age-related decline in antigen specific T cell proliferative response: IL-2 receptor expression and recombinant IL-2 induced proliferative response of purified TAC-positive T cells. Mech Ageing Dev 1986; 36:223–241.
32. Gillis S, Kozak R, Durante M, Weksler ME. Immunological studies in aging. Decreased production of and response to T cell growth factor by lymphocytes from aged humans. J Clin Invest 1981; 67:937–942.
33. Ershler WB, Moore AC, Roessner K, Ranges GE. Interleukin-2 and aging. Immunopharmacology 1985; 10:11–17.
34. Traill KN, Schonitzer D, Jurgens G, et al. Age-related changes in lymphocyte subset proportions, surface differentiation antigen density and plasma membrane fluidity: application of the Eurage Protocol Admission criteria. Mech Ageing Dev 1985; 33:39–66.
35. Ligthart GJ, Vlokhoven PC, Schuit HRE, Hijimans W. The expanded null cell compartment in ageing: increase in the number of natural killer cells and changes in T-cell and NK-cell subsets in human blood. Gerontology 1986; 59:353–358.
36. Nagel JE, Chrest FJ, Adler WH. Enumeration of T-lymphocyte subsets by monoclonal antibodies in young and aged humans. J Immunol 1981; 127:2086–2088.
37. Burton RC, Ferguson P, Gray M, Hall J, Hayes M, Smart YC. Effects of age, gender and cigarette smoking on human immunoregulatory T-cell subsets: establishment of normal ranges and comparison with patients with colorectal cancer and multiple sclerosis. Diagn Immunol 1983; 1:216–223.
38. Bender BS, Nagel JE, Adler WH, Andres R. Absolute peripheral blood lymphocyte count and subsequent mortality of elderly men. J Am Geront Soc 1986; 34:649–654.
39. Bender BS, Chrest FJ, Adler WH. Phenotypic expression of natural killer cell associated membrane antigens and cytolytic function of peripheral blood cells from different aged humans. J Clin Lab Immunol 1986; 21:31–36.
40. Wolf GT, Lovett EJ, Peterson KA, et al. Lymphokine production and lymphocyte subpopulations in patients with head and neck squamous carcinoma. Arch Otolaryngol 1984; 110:731–735.

41. Balch CM, Tilden AB, Dougherty PA, et al. Depressed levels of granular lymphocytes with natural killer (NIC) cell function in 247 cancer patients. Proc Am Assoc Cancer Res 1983; 23:905.
42. Wustrow TPU, Zenner HP. Natural killer cell activity in patients with carcinoma of the larynx and hypopharynx. Laryngoscope 1985; 95:1391–1400.
43. Schantz SP, Shillitoe EJ, Brown B, et al. Natural killer cell activity and head and neck cancer: a clinical assessment. Natl Cancer Instit 1986; 77:869–875.
44. Schantz SP, Goepfert H. Multimodality therapy and distant metastases. Arch Otolaryngol Head Neck Surg 1987; 113:1207–1213.
45. Wolf GT, Schmaltz S, Hudson J, et al. Alterations in T-lymphocyte subpopulations in patients with head and neck cancer: correlations with prognosis. Arch Otolaryngol Head Neck Surgery 1987; 113:1200–1206.
46. Wu W, Pahlavani M, Cheung HT, Richardson A. The effect of aging on the expression of interleukin 2 messenger ribonucleic acid. Cell Immunol 1986; 100:224–231.
47. Indiveri F, Pierri I, Viglione D, Rende D, Russo C, Pellegrino MA, Ferrone S. Human T lymphocytes in aging and malignancy: abnormalities in PHA-induced Ia antigen expression and in functional activity in autologous and allogeneic MLR. Cell Immunol 1983; 76:224–231.
48. Wolf GT, Chretien PB, Weiss JF, Edwards BK, Spiegel HF. Effects of smoking and age on serum levels of immune reactive proteins. Otolaryngol Head Neck Surg 1982; 90:319–326.
49. Thoman M, Weigle W. Reconstitution of in vivo cell-mediated lympholysis responses in aged mice with interleukin 2. J Immunol 1985; 134:949–952.
50. Yamashita N, Suzuki H, Maruyama M, Sugiyama E, Yano S. Effects of aging on the in vitro response of human lymphocytes to interleukin 2. Jpn J Med 1984; 23:213–221.
51. Sauder DN. Effect of age on epidermal immune function. Dermatol Clin 1986; 4:447–454.
52. Wolf GT, Hudson JL, Peterson KA, et al. Lymphocyte subpopulations infiltrating squamous carcinomas of the head and neck: correlations with extent of tumor and prognosis. Otolaryngol Head Neck Surg 1986; 95:142–152.
53. Henney CS, Kuribayaski K, Kern DE, Gillis S. Interleukin 2 augment natural killer cell activity. Nature 1981; 291:335–338.
54. Wanebo HJ, Pace R, Hargett S, et al. Production of and response to interleukin 2 in peripheral blood lymphocytes of cancer patients. Cancer 1986; 57:656–662.
55. Sato M, Yoshida H, Yanagawa T, et al. Interferon activity and its characterization in the sera of patients with head and neck cancer. Cancer 1984; 54:1239–1251.
56. Wolf GT, Amendola BE, Diaz R, et al. Definitive vs. adjuvant radiotherapy: comparative effects on lymphocyte subpopulations in patients with head and neck squamous carcinoma. Arch Otolaryngol Head Neck Surg 1985; 111:716–726.
57. Gray WC, Chretien PB, Suter CM, et al. Effects of radiation therapy on T-lymphocyte subpopulations in patients with head and neck cancer. Otolaryngol Head Neck Surg 1985; 93:650–660.
58. Rosenberg SA, Lotze MT, Muul LM, et al. A progress report on the treatment of 157 patients with advanced cancer using lymphokine-activated kiler cells and interleukin-2 or high dose interleukin-2 alone. N Engl J Med 1987; 316:889–897.
59. West WH, Tacer KW, Yonnelli JR, et al. Constant infusion recombinant interleukin-2 in adoptive immunotherapy of advanced cancer. N Engl J Med 1987; 316:893–905.
60. Goldstein AL, Low TLK, Hall N, Naylor PH, Zatz MM. Thymosin: can it retard aging by boosting the immune capacity? In: Regelson W, Sinex FM, eds. Intervention in the aging process. Part A: Quantitation, epidemiology and clinical research. New York: Liss, 1983:169.
61. Low TLK, Thurman GB, McAdoo M, et al. The chemistry and biology of thymosin. Isolation, characterization and biological activities of thymosin α_1 and polypeptide B_1 from calf thymus. J Biol Chem 1979; 254:981–986.
62. Gray WC, Hasslinger BJ, Suter CM, et al. Suppression of cellular immunity by head and neck irradiation: precipitating factors and reparative mechanisms in an experimental model. Arch Otolaryngol Head Neck Surg 1986; 112:1185–1190.
63. Wolf GT, Peterson KA, Lovett EJ. In vitro immune modulation by thymosin alpha-1 in patients with head and neck squamous carcinoma. Head Neck Surg 1985; 7:350–356.
64. McClure JE, Lameris N, Wara DW, Goldstein AL. Immunochemical studies on thymosin: radioimmunoassay of thymosin α_1. J Immunol 1982; 128:368–371.
65. Zatz MM, Oliver J, Samuels C, et al. Thymosin increases production of T-cell growth factor by normal human peripheral blood lymphocytes. Proc Nat Acad Sci USA 1984; 81:2882–2885.
66. Meroni PL, Barcellini W, Frasca D, et al. In vivo immunopotentiating activity of thymopentin in aging humans: increase of IL-2 production. Clin Immunol Immunopathol 1987; 42:151–159.
67. Sztein MB, Serrate SA, Goldstein AL. Modulation of interleukin 2 receptor expression on normal human lymphocytes by thymic hormones. Proc Natl Acad Sci USA 1986; 83:6107–6111.
68. Serrate SA, Schulof RS, Leondaridas L, et al. Modulation of human natural killer cell cytotoxic activity, lymphokine production and interleukin 2 receptor expression by thymic hormones. J Immunol 1987; 139:2338–2343.
69. Hayaski Y, Yoshida H, Furumoto N, et al. Monoclonal antibody analysis of peripheral blood lymphocyte subpopulations in squamous cell head and neck cancer. Cancer 1986; 1:25–30.
70. Schuff-Werner P, Lohr G, Rauschning W, et al. Longitudinal assessment of lymphocyte subpopulations in patients with squamous cell carcinoma of the head and neck. Serono Symp 1986; 28:425–431.

FACIAL PLASTIC AND RECONSTRUCTIVE SURGERY IN AN AGING POPULATION: A CRITICAL OVERVIEW

Chapter Twenty-Four

FACIAL PLASTIC AND RECONSTRUCTIVE SURGERY IN AN AGING POPULATION: A CRITICAL OVERVIEW

M. EUGENE TARDY Jr., M.D., F.A.C.S.
DEAN TORIUMI, M.D.
DAVID BROADWAY, M.D.

To most individuals, the prospect of living longer holds appeal only if good health graces advancing years. A sense of well-being, essential to the enjoyment and productivity of the aging population, is derived principally from the retained ability to function in a healthy and relatively normal manner. Not surprisingly, older individuals commonly seek to *look* as good as they *feel*. Concern about body image and appearance persists vividly, even in octogenarians (Fig. 24–1). The head and neck surgeon devoted to plastic and reconstructive surgery has substantial challenges and opportunities to improve both the normal function and the appearance of the enlarging population referred to as "geriatric" (Fig. 24–2). These challenges are by no means unique to the end of the 20th century; surgeons struggled to improve the quality of life in a similar fashion over 100 years ago. Today, however, the 30 million persons aged 65 and over constitute a more substantial opportunity for service than ever before.

At present, more suitable tools, time tested techniques, and a rededication to fundamental principles of plastic surgery coalesce to improve quality of life meaningfully by restoring function and improving facial form. These venerated principles of plastic surgery apply throughout all the age groups of life, but require modification when dealing with aging inelastic skin, ptotic head and neck structures, reduced blood supply, more frail skeletal supporting structures, and a reduced collagenous healing response. The last phenomenon, however, like other aging characteristics, may be turned to the surgeon's advantage by creating more delicate and better camouflaged scars.

From an emotional standpoint, the equanimity possessed by most older patients, seasoned by life's experiences, creates an especially gratifying

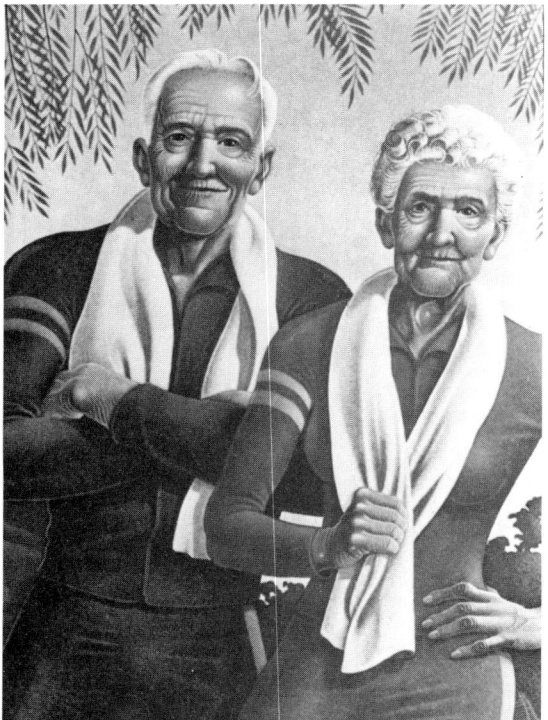

Figure 24–1 Aging individuals in the present era seek to look as good as they feel. Bodily physical fitness is increasingly common among older individuals who understandably seek to improve their facial appearance as well.

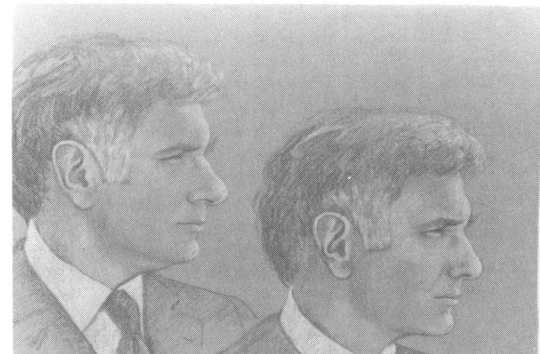

Figure 24–2 The level of sophistication in the aging population has increased to the level of providing the surgeon with an extremely precise artist's sketch of anticipated results of facial surgery.

surgeon-patient experience. Individuals in this age group have generally respected and trusted their physician's judgment and recommendations since childhood, an attitude shared to a much lesser degree by a younger population bombarded by media distortions and with an all-consuming urge to reward less-than-perfect treatment outcomes with accusatory litigation.

It is impractical if not impossible to examine the wide spectrum of useful plastic procedures unique to an aging patient population. Instead we shall endeavor to demonstrate visually a number of refinements and advances in facial plastic and reconstructive surgery that possess reliability and safety (Figs. 24-3 to 24-43).

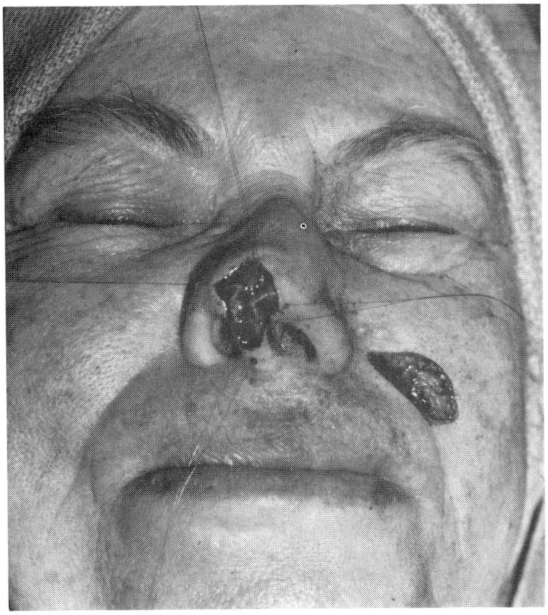

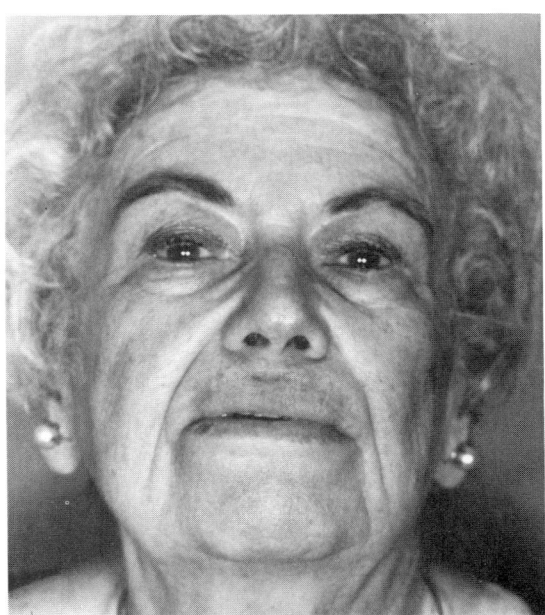

Figure 24-3 Basal cell carcinomas of the immobile nasal tip skin are ideally repaired by total resection and reconstruction with full-thickness skin grafts from the adjacent cheek-lip fold. This skin is of a superb color match and has similar texture to the nasal tip skin.

Figure 24-4 Six months following repair of a nasal tip defect with full-thickness nasolabial fold skin graft.

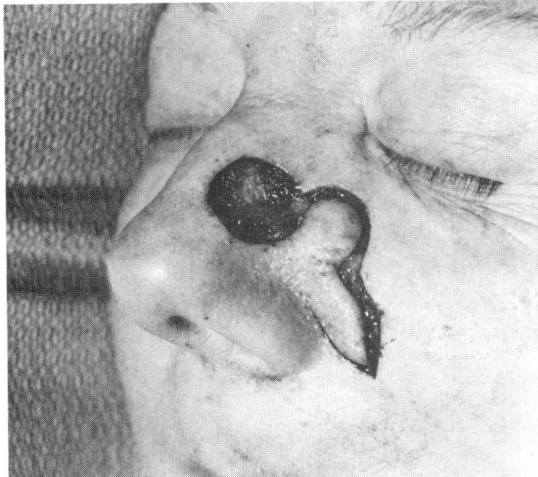

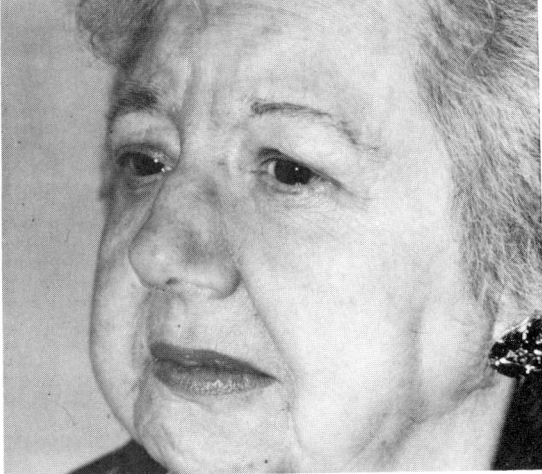

Figure 24-5 Defects of the lateral surface of the nose may be repaired favorably with the bilobular transposition flap with the secondary lobe derived from redundant skin of the nasolabial fold.

Figure 24-6 One year following lateral nasal repair with the bilobed transposition flap.

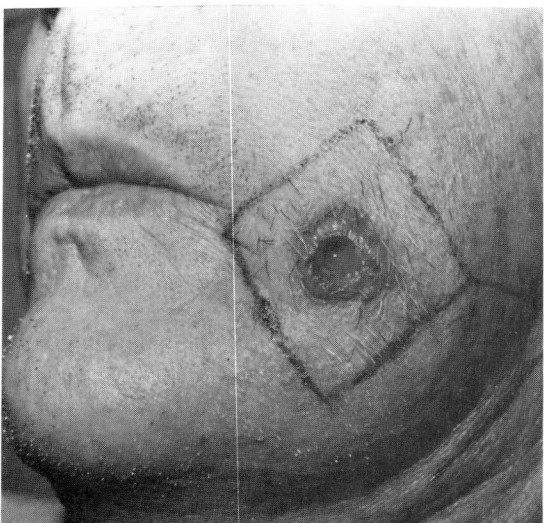

Figure 24–7 Defects resulting from resection of squamous cell carcinomas of the exposed lateral cheek are favorably repaired with rhomboid flaps derived from the redundant submental skin. The skin texture is ideal, and the hair-bearing skin favorably camouflages the defect.

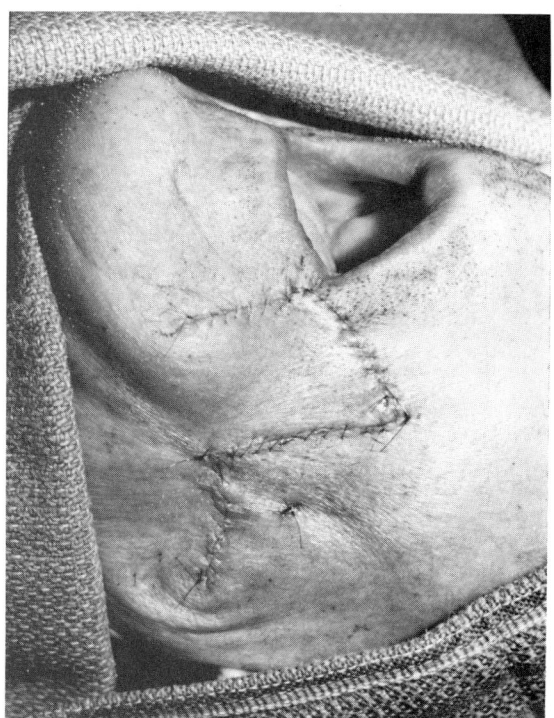

Figure 24–8 Rhomboid flap reconstruction completed.

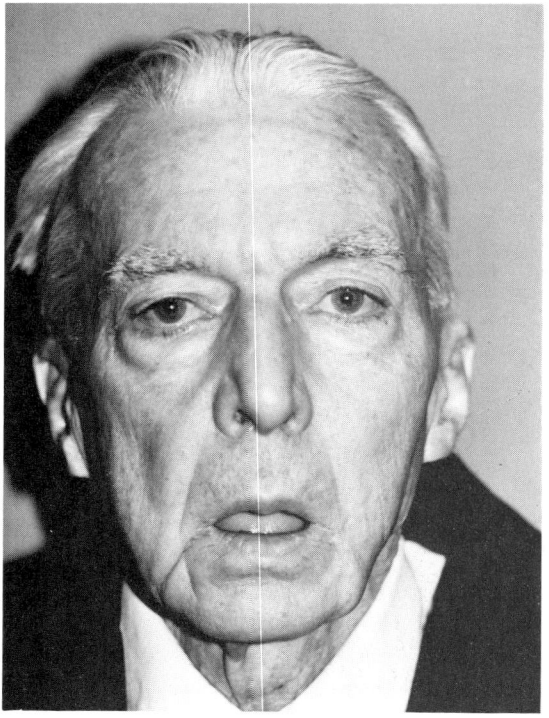

Figure 24–9 Six months following cheek repair with submandibular rhomboid flap procedure.

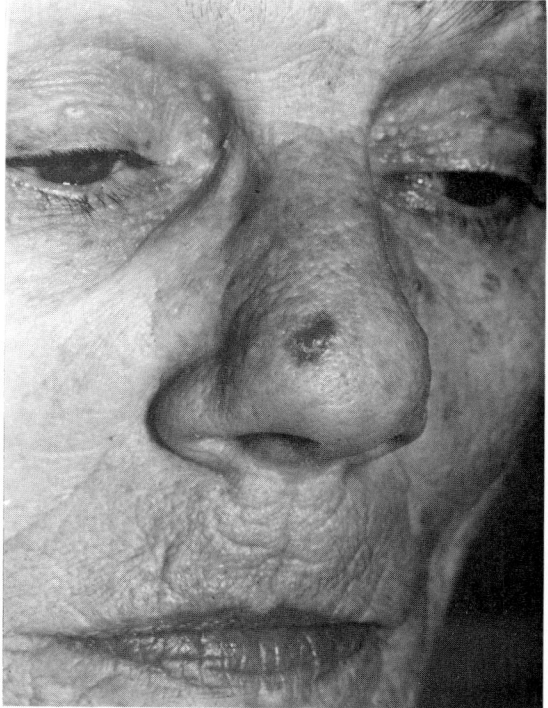

Figure 24–10 A leiomyosarcoma of the nose in an aging patient.

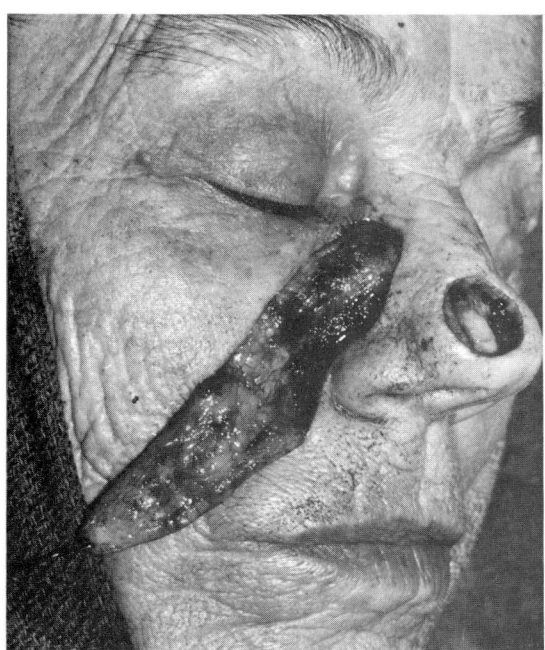

Figure 24–11 The defect resulting from total excision is ideally repaired with an inferiorly based flap derived from the redundant nasolabial fold.

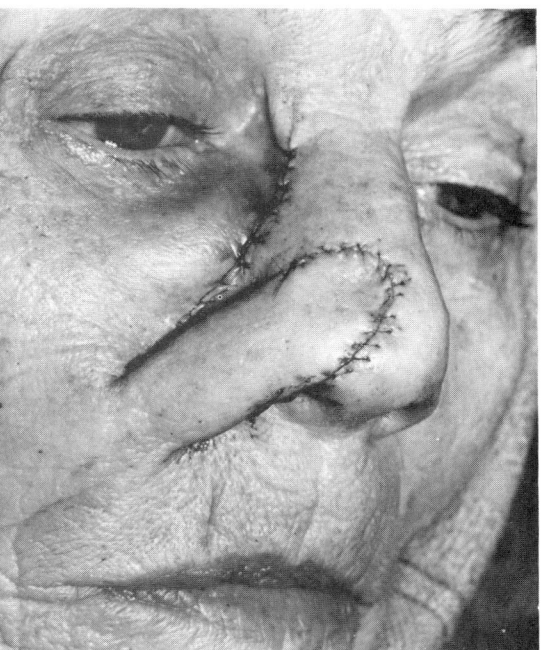

Figure 24–12 The nasolabial flap is interposed into the defect and the donor site closed primarily.

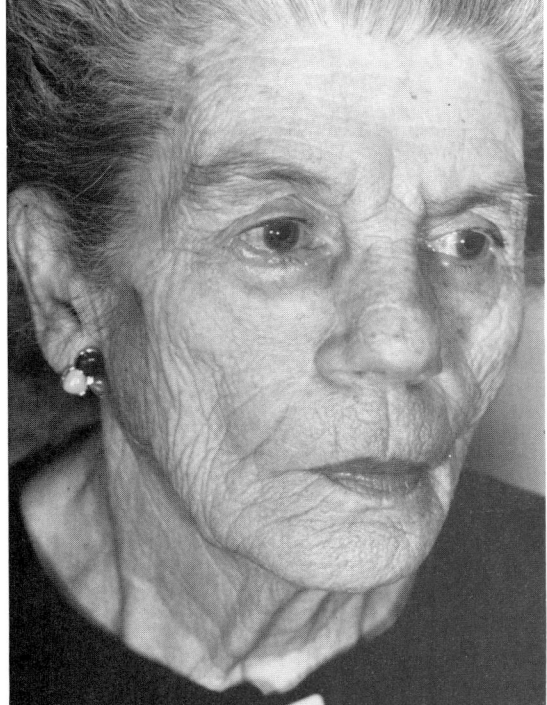

Figure 24–13 Four years following repair of the nasal defect. Similar texture of the surrounding skin and ideal camouflage of the donor site area are illustrated.

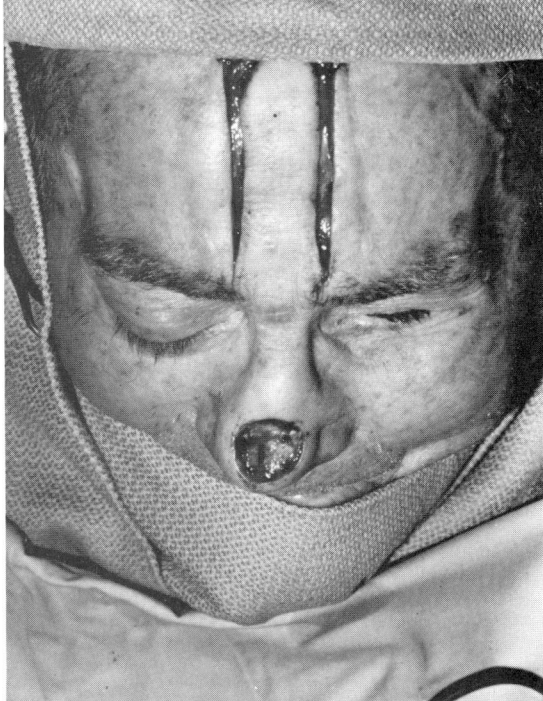

Figure 24–14 A large nasal dorsal defect in an aging individual may be favorably repaired with the precise midline forehead interposition flap.

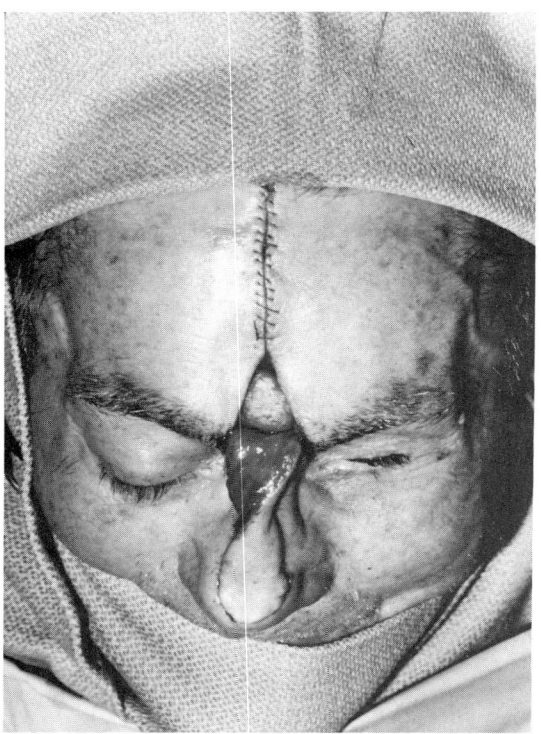

Figure 24–15 Precise midline forehead flaps are ideal because of similar skin color and texture and have the additional advantage of immediate and simple closure of the midline forehead donor site.

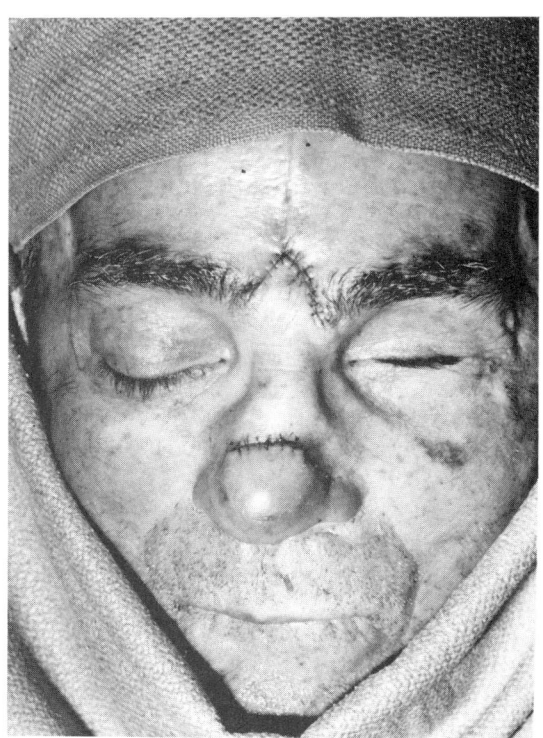

Figure 24–16 Final stage reconstruction of the nasal defect at 12 days after surgery with repair only of the interbrow area in the oblique glabellar creases.

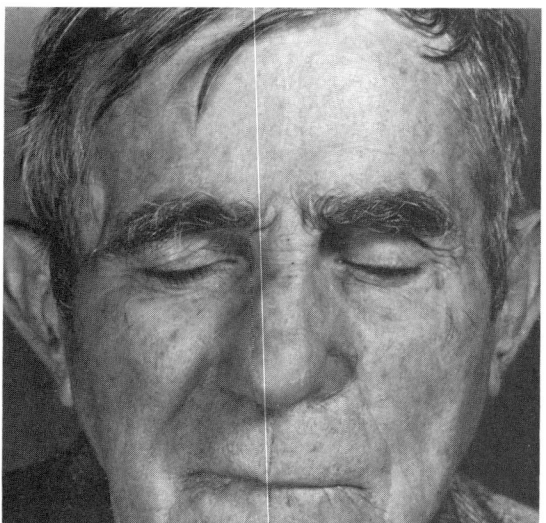

Figure 24–17 Six months following nasal dorsal repair, the midline forehead scar is minimal and the defect is well camouflaged from the standpoint of color and texture.

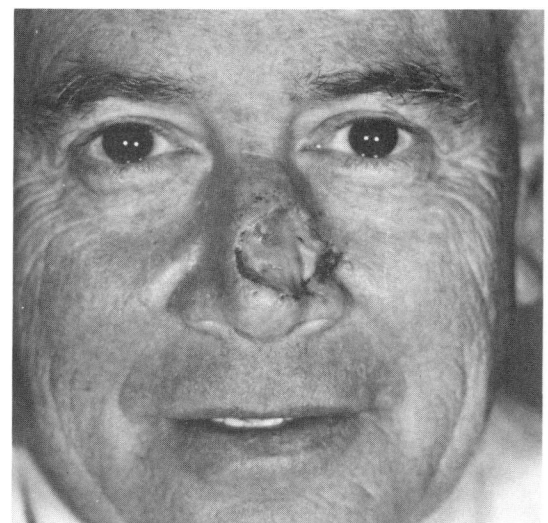

Figure 24–18 A large dorsal nasal defect inadequately repaired with a split-thickness skin graft. The irregular contour, inadequate effacement, and poor color match reveal the inadequacies of this type of repair.

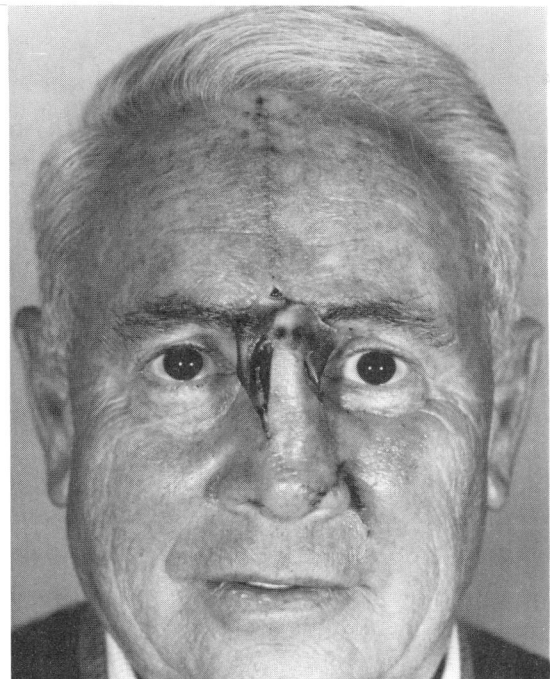

Figure 24-19 Midline forehead flap pictured 5 days after interposition.

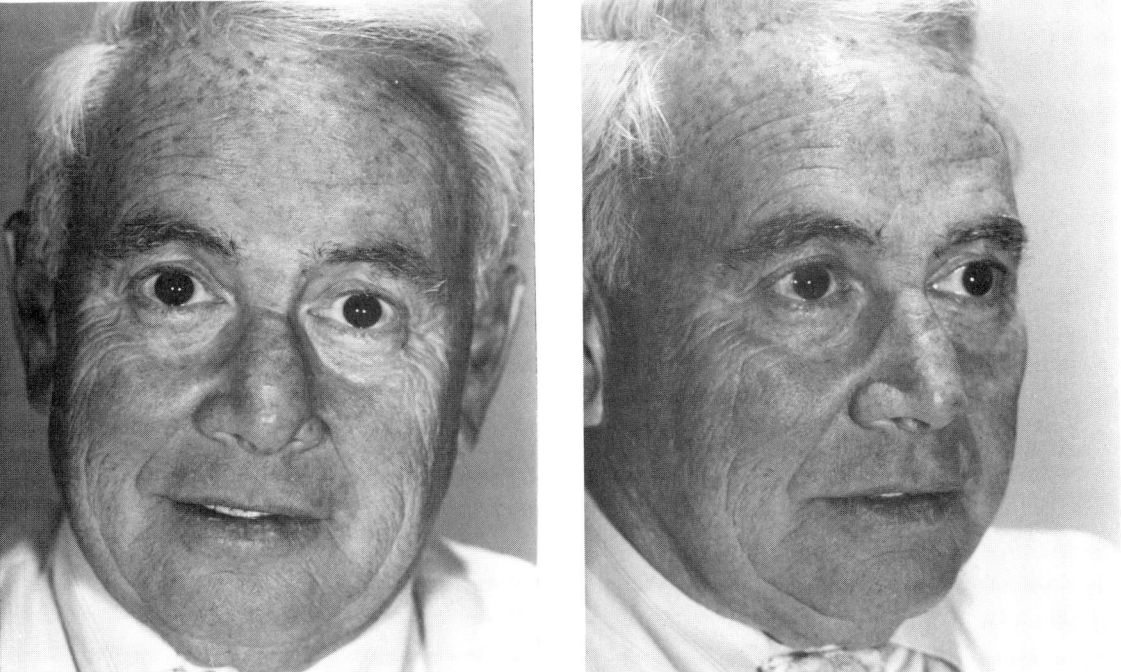

Figure 24-20 and 24-21 Six months following nasal dorsal reconstruction with a midline forehead flap, the midline scar is negligible and the nasal defect is well effaced with good texture and color match.

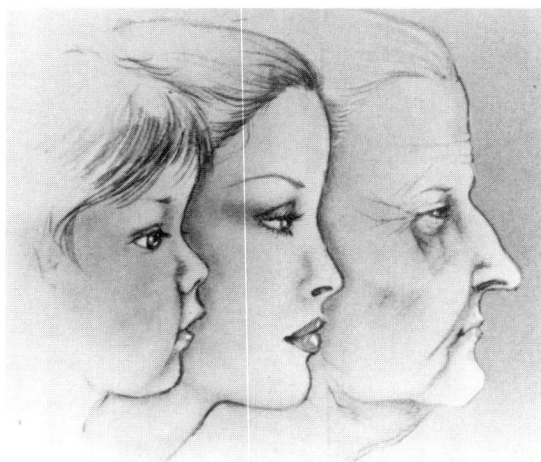

Figure 24–22 As aging progresses, all facial features become ptotic and less well supported as the underlying facial skeleton shrinks, thereby allowing the overlying skin and musculature to be less well supported and to descend in redundant folds.

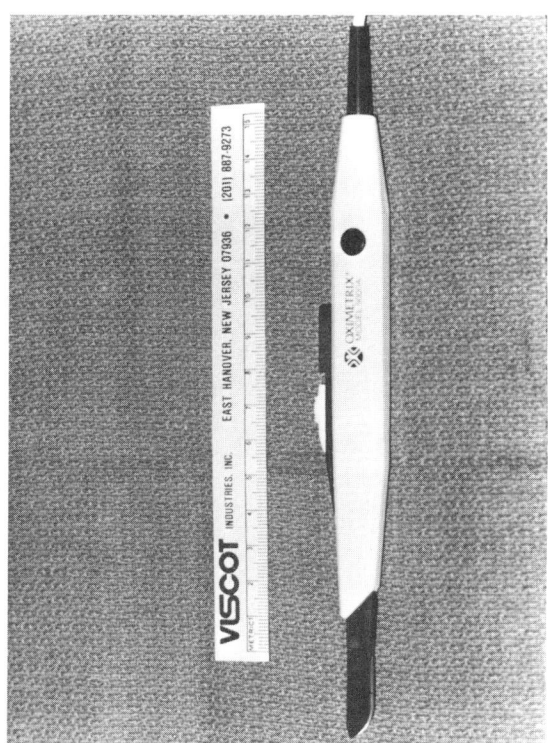

Figure 24–23 A significant advance in facelift surgery has been the employment of the Shaw hemostatic scalpel, which thermally seals small blood vessels during direct vision undermining of facial skin. The significant advantages of this approach have been demonstrated over the past 8 years and include decidedly less swelling, ecchymosis, and patient discomfort.

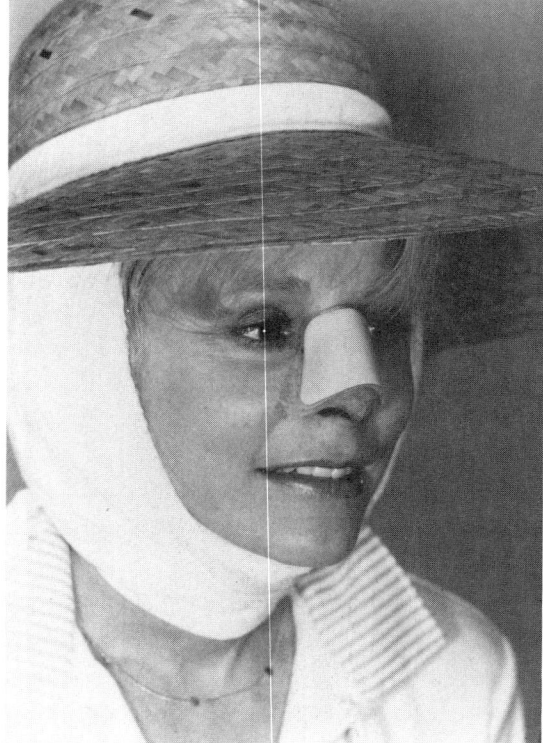

Figure 24–24 The advantages of the Shaw hemostatic scalpel are apparent in this patient photographed 3 days following total facelift and rhinoplasty. There is minimal swelling, little bruising, and rehabilitation develops much more quickly as a result of the dry surgical field.

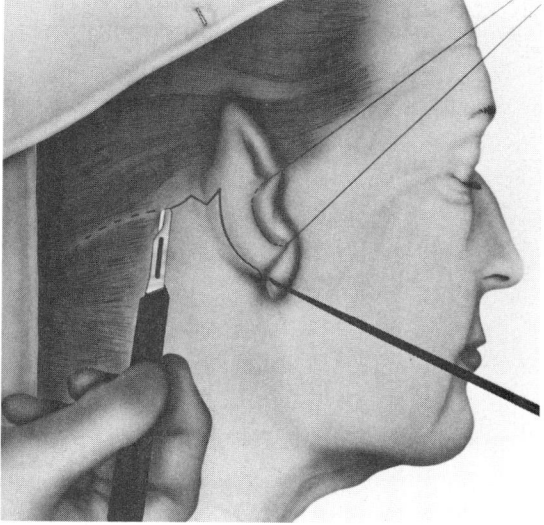

Figure 24–25 The postauricular incision in facelift surgery is facilitated if a small offset is created as the incision traverses the auriculomastoid sulcus. Since all incisions that directly cross a concavity result in a retracted bridle scar, irregularizing the incision at this point leads to a flat, camouflaged, and bandless scar.

Facial Plastic and Reconstructive Surgery in an Aging Population: A Critical Overview / 175

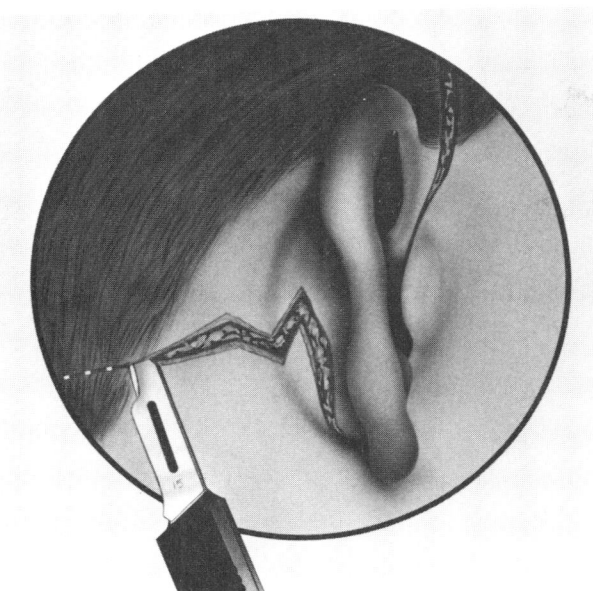

Figure 24–26 A close-up view of the irregularization of the postauricular incision.

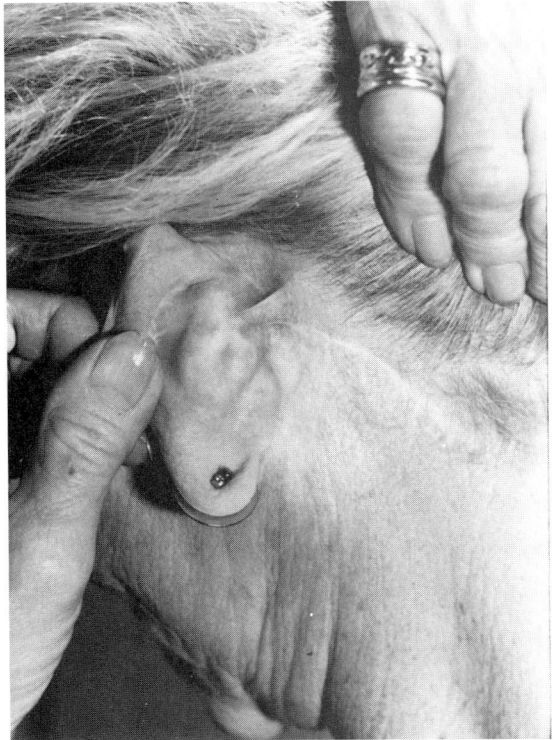

Figure 24–27 A contracted scar, poorly healed, in a patient whose incision has been created directly across the auriculomastoid sulcus and carried inferiorly in front of the posterior hairline. A significantly apparent scar develops along with a palpable contracted band at the auriculomastoid sulcus.

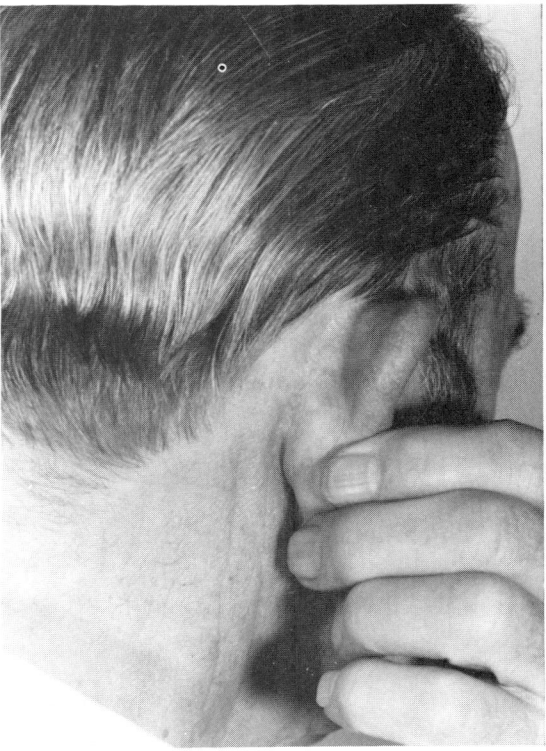

Figure 24–28 Irregularization of the postauricular scar crossing the auriculomastoid sulcus results ordinarily in a nicely camouflaged scar shown here 6 months following surgery.

176 / Geriatric Otorhinolaryngology

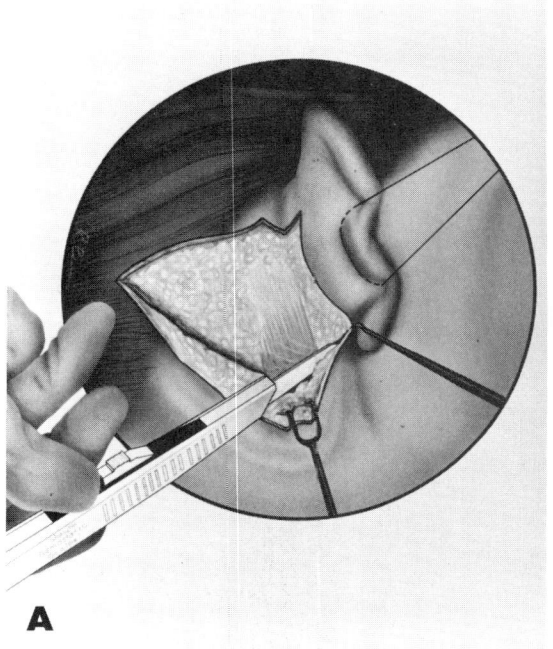
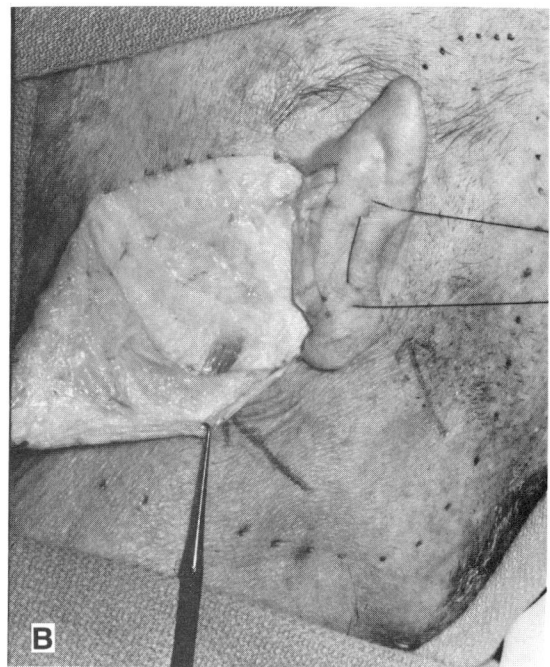
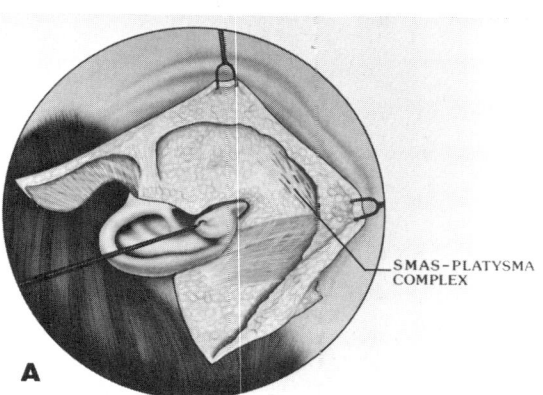
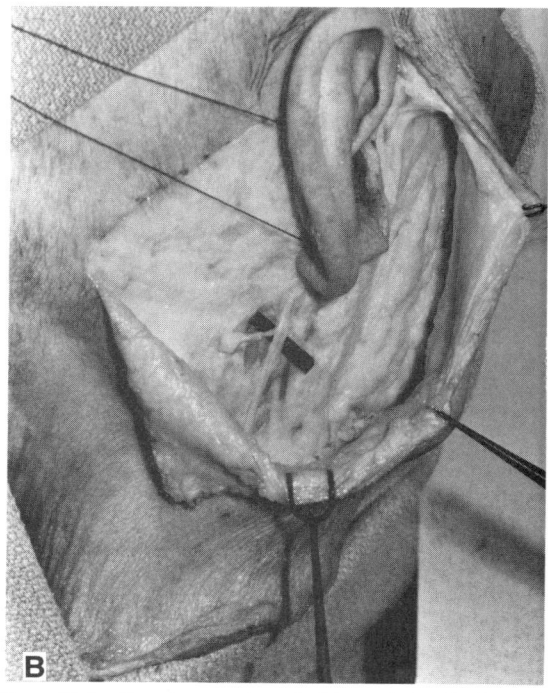

Figure 24–30 *A* and *B*, Elevation of the temporal and preauricular flap with the Shaw hemostatic scalpel is carried as far forward as necessary to achieve appropriate advancement rotation of the skin flap and to identify the superficial musculoaponeurotic system (SMAS)-platysmal complex of tissue to be posteriorly and superiorly repositioned.

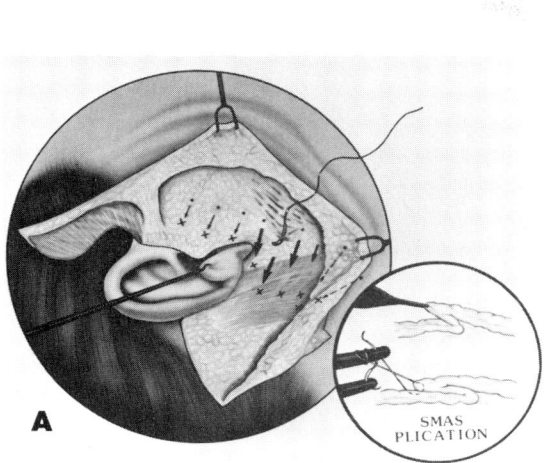
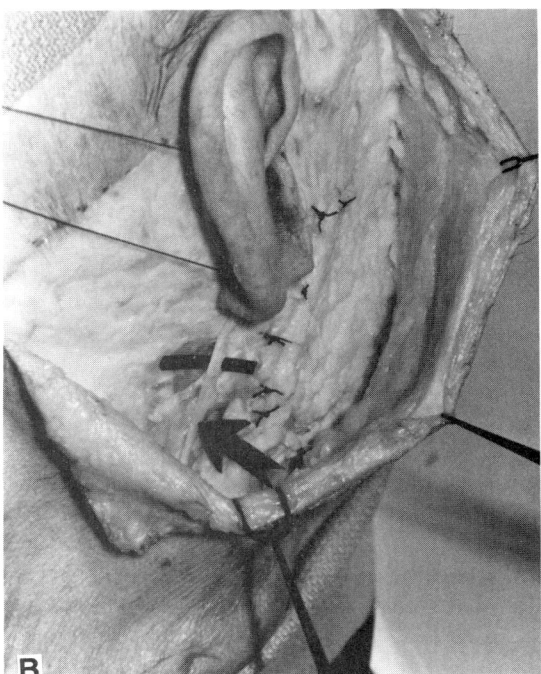
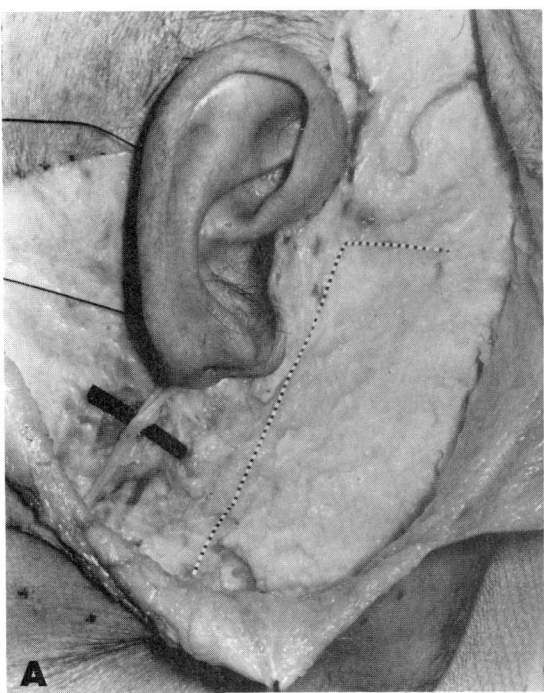
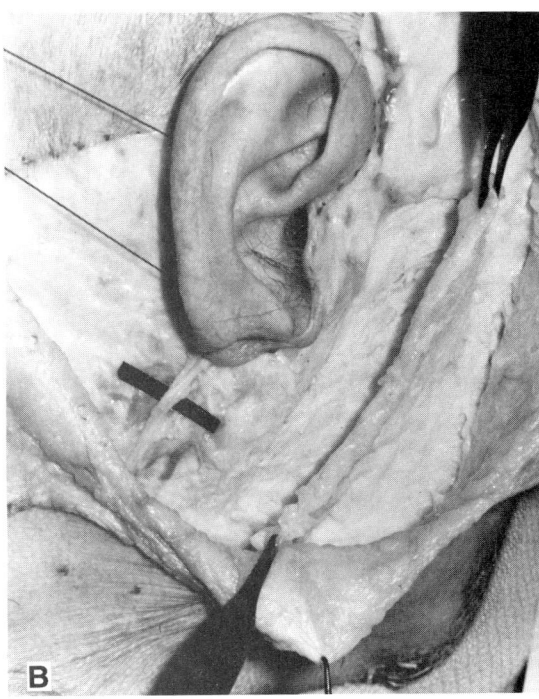

Figure 24–32 *A* and *B*, If the underlying SMAS-platysmal muscle complex is relatively immobile, improvement in facial contour can be gained by incision of the SMAS-fascia as indicated by the dotted line (*A*), development of a separate SMAS-platysmal flap, and advancement rotation of a separate flap for underlying musculofascial support.

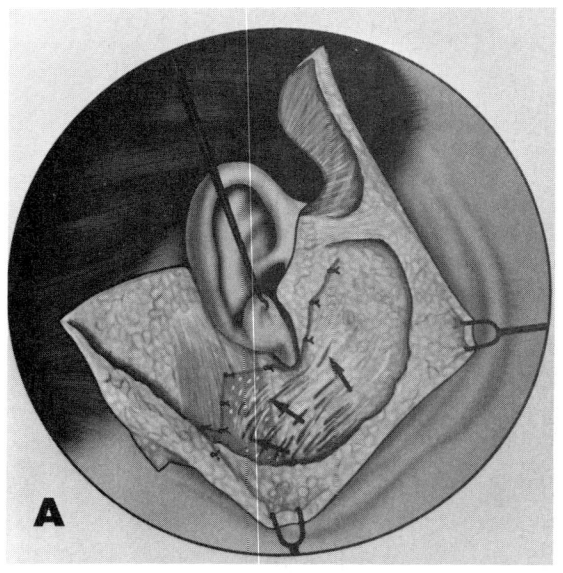

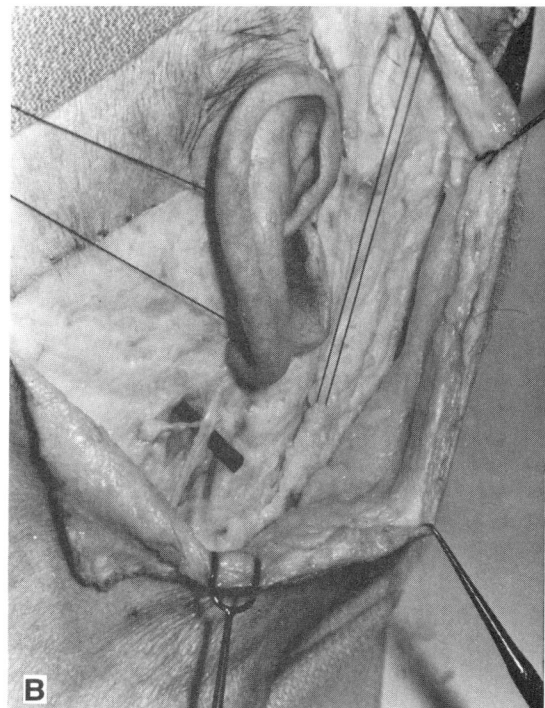

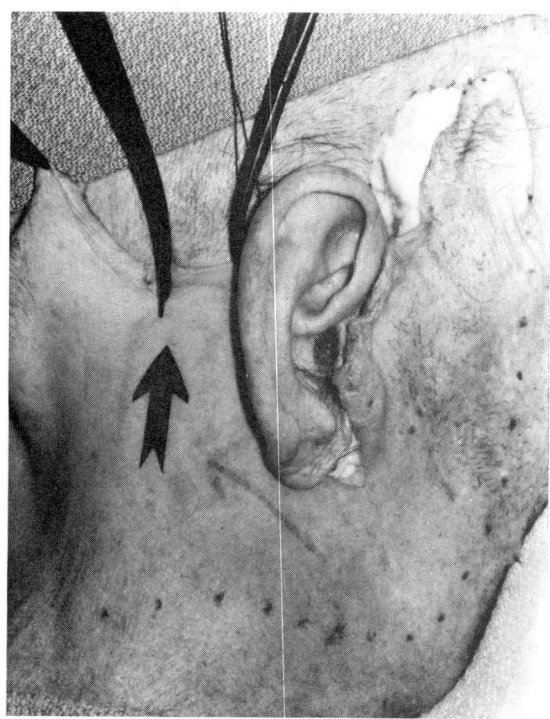

Figure 24–34 The elevated skin flap may now be advanced and rotated without tension and the excess trimmed and discarded.

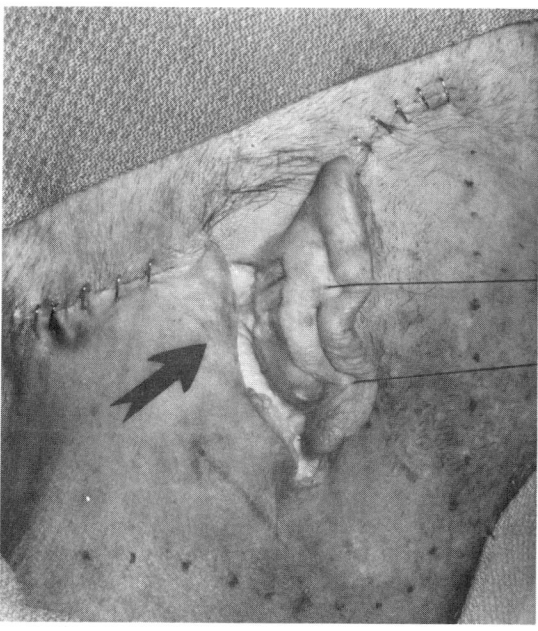

Figure 24–35 An important factor in postauricular flap repositioning is the anterosuperior positioning of the flap to recreate the auriculomastoid sulcus. In this area, very little skin needs to be excised in order to totally reconstruct this important landmark. Blunting of the auriculomastoid sulcus is a common complication following facelift surgery and is easily avoided.

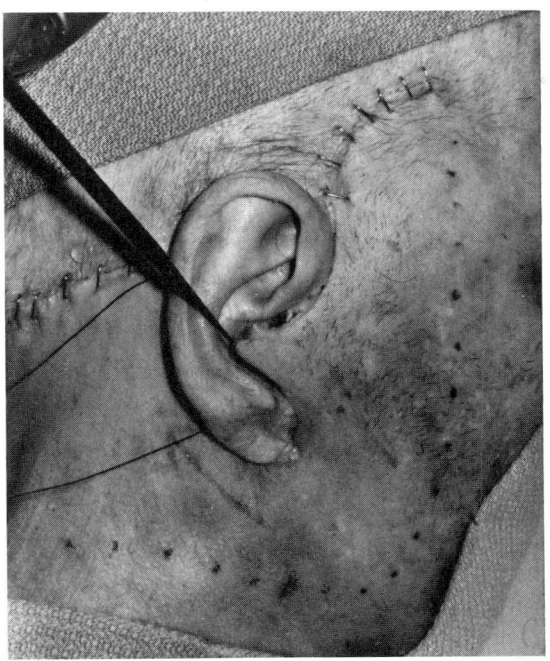
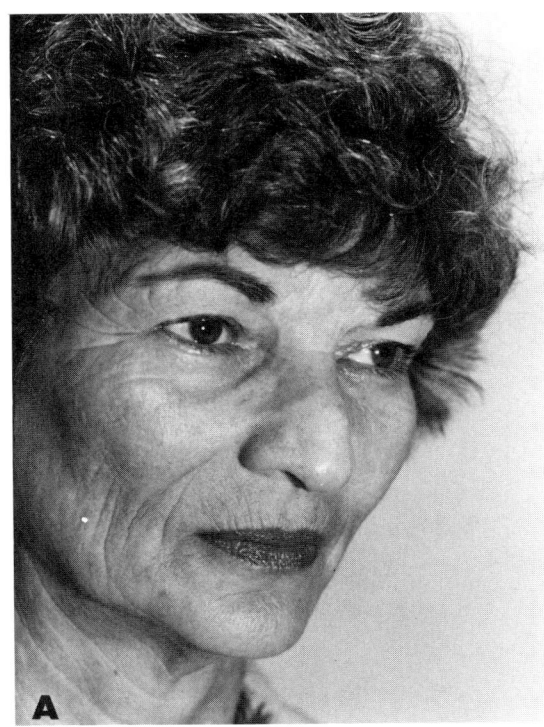
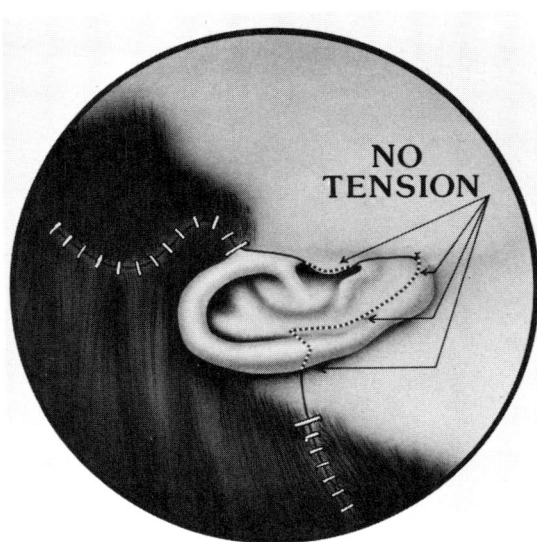
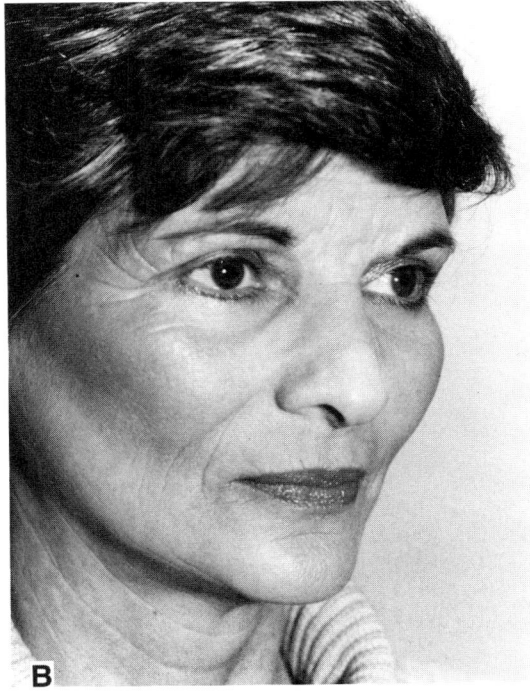

Figure 24–37 A completed repair with surgical staples in the hairline and nonabsorbable fine sutures in the periauricular incisions is finalized under no tension. The support of the facial flap is provided entirely by the repositioned SMAS-platysmal complex, thus facilitating the development of well-camouflaged incisions.

Figure 24–38 *A* and *B*, Rejuvenation and freshening of the entire facial appearance are accomplished by bilateral upper and lower lid blepharoplasty, cervicofacial lift, and subtle rhinoplasty in this aging patient.

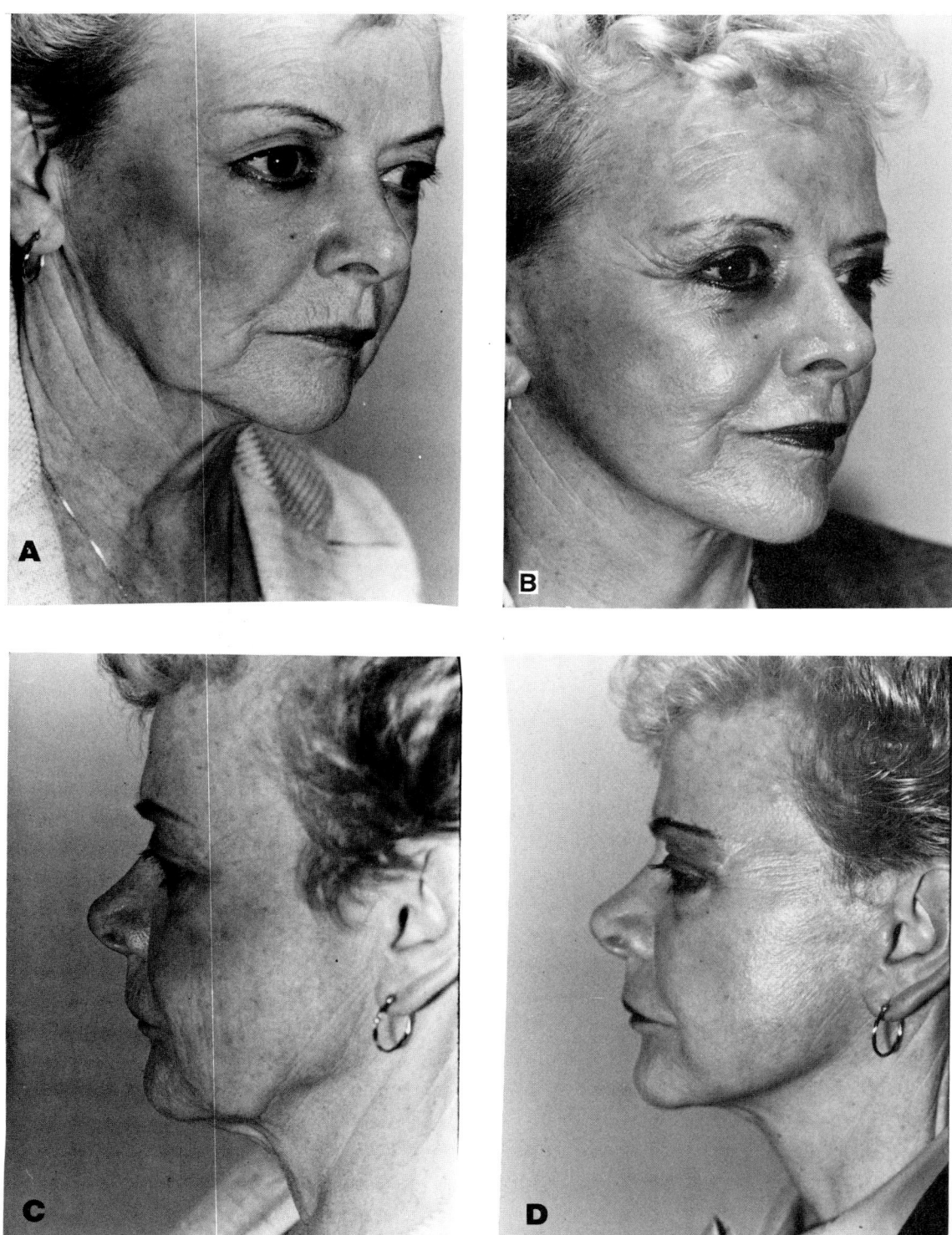

Figure 24–39 *A, B, C,* and *D,* Improvement in the appearance of this patient's eyes and face is accomplished with bilateral upper and lower lid blepharoplasty combined with a cervicofacial lift with SMAS-platysmal plication. Note the improved jawline, the more youthful cervicomental profile line, and the well camouflaged preauricular scars.

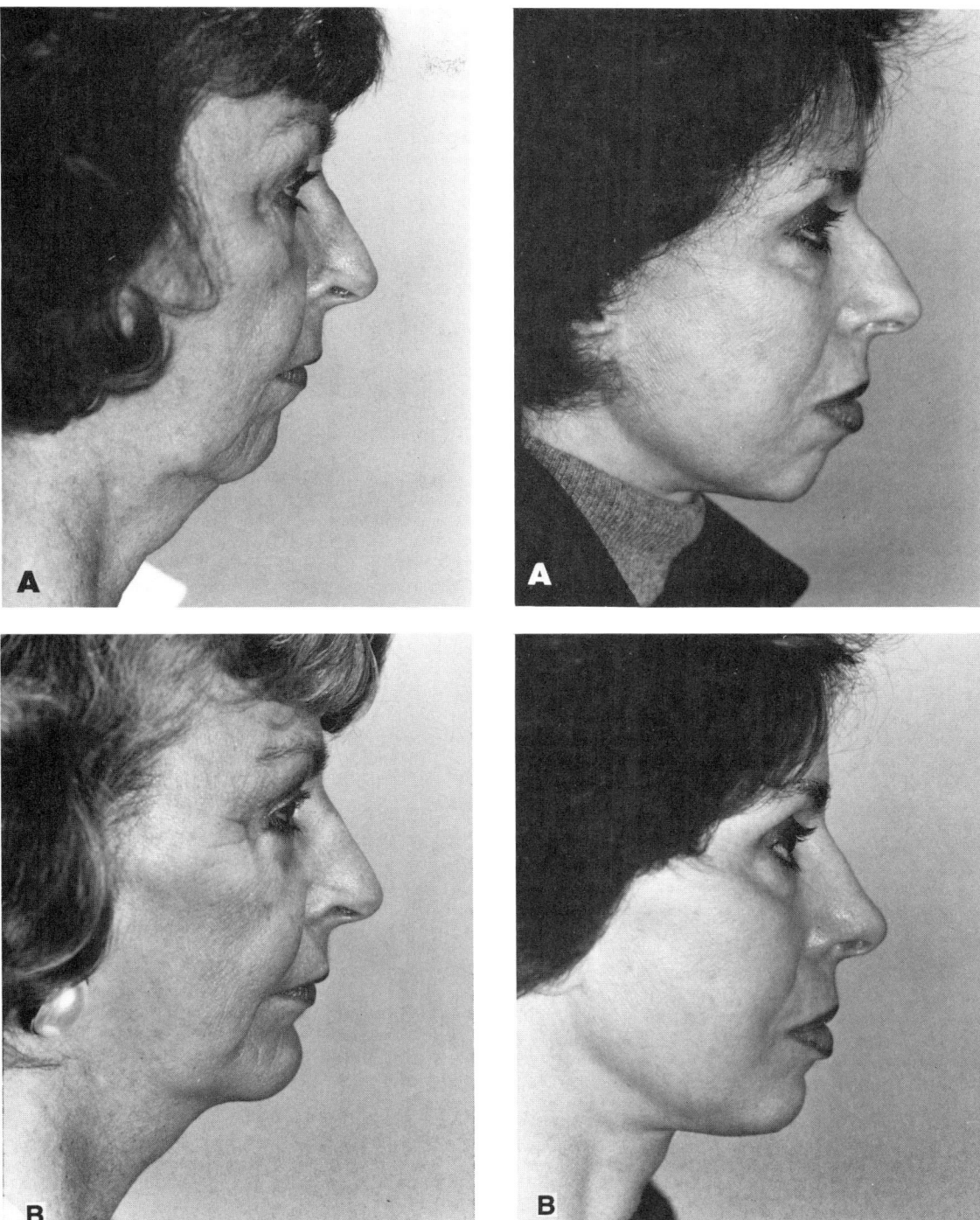

Figure 24–40 *A,* This aging patient represents an individual with significant retrognathia, a low-lying hyoid-thyroid complex, and redundant submental fat and skin. *B,* Rejuvenation is accomplished with a cervicofacial lift, augmentation of the chin, excision of submental fat, and subtle rhinoplasty. The profile improvement is profound when these procedures are combined.

Figure 24–41 *A* and *B,* Improvement of the entire facial profile skeleton is accomplished in this instance with chin augmentation.

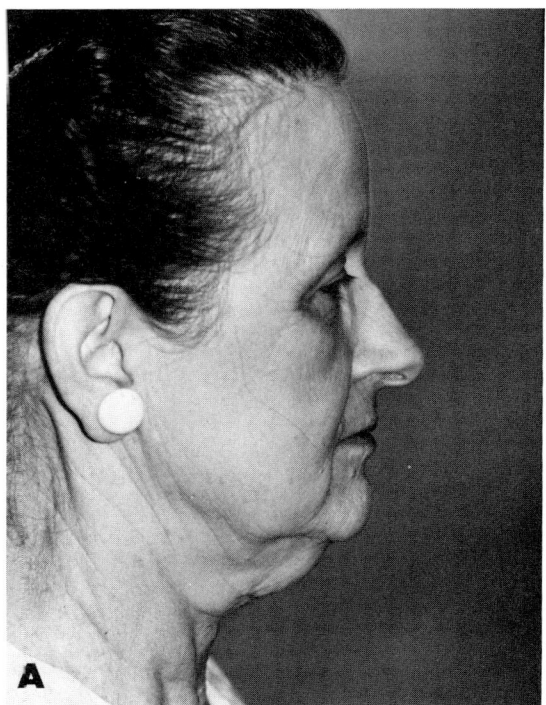

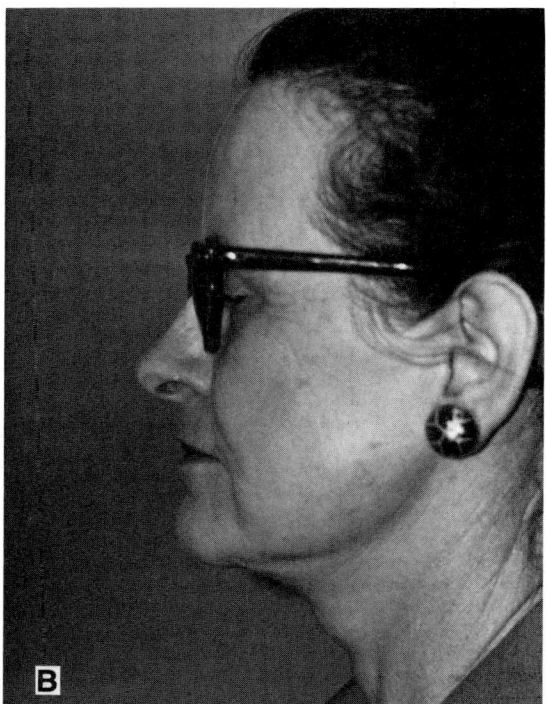

Figure 24–42 *A*, Significant facial skin excess is apparent in this patient as a result of prominent weight loss. *B*, Cervicofacial lifting with SMAS-platysmal plication combined with submentoplasty has been helpful in restoring this patient's appearance and self-confidence.

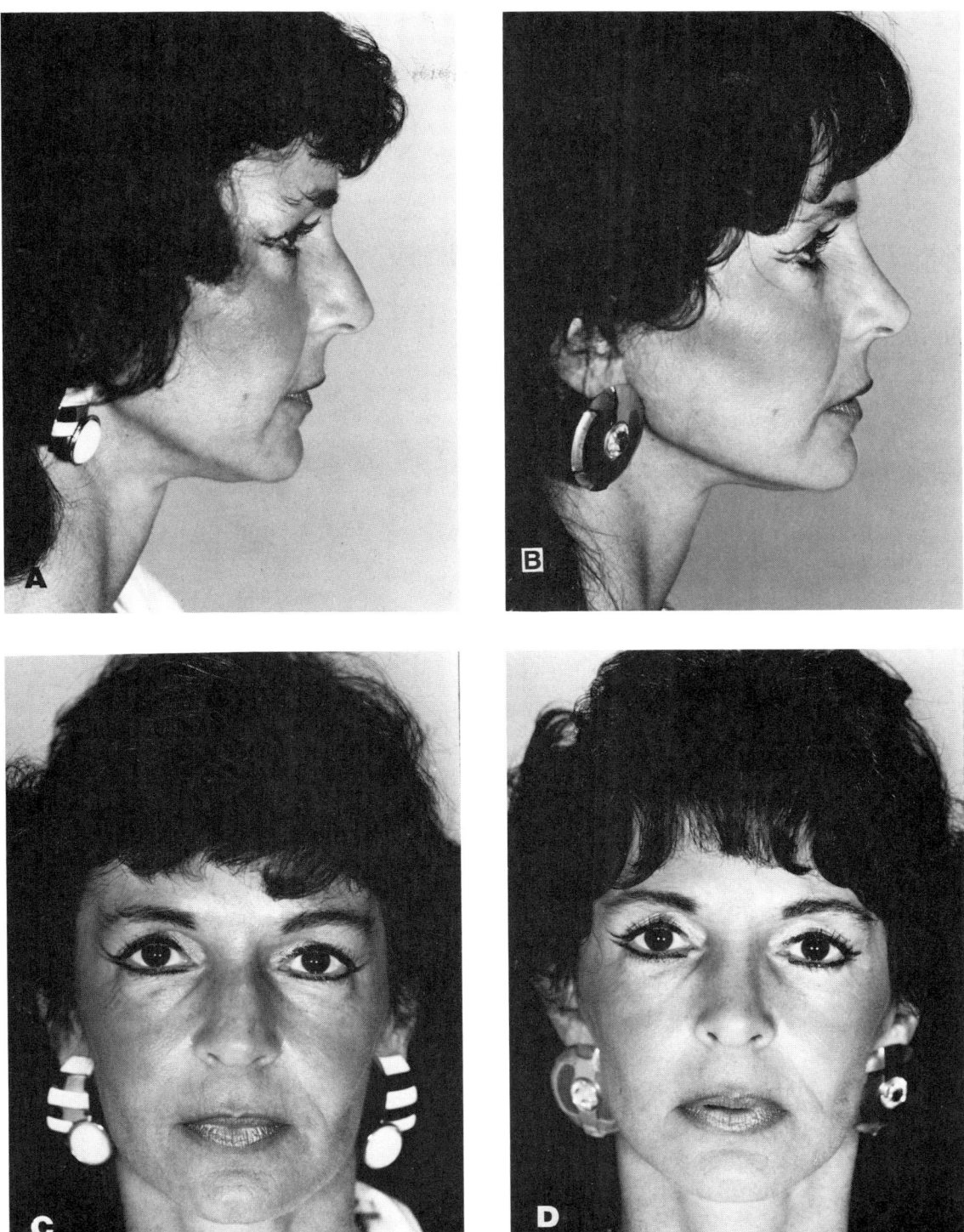

Figure 24–43 *A, B, C,* and *D,* Softening and improvement of the entire facial appearance are accomplished in this patient following subtle rhinoplasty, a cervicofacial lifting procedure, and bilateral upper and lower lid blepharoplasty. The appearance is one of a more rested and sculptured face with a more youthful aspect.

Chapter Twenty-Five

PATHOLOGY OF THE SKIN IN AGING

FRANK JOHNSON, M.D.

As Kligman et al[1] point out in their excellent review on aging of human skin, "After all, no one dies of old skin! The skin never really wears out or falls off. There is heart failure, but no skin failure." Even the most common malignant skin tumors are fairly nonaggressive,[2-4] particularly if treated early. Nevertheless, skin conditions can be among the most distressing and externally obvious signs of old age.[5-8] Hollingsworth et al[9,10] reported from comprehensive studies of the Atomic Bomb Commission in Hiroshima that simple observations on the skin were reliable indicators of chronologic age and that radiation from the atomic bomb did not accelerate aging. It is difficult to separate the consequences of the passage of time from the effects of the actinic rays of the sun.[6-8,11-17]

Let us consider some of the various possible causes of the aging process. The first cause is genetics. Dr. Hayflick[18] has done exciting work on this subject. It is apparent that organisms are bound by genetic factors to a finite life, and that mitoses, except in certain tumor cell lines, cannot go on forever. Diminution of mitotic activity leads to atrophy, and aberrant mitoses can lead to neoplasia. Some syndromes of premature aging are inherited.[19-21] These include progeria of the Hutchinson-Gilford type, of Werner's syndrome, and of Down's syndrome. The latter two are both marked by the early appearance of skin cancers. These rare conditions deserve further study.

Cross linking is an important phenomenon in aging, particularly in regard to fibrous proteins and nucleic acids. Cross linking of strands of nuclear DNA can cause genetic abnormalities in dividing cells and can induce neoplasms. Free radicals, highly reactive, self-propagating chemical groups, may lead to the formation of epoxides, which are potent cross linkers. Free radical formation is favored by oxidation of unsaturated lipids and acids, but free radical formation can be lessened by a number of reducing agents including vitamin E. Radiant energy, especially ionizing radiation, triggers free radical chain reactions. The sun screen agents offer protection from ultraviolet radiation to the skin. Of course melanin pigment also helps, but need not offer complete protection.[22]

Cell-mediated and humoral immunologic deficiencies are widely believed to be responsible for the poor defense of the aging skin against infections and neoplasms. However, Beeson[23] cautions against this assumption and states that more information is needed. In patients who are having reexcision of previous sites of skin pathology, I have noticed no failure of healing in the aged that could be attributed to infection. My experience as a reviewer of biopsy specimens gathered from an aging veteran population shows that the following are frequently occurring pathologic conditions in the skin of the head and neck region: wrinkles, solar elastosis, solar (actinic) keratosis, seborrheic keratosis, sebaceous gland hyperplasia, pigmented nevi, basal cell carcinomas, squamous carcinomas, and melanomas. These entities are almost invariably associated with evidence of actinic damage. Particularly noticeable is the presence of altered connective tissue with an increase in material staining that resembles coarse elastic tissue. Vasculature is diminished and low-grade chronic inflammation is seen, even though general capillary vasculature may be dilated.

The veterans in our patient population did not have elective cosmetic surgery for wrinkles, so I have no specific experience with such specimens. Tsuji et al[24-26] have performed studies of wrinkles in the skin of elderly persons by using the light microscope and the scanning and transmission electron microscope. They report that there are two types of wrinkles. There are shallow wrinkles that disappear on stretching. These develop in sun-protected skin. There are deep wrinkles that develop in sun-exposed skin and that do not disappear on stretching. Elastotic changes in the area of the deep wrinkle are less severe than in the surrounding area. The fundamental changes in actinic damage to the skin are still not completely understood.

Considerable research is being done on alterations in collagen and/or elastic tissue, the ground substance of enzymes of the skin.[6,12,15,27-33] I have not attempted to detail the histopathology of the skin, which is available in textbooks of pathology. My effort has been to provide information on mechanisms and to provide some recent references.

References

1. Kligman AM, Grove GL, Balin AK. Aging of human skin. In: Finch CE, Schneider E, eds. Handbook of the biology

of aging. 2nd ed. New York: Van Nostrand Reinhold, 1985:820.
2. Kao GF, Graham JH. Premalignant cutaneous disorders of the head and neck. In: English GM, ed. Otolaryngology. Vol. 5. Philadelphia: Harper and Row, 1986: Section 58:1.
3. Pollack SV. Skin cancer in the elderly. Clin Geriatr Med 1987; 3:715-728.
4. Shockley WW, Stucker FJ Jr. Squamous cell carcinoma of the external ear: a review of 75 cases. Otolaryngol Head Neck Surg 1987; 97:308-312.
5. Denes Z. Age and the neck's "decollete syndrome." ZFA 1985; 40:159-164.
6. Fenske NA, Lober CW. Structural and functional changes of normal aging skin. J Am Acad Dermatol 1986; 15:571-581.
7. Grove GL. Physiologic changes in older skin. Dermatol Clin 1986; 4:425-432.
8. Larrabee WF Jr, Caro I. The aging face. Why changes occur, how to correct them. Postgrad Med 1984; 76:37-39, 42-46.
9. Hollingsworth JW, Hazhizume A, Jablon S. Correlations between tests of aging on Hiroshima subjects, an attempt to define "physiological age." Yale J Biol Med 1965; 38:11-26.
10. Hollingsworth JW, Ishi G, Conrad RA. Skin aging and hair graying in Hiroshima. Geriatrics 1961; 6:27-36.
11. Frentz G, Munch-Perersen B, Wulf HC, Niebuhr E, da-Chunha Bang F. The nevoid basal cell carcinoma syndrome: sensitivity to ultraviolet and x-ray irradiation. J Am Acad Dermatol 1987; 17:637-643.
12. Gomez EC, Berman B. The aging skin. Clin Geriatr Med 1985; 1:285-305.
13. Kligman LH. Photoaging. Manifestations, prevention and treatment. Dermatol Clin 1986; 4:517-528.
14. Lin AN, Carter DM. Skin cancer in the elderly. Dermatol Clin 1986; 4:467-471.
15. Oikarinen A, Karvonen J, Uitto J, Hannuksela M. Connective tissue alterations in skin exposed to natural and therapeutic UV-radiation. Photodermatol 1985; 2:15-26.
16. Sams WM Jr. Sun-induced aging. Clinical and laboratory observations in man. Dermatol Clin 1986; 4:509-516.
17. Scotto J, Fears TR. The association of solar ultraviolet and skin melanoma incidence among caucasians in the United States. Cancer Invest 1987; 5:275-283.
18. Hayflick L. Cell biology of human aging. In: Goldstein JC, Kashima HK, Koopmann CF Jr, eds. Geriatric otorhinolaryngology. Toronto: BC Decker, 1989:8.
19. Beauregard S, Gilchrest BA. Syndromes of premature aging. Dermatol Clin 1987; 5:109-121.
20. Gawkrodger DJ, Priestly GC, Vijayalaxmi, Ross JA, Narcisi P, Hunter JA. Werner's syndrome. Biochemical and cytogenetic studies. Arch Dermatol 1985; 121:636-641.
21. Goldstein S. Human genetic disorders that feature premature onset and accelerated progression of biological aging. In: Schneider EL, ed. The genetics of aging. New York: Plenum Press, 1978: 171.
22. Altman A, Rosen T, Tschen JA, Hoffman T, Bruce S, Siegel DM, Levey ML, Schaefer D, Goldberg LH. Basal cell epithelioma in black patients. J Am Acad Dermatol 1987; 17:741-745.
23. Beeson PB. Alleged susceptibility of the elderly to infection. Yale J Biol Med 1985; 58:71-77.
24. Tsuji T, Yorifuji T, Hayashi Y, Hamada T. Two types of wrinkles in aged persons. Arch Dermatol 1986; 122:22-23.
25. Tsuji T, Yorifuji T, Hayashi Y, Hamada T. Light and scanning electron microscopic studies on wrinkles in aged persons. Br J Dermatol 1986; 114:329-335.
26. Tsuji T. Ultrastructure of deep wrinkles in the elderly. J Cutan Pathol 1987; 14:158-164.
27. Edelstein SB, Breakefield XO. Monoamine oxidases A and B are differentially regulated by glucocorticoids and "aging" in human skin fibroblasts. Cell Mol Neurobiol 1986; 6:121-150.
28. Lippman RD. Rapid in vivo quantification and comparison of hydroperoxides and oxidized collagen in aging mice, rabbits and man. Exp Gerontol 1985; 20:1-5.
29. Robert L, Jacob MP, Frances C, Godeau G, Hornebeck W. Interaction between elastin and elastases and its role in the aging of the arterial wall, skin and other connective tissues. A review. Mech Ageing Dev 1984; 28:155-166.
30. Schmiegelow P, Nussgen A, Grasedych K, Lindner J. Hautveränderungen im hohen Lebensalter—korrespondieren biochemische Befunde zur Morphologie? Z Gerontol 1986; 19:179-189.
31. Uitto J. Connective tissue biochemistry of the aging dermis. Age-related alterations in collagen and elastin. Dermatol Clin 1986; 4:433-446.
32. Uitto J, Shamban A. Heritable skin diseases with molecular defects in collagen or elastin. Dermatol Clin 1987; 5:63-84.
33. Vogel HG. Biochemical studies of human and animal skin in vivo and in vitro. Z Hautkr 1984; 59:1098-1100.

Chapter Twenty-Six

RHINOPLASTY, BLEPHAROPLASTY, AND RHYTIDECTOMY IN THE AGING PATIENT

FRANK M. KAMER, M.D., F.A.C.S.

INTRODUCTION

As an otolaryngologist specializing in facial plastic and reconstructive surgery for almost 20 years, I have been witness to a burgeoning growth in my specialty. The American Academy of Facial Plastic and Reconstructive Surgery has responded to the great demand for facial plastic surgery by helping to educate and train an ever-growing supply of otolaryngologists. From a nidus of a few eye, ear, nose, and throat trained surgeons who primarily were interested in rhinoplasty, the Facial Plastic Academy now has 3,000 members from various disciplines all over the world. In the 25 years since its inception, there has been a corresponding graying of America. There are more older people today living active and healthy lives who seek elective surgery to enhance and improve the quality of their lives.

In its cover story about cosmetic surgery 2 years ago, Newsweek magazine chronicled the increase in cosmetic surgery in this country. It is remarkable that a major magazine should feature this subject on its front page, whereas only a few years before, most patients and their surgeons were hesitant to even discuss the subject in public as it remained a somewhat private and often guilt-provoking acquiescence to vanity. Patients enjoyed the benefits of the procedures, but rarely acknowledged its existence, while specialists who pursued the art were often ridiculed by their colleagues as beauty parlor surgeons.

Times have changed. Each week some recognizable person or another talks in the media about the personal benefits of cosmetic surgery. According to Newsweek, plastic surgery is booming, up 61 percent between 1981 and 1984. Over 500,000 operations are performed each year and that number is increasing. In part, this reflects the decline in occupations for which appearance is pretty much irrelevant, such as farming, and a corresponding rise in the number of jobs for which a primary qualification is to be able to look the part, such as sales and management. As the baby boom generation has come of age, the hard working, fit-looking yuppies are breathing down the wrinkled necks of the middle-aged executives ahead of them. These baby boomers see young people hired over older ones and people their own age being laid off. To be competitive, they just want to look themselves, the way they did years ago. Plastic surgery is no longer regarded as an indulgence of vain old women and spoiled high school girls. Patients come from all socioeconomic levels and backgrounds.

GENERAL CONSIDERATIONS

Facial plastic surgery done well demands a high level of technical skill, a rare esthetic sensibility, and a degree of empathy not always found in more abstract medical disciplines. In treating an ever-aging population, the otolaryngologist who performs facial plastic surgery must possess these general qualifications as well as a detailed knowledge of each specific procedure.

This discussion is limited to rhinoplasty, blepharoplasty, and rhytidectomy in the older age groups. Obviously, elective surgery is not indicated if the patient's general health is not optimal. A complete work-up by an internist, with appropriate preoperative laboratory, x-ray, and ECG analysis, is suggested. If any problems arise, surgery is delayed until full clearance is obtained. Local anesthesia is desired, with an anesthetist providing the sedation and monitoring. The surgeries can be performed either in a well-equipped outpatient facility or in a hospital.

RHINOPLASTY

Rhinoplasty is more frequently performed in the older patient. In my earlier training, it was taught not to operate on the external pyramid in any patient after the age of 40 except for trauma, tumor, or infection. Today, 50-, 60-, and even 70-year-old people seek consultation for esthetic rhinoplasty, either alone or in conjunction with other facial plastic surgical procedures. Some have functional problems. Many have contemplated the surgery at an earlier age, but only when the effects of age compound the functional or esthetic deformity do they actually decide to undergo the procedure. These changes involve the skin, cartilage, and bone. Skin becomes more inelastic, cartilage less resilient, and bone more brittle. If the tip is ptotic, it becomes more obvious with age. Nasal humps become more prominent as the overlying skin thins and the tip descends. The weight of a more prominent lower lateral cartilage adds to the deformity. Patients often state that they can breathe better if they raise their nasal tips.

Surgery must be done conservatively. Radical esthetic changes are better left for the younger patient. Older patients desire a more refined nose with a smaller hump and a less prominent tip. They want to be restored, not remade. Minimal excision and contour changes are desirable. Techniques vary according to the perceived deformity. Forman's rotation technique is helpful for the ptotic tip. Subperiosteal rasping, rather than chisel or saw excision, is useful for the more brittle hump. Lateral osteotomies should be appropriate to return the nasal pyramid to its normal anatomical position. Upper and lower cartilaginous vault changes should be minimal since overzealous excisions can lead to functional as well as to esthetic problems in the internal and external nasal valves. Septal and turbinate surgery is performed when indicated.

Healing takes longer. The skin drapes slowly, especially in the glabellar regions. Although cutaneous sebaceous activity is notably less than in younger patients, the inelastic skin can present a problem as the rhytides become more prominent and expressive lines remain, even in repose. If these limitations and expectations are understood, most patients are pleased with their results. Some are thrilled and become as happy as a teenager with an improved self-image. Complications are few, as with most well-performed nasal surgeries.

BLEPHAROPLASTY

Blepharoplasty has become one of the most frequently performed operations for the otolaryngologist-facial plastic surgeon. The eyes are said to be the center of expression and, as they age, come to look tired and listless. Redundant skin, especially exacerbated by prolonged sun exposure, can weigh on the upper lid, thus creating a functional pseudoptosis and causing the patient to complain of heaviness or tearing. Sacs of herniated supra- and/or infraorbital fat appear as the septum orbitale loosens. Patients look tired even after a restful vacation. Muscle hypertrophy or redundancy creates ridges and folds as the lines of expression deepen. Crow's feet become more prominent and obvious on repose.

The surgery should address these problems without removing or changing the natural eye contour or expression. Radical techniques to drastically alter these components are best reserved for the functional necessities such as ptosis repair or senile ectropia. Upper lid tarsal fixation by creating a higher levator attachment to the tarsus can create a permanent deeper upper lid fold. Although esthetically pleasing, this can often be too striking and radical a change for older patients who simply want to restore, and not alter, their appearance. As in rhinoplasty, conservatism should be the rule in skin, muscle, and fat excision. A subtle deepening of the upper lid can be accomplished with conservative orbicularis muscle resection, rather than the more radical tarsal fixation procedures. Deep suturing is unnecessary in skin closure utilizing fast absorbable catgut, and there is no need for suture removal. The incision is brought out laterally within an available crow's foot. M or Z plasties in attempts to shorten the incision laterally can leave unsightly scars and should be avoided.

It is advisable to maintain support of the lower lid by not interrupting the integrity of the pretarsal obicularis. Skin muscle flaps that transect the lateral attachment routinely necessitate resuturing of the transected muscle to a higher level or more radical vertical lid shortening procedures in hopes of preventing a rounding or downward pull of the aging lower lid. If left intact or if imbricated without transection, the obicularis adequately maintains support. Skin and fat excision should be conservative. Excess skin can be removed by lateral flaps or by pre-excision. Transconjunctival techniques that safely maintain the interior lamella and prevent scleral show are rarely used in the older patients because of the need for skin excisions.

The complications of blepharoplasty are few if adequate preoperative ophthalmologic analysis is performed and if these principles are followed. This surgery can do much to rejuvenate an aging face and to give great pleasure to those who elect to undergo the procedure. It does not, however, remove lines, discolorations, or edema within the skin or subcutaneous tissue. Brow ptosis, which often accompanies the aging eye, must be dealt with by suitable lifting, usually in conjunction with rhytidectomy.

RHYTIDECTOMY

Although patients are face-lifting at earlier ages today, the operation is mainly performed on an aging population. It requires the most extensive surgery and, with up-to-date techniques, can produce the most dramatic results. Radical undermining surgery is often required to accomplish a natural unoperated appearance. Excess fat in the jowl or submental area can be removed by suction-assisted lipectomy, an innovative and now the single most frequently performed plastic surgical procedure. It was developed in France only 10 years ago. The superficial musculoaponeurotic system flap, in conjunction with anterior and posterior platysmal surgery, can create a firm and natural-appearing facial and cervical area effectively supporting the underlying tissues to allow the skin to drape more confluently. Skin incisions and excisions should be tailored to the individual anatomy, well-hidden within the folds and convolutions of the ear, and closed meticulously without undue tension. Coronal-lifting not only can correct the ptotic brow to further improve the results of a blepharoplasty, but by appropriate myotomy can improve forehead and glabellar furrows caused by overactive procerus corrugator or frontalis. Contour changes in the cheeks and mentum can be accomplished where indicated by suitable malar and chin augmentation.

Rhytidectomy patients may be older, but they must be healthy to ensure adequate wound healing. Proper preoperative mental and physical evaluation is important to help eliminate potential problems postoperatively. Cigarette smoking, alcohol use, and aspirin use should be discontinued 2 weeks before surgery. Patients must lose weight if obese. An internist's clearance after a complete history, physical, laboratory analysis, ECG, and chest x-ray are performed is strongly advised. With these conditions met, suitable face-lift candidates can be in their late seventies or early eighties although most of these patients have usually had previous surgery.

The procedure requires technical skill to esthetically restore and rejuvenate a face without drastically altering its character and individual human expression. Complications such as hematoma, hypertrophic scarring, and numbness are not uncommon, but fortunately only rarely detract from the final result. Motor nerve damage, skin slough, and overzealous tightening is usually preventable by adequate surgical training and experience. This procedure is becoming ever more popular, having increased by 38 percent between 1981 and 1984. Most patients are extremely pleased with the results and grateful to the facial plastic surgeon, whom they feel is responsible for making them look well and, more significantly, feel better about themselves.

CONCLUSION

Otolaryngology has historically evolved as a specialty. As we enter the future of an aging population desiring to improve the quality of their lives by good nutrition and exercise, facial plastic surgery will remain an important area for research, development, and growth. Most people feel better when they look better. The challenge to otolaryngology is to continue to train compassionate, highly skilled, and knowledgeable surgeons able to meet the demands of the ever-growing number of patients who desire this surgery.

Summary

PERSPECTIVES ON HEALTH CARE FOR THE ELDERLY

BYRON J. BAILEY, M.D., F.A.C.S.

INTRODUCTION

I am honored to have the privilege of summarizing this outstanding meeting, which has focused attention on our newest subspecialty, Geriatric Otolaryngology. The planning and presentation of this conference have been conducted at an extremely high level and have served to establish a clear presence for geriatric otolaryngology within our specialty. It has also raised our consciousness in this important area by highlighting problems we have not considered previously as a group. The program participants have acquainted us with the status of research in several key areas and have shown us glimpses of the exciting prospects for future investigation. In addition, some of the presentations have reviewed important aspects of diagnosis and treatment for conditions that affect our elderly patients.

In summarizing this meeting, it is important to deal not only with the issues presented during the scientific sessions, but also to comment on the equally important topics of conversation from the coffee breaks, lunches, and cocktail hours, because there is a tremendous interest in the matter of putting this major issue into a broader social and philosophical perspective.

OPPORTUNITIES IN GERIATRIC OTOLARYNGOLOGY

During the past 2 days we have been introduced to a great many facts and findings that are relevant to the health of senior citizens in the United States. We have been told that otolaryngologists–head and neck surgeons have a major role to play within the broad field of geriatrics. The previous speakers have identified for us at least eight major areas of opportunity for our involvement, and these include such broad categories as the following:

1. Prevention of premature death by the early detection of head and neck cancer, improved management of trauma, and programs directed at smoking and ethanol cessation
2. Prevention of disability, particularly through programs of hearing conservation and the improved treatment of hearing loss
3. Control and management of annoying to disabling symptoms such as nasal congestion, chronic sinusitis, tinnitus, and vertigo
4. Treatment of common and usually benign diseases such as upper respiratory infections, acute sinusitis, otitis media, and pharyngitis
5. Management of conditions that limit mobility and promote isolation among the elderly, such as hearing loss, disequilibrium, and voice changes
6. Improvement of the quality of life, for example with facial plastic and reconstructive surgical techniques
7. Treatment of sometimes fatal conditions such as head and neck cancer
8. Providing informed participation in the societal deliberations concerning the social and economic aspects of the disproportionate growth of the elder segment of our population.

THE IMPACT OF CHANGE

We do not live, nor do we practice, in a vacuum. The society around us is changing dramatically, and we are beginning to feel many of the vibrations of this change. During the past 50 years, the concept of "Medicine" has changed from "caring" to "caring and curing". The concept of "health" has changed from simply having the good fortune not to be sick or to have died to a feeling on the part of individuals that it is the responsibility of society to honor the right of everyone to have everything possible done to maintain one's happiness and mental and physical well-being at an extremely high level. The medical hopes of the elderly have been formally and prominently enfranchised by government. Through a variety of existing federal and state programs and many more that are proposed, our society has made major commitments to our citizens. Much of this is entirely appropriate, because it has been said since the time of ancient Greece that a society is judged by how it cares for its young and its elderly.

The basic concept of "life" has changed from simply the status of being alive to a sense that modern biomedical resources can guarantee many active, vital years following the time of retirement from active work. There is also an expectation that old age will not be a period of illness and an expectation that cancer, heart disease, stroke, dementia, infections, and most of the conditions that have historically been associated with old age can be either controlled individually or eradicated, like small pox. In other words, the prevailing societal expectation is for a long, healthy life that ends with death from "old age" at about the age of 100 years.

But this new world and this new vision bring sizable challenges and many new fears. Older citizens worry that their money will run out before their life does. They worry about ending up in a nursing home, and at the present time more than 5 percent of them do. They are fearful that Alzheimer's disease, or some other condition, will make their life useless or burdensome or will bankrupt them and their children. They worry that they will be sick, shut in, uncomfortable, or in pain for years. All of these problems present increased risks and growing probability of some adverse outcomes as the life span of individuals in the United States increases.

We have seen how the scope of the problem is clearly related to changing demographics in our society. Between the year 1900 and the present time, the population over 65 has increased 9-fold from 3 million to 28 million. Those among us who are older than 85 have increased 21-fold. At the present time there are now 3 million people 85 years of age or older and by the year 2050 there will be 15 million people older than 85. For the first time in the history of our country, we have more citizens who are over 65 than 18 years of age and under.

The impact of this disproportionate growth of our older population is now being felt in our pocketbooks. During the early 1960s, less than 15 percent of all of the federal dollars went to those citizens who were over 65 years of age. By 1985, 28 percent of the federal dollars went to that same group.

There are many more statistics that underscore the social change that we are now experiencing. They all support the observation that we are hearing more overt complaints and growing concerns than ever before about the fact that we are spending more for the elderly and relatively less for the young in our society. Some of these complaints address the issue that a disproportionate amount of our health care dollars are being spent for the elderly who are dying, and that a disproportionate amount of our research and technology is being directed toward the elderly at the expense of the young. These observations have caused some to conclude that the health care needs of the growing elderly population in the United States pose an economic threat to our health care system and eventually will spill over to other areas of our economy.

We ask ourselves, how did we get to this point? Actually, physicians cannot take all of the credit for the fact that during the past century there has been a dramatic extension of the average lifespan in the United States. The key factors include improved housing, nutrition, water supplies, and sanitation. There have been massive immunization and public education programs that have eliminated polio, small pox, and other serious diseases. Major strides have been made in the prevention of premature deaths by the introduction of antibiotics and by advances in anesthesia, blood transfusion technology, and surgical procedures. Preventive medicine and health maintenance have been factors in reducing somewhat the national passion for smoking and for increasing our tendency to exercise more and to drive more safely. In addition there clearly have been important advances in the area of diseases commonly associated with death, namely better control of hypertension, cardiac arrythmias, and the treatment of myocardial infarction. As a result of this broad progress, many more of our citizens are reaching the ripe old age of 65.

At the present time much of our work, our living, and our planning is organized around the age of 65 years. We define a "premature death" as any death occurring before age 65, and we have traditionally looked at that age as a time of retirement. However, it is an arbitrary figure and it dates back to the time of the establishment of the first social security system by Bismark in Germany during the 19th Century.

At the turn of the century, the average American who reached the age of 65 survived for another 12 years. Now a comparable individual can expect to live for 17 years and, within another 25 years, it will probably be more than 20 years. The economic impact of extended survival and prolonged retirement years raises some economic issues that may require us to rethink the age of 65 for retirement, both as physicians and as a society in general. We must ask ourselves whether or not we are planning the best use of our health care resources and our research resources by pursuing our present course. We must ask whether the politics of these issues as they are currently framed are fair and just. Many of these issues are addressed in an extremely provocative way by the new book entitled *Setting Limits*,[1] and I believe that it should be required reading for every responsible physician. I do not believe that it provides the proper answers for the questions that we are going to have to face, but I do feel that it raises the right questions.

WHO WILL ANSWER THESE QUESTIONS?

The American public through its Congress has made a series of far-reaching changes in medical practice in the United States. I believe firmly that health policy in this country is ordinarily set in motion by the public's perception of the care that is available to them. During the 1950s there was a public perception of physician inaccessibility, and as a result of this perception, a few years later there was legislation that has led to policies that have doubled the number of doctors practicing in this country in the last 25 years. During the 1960s the public perception of medical care was that it was beginning to cost too much and might not be affordable to our senior citizens. Subsequently, we have seen the solutions brought about through the implementation of the Medicare program and DRGs. The public's perception has also fueled the growth in popularity of HMOs and PPOs. The public now seems to want high quality medical care and I believe that public perceptions are related to the early efforts to require recertification through a variety of techniques. One is reminded of the story about a sign that was displayed in a Chinese laundry. It said "High quality work, fast service, low cost—pick any two of the above." There is a great deal of truth in that concept, because it is virtually impossible to design a system in which all three of those elements are conspicuous.

The political process whereby the cost for retirement income and health care for the elderly was transferred from their children to the government is now having far-reaching consequences and it is likely that these will be magnified during the next few decades. One can quickly see that ideal solutions are not readily available and that it is not yet time to arrive at any conclusions. The approach one would take at this time would simply be a reflection of the individual's view of the world. Some see the world as being comparable to a lifeboat in which the boundaries are finite, the resources are limited, and if we give to one we must take from another. It is a system that is not expandable.

At the other end of the spectrum is the view of the world that could be termed "the Balloon Concept." It has the attractive feature of a vision that conceives any system as capable of being expanded and simply asks that we all blow a little harder in order to accomplish the required expansion. Reality lies somewhere between these two extremes, and if we bring the analogy back to the issue of a growing elderly population, we come face to face with some present and future facts that are attracting the attention of economists, politicians, and physicians.

For example, as of the year 1984, the elderly comprised 11 percent of our population and consumed 29 percent of our health care expenditures. It is projected that, in another 50 years, the elderly will comprise 21 percent of our population and will consume 45 percent of the nation's health care expenditures.

This type of projection forces us to ask whether there is a real and growing problem or whether there is not such a problem. If there is a problem, will the demand for services outstrip the supply or the capacity of the health care system or will it not?

Those who argue against the presence of a serious problem point to the heterogeneity of the elderly as a population and to the long-term projections in regard to their general state of health. It is noted that many of the elderly are not ill, and that a growing proportion of our senior citizens require little health care until just prior to their death. The statisticians refer to this phenomenon as a "squaring of the curve" of dying. Like the wonderful one horse shay of poetic fame, the optimistic among this group foresee a society in which we have many healthy, elderly patients who are active and well until a short time before they die quickly (and less expensively) from "old age." The argument continues by stating that health care rationing will probably not become necessary and that it certainly is premature to try to answer such questions. Surely we can spend less for defense, for tobacco, for cosmetics, and for other unnecessary commodities than we are at present. This view is based on the principle that we all have a common stake in providing for the elderly, and that there are many strategies that have not been implemented, such as an expanded hospice program that would drastically reduce expenses for the dying elderly. It is also possible that physicians and hospitals could expand the volume of their charitable care for elderly patients.

But what if these efforts are not sufficient to meet the need? Callahan[1] proposes that age should be established as a criterion for resource allocation. His argument is that suffering must be relieved in all instances, but that life-extending, costly, high technology measures should be rationed because they are excessively expensive and return little to the society. He feels that quality of life should be given a higher priority and that prolonging maximally the time that it takes for an individual to die should be given a lower priority. In his view, patient status and types of treatment should be stratified, and agreement should be sought that certain levels of patient debility would disqualify some individuals from eligibility for the highest level of medical technology, at least at public expense.

In the meantime, while the rest of us await clarification of some of these fundamental issues, there are a number of opportunities for providing better service to our elderly patients. We can work quite cost-effectively on the prevention of pathologic conditions that cause disability and premature death. We can improve our ability to treat conditions that annoy, disable, or limit the elderly in terms of their mobility and the quality of their lives.

Through a variety of surgical and rehabilitative approaches, we may increase our efforts to improve the quality of life for the aging segment of our population. Cosmetic surgery, smaller and better hearing aids, and improved management of disequilibrium and dysphagia are prime examples of opportunities for better service to this group.

In addition to our patient care activities, we can work in a more general sense to develop a better-balanced health care system. It could well be that, by spending fewer dollars for high technology intensive care units and expensive terminal care programs, that we could divert these resources toward the improvement of standards and conditions in the nation's nursing homes. By becoming better informed participants in the upcoming societal debates and the tough decisions that are on the table, we will be able to fulfill more effectively our role as citizens and voters.

To effectively address these challenges, we may have to start from the bottom up and deal with some unrealistic public expectations as we redefine the nature of appropriate health care programs and policies for the elderly. Whatever we do, we must not promise more than we can deliver, but we must deliver what is necessary and we must be certain that we are committed to provide all that we can afford.

CONCLUSION

As a final observation in trying to place these issues into perspective, it appears to me that we find ourselves facing a classical dilemma with a new twist. The classical dilemma is that if we devote more resources to health care for the elderly we must decide where we are to devote *fewer* resources. Will it be to the health care of other age groups? Will it be a matter of spending less money on defense or less money on education?

The new twist that we are encountering in this dilemma involves the issue of fairness. Is it more fair to approach these problems from the standpoint of society at large, or from the standpoint of the individual? As Canon Moore pointed out in his presentation, Western medicine has two points of origin, Platonic and Socratic, and occasionally one finds an element of tension between these two different perspectives. Plato developed a philosophy based on the greatest good for the society while Socrates and Hippocrates established medical traditions and ethics that were focused on the greatest good for the individual.

If we are to find answers to these complex questions, we will have to begin by educating the public, and in particular our patients. They are far more numerous than are we, and their political clout must be linked to a better awareness of the issues that must be confronted. As the technical progress of medicine continues to march forward and the political debate grows louder in the background, we must, as individual physicians, continue to provide the highest possible level of care to each patient, regardless of other factors. Additionally, we must take on further responsibilities as advocates of the best interests of individual patients and of society in general.

Reference

1. Callahan D. Setting limits: medical goals in an aging society. New York: Simon & Schuster, 1987.

INDEX

A

Adenosine monophosphate (AMP), 114
Aging
  and animals, 8, 16-17
    chick heart tissue, 9-10, 11
    Galapagos tortoise, 12
  and cancer. *See* Cancer
  and cell biology, 8-18
    entropy, 16
    error theory, 15
    genes, 16-17
    immortal cells, 9-11
    normal human cells, 12-14
    Phase III, 13
    population doublings, 11-12
    program theory, 15-16
    somatic mutation theory, 14-15
  and demographics, 19-23
    chronic conditions, 21-23
  and depression, 45-48
  and dysequilibrium, 27-28
  and epidemiology, 23-25
  and falling, 27, 58-61
  future research, 4-7
  health care overview for, 189-192
  and medical/surgical care, 36-37
  and plastic surgery. *See* Plastic surgery
  related to head and neck, 138-143
  and the skin, 184-185
  and smell, 92-96, 97-101
    in age-related diseases, 100-101
    odor detection, 97
    odor discrimination, 99
    odor hedonics, 99-100
    odor identification, 98
    odor intensity perception, 98-99
  and speech understanding, 32-35
  and taste, 92-96, 101-103
    taste detection, 101-102
    taste hedonics, 103
    taste intensity perception, 103
  See also specific complications associated with aging
Alzheimer's disease, affecting olfaction, 100-101
American Association of Retired Persons (AARP), 1-2
American Cancer Society, 155
Animals. *See* Aging, and animals
Antibodies. *See* Immune deficiency

Antigen-presenting cells (APC), 107
  See also Major histocompatibility complex (MHC)
Aspiration, 124-133
  and laryngeal dysfunction, 127-130
    glottic prosthesis to correct, 128-129
    glottic and supraglottic laryngeal closure to correct, 129
    laryngeal diversion to correct, 130
    laryngectomy to correct, 129
    partial cricoid resection to correct, 130
    tracheotomy to correct, 128
    vocal cord augmentation to correct, 128
  pulmonary consequences of, 124-125
  See also Swallowing disorders
Ataxia, 58-62
  case studies, 59-60
  causes of, 59
Audiograms, of elderly with high-tone hearing loss, 41, 44
Auditory system disorders. *See* Hearing disorders

B

Balance. *See* Presbyastasis
Baltimore Longitudinal Study on Aging (BLSA), 25
Basal cell carcinoma. *See* Cancer
Basilar membrane, thickening of, 43
B cells. *See* Immune deficiency
Blepharoplasty, 187
  See also Plastic surgery
Burkitt's lymphoma, 150-151

C

Cancer
  etiologic factors, 148-157
    alcohol, 153
    carcinogen exposure, 149-150
    cigarette smoking, 150, 151-153
    and epidemiology, 151
    genetic, 150
    infectious agents, 150-151
    known human carcinogens, 153-155
    meat consumption, 151, 152

    multiple, 150
    unproven human carcinogens, 154-155
  head and neck, 158-165
    B cell differentiation, 159
    and immune deficits, 161-162
    and immune restoration, 162-164
    and reconstructive plastic surgery, 169-173
    T cell differentiation, 159-160, 161
    transplanting of cells, 14
Carrel, A., on heart cells, 9-10, 11
CD8 cells, 162-163
Cell biology. *See* Aging, and cell biology
Cells. *See* Aging, and cell biology
Cerebellar damage, 56-57
Cerebellar sulci, 60
Chemotherapy. *See* Cancer
Chromosomes. *See* Major histocompatibility complex (MHC)
Cochlear neurons, loss of, 40-42, 44
Collagen, 13, 184
Computerized tomographic (CT) scan, 60
Concanavalin A (Con A), 109
Cricopharyngeal myotomy, 126
Cupulolithiasis, 55
Cytogerontology, 9-10
  See also Aging, and cell biology
Cytohistograms, of elderly with hair cell loss, 41, 44

D

Dentists, statistics for use of, 23
Depression, and tinnitus, 45-48
Diabetes, type I, 119
Diploid cells, 12-13
  See also Aging, and cell biology
Disease, and aging, 8
  See also specific types
DNA, effects on aging, 15, 109
Doctors. *See* Physicians, statistics for use of
Drugs. *See* Prescription drugs
Dysphagia. *See* Swallowing disorders
Dysphonia. *See* Voice disorders

E

Electroglottography, 72, 73, 74, 75, 76, 77, 127

Electromyography, in examining pharyngeal swallowing, 135, 136
Entropy, and aging, 16
Epstein-Barr virus, 150–151
Eye disorders, 55–57

F

Fibroblasts, embryonic, 12

G

Ganglion cells, 41
  decrease of, 55
Gastroesophageal reflux, 68, 69
Genes
  See also Immune deficiency, gene expression
Genes, and aging, 16–17
Genetics, and HLA, 113
Geriatrics. *See* Aging
Gerontology. *See* Aging, and cell biology
Gustation
  anatomy, 93
  disorders affecting, 95–96
    treatment, 96
  pathology, 94
  physiology, 93–94
  See also Aging, and taste
Gyral atrophy, 60

H

Habrobracon, 14–15
Hamilton Depression Scale, 46
Haploid cells, 14–15
  See also Aging, and cell biology
Haplotype B8/DR3, immunologic abnormalities associated with, 118
Hashimoto's disease, 119
Head, related to swallowing disorders, 138–143
Health care. *See* Aging, health care overview for; Hospitals; Medicaid; Medicare; Nursing homes
Hearing aids. *See* Hearing disorders, communication assistive devices for
Hearing disorders, 29–31, 115–119
  communication assistive devices for, 49–51
    listening in public places, 50
    the professional, 50–51
    signaling, 50
    telephone amplifiers, 49
    telephone devices for the deaf, 49
    television, radio, and stereo amplifiers, 49–50
  See also Presbycusis; Tinnitus
Heart cells, 9–10
Histocompatibility. *See* Major histocompatibility complex (MHC)
Hospital Cost and Utilization Project (HCUP) Survey, 24, 25
Hospitals, 23
  costs, 26
  statistics for use of, 24

average length of stay (ALOS), 25–27
diagnosis-related groupings (DRGs), 25, 26–28
treatment of swallowing disorders, 122
Human cell population. *See* Aging, and cell biology
Human leukocyte antigens (HLA), 106, 112–120
  and temporal bone disorders, 115–118
  typing of, 112–113
  DR, 116
  viral, 114
Human papillomavirus (HPV), 151

I

Immune deficiency, 106–111
  and antigen-presenting cells (APC), 107
  decrease in Interleukin-2 (IL-2) production, 108
  gene expression, 109
  T and B cell changes, 106–107
  T cell function deficits, 107
  and thymus gland shrinking, 107
  T lymphocyte activation, 109, 110
  See also Human leukocyte antigens (HLA)
  See also specific diseases
Immunology. *See* Immune deficiency
Interleukin-2 (IL-2), 108, 159–163
Ischemic brain disease, 59

L

Laryngeal nerve paralysis, 75
Laryngectomy, to avoid aspiration, 129
Larynx. *See* Laryngeal nerve paralysis; Voice disorders
Lipofuscin, increase of, 55, 56
Lymphocytes. *See* Immune deficiency

M

Major histocompatibility complex (MHC), 112–115
  function of, 114–115
Manometry, in study of swallowing, 126, 134–135
Medicaid, 1
Medicare, 1–2, 24, 25, 26, 191
Meniere's disease, 40, 59, 61, 116–117, 119
Messenger ribonucleic acid (mRNA), and immune deficiency, 109
Minnesota Multiphasic Personality Inventory (MMPI), 45
Mitotic failure, 13
Myasthenia laryngis, 74–75

N

Nasal cavities. *See* Olfaction, pathology
National Academy of Sciences, 6

National Advisory Council on Aging, 4
National Ambulatory Medical Care Survey (NAMCS), 24–25, 27–28
National Cancer Program, 155
National Health Interview Survey, 21–22
  Supplement on Aging (NHIS-SOA), 24, 27
National Hospital Discharge Survey (NHDS), 24, 25, 26
National Institute on Aging (NIA), 4–7
  research on auditory system disorders, 29–30
National Institute of Dental Research (NIDR), 29
  research on swallowing and voice disorders, 31
National Institute of Neurological and Communicative Disorders and Stroke (NINCDS), 29
  research on hearing and laryngeal disorders, 30–31
National Institutes of Health (NIH), 4, 5, 29
Natural killer (NK) cells, 160, 161
Neck, related to swallowing disorders, 138–143
Neurologic disorders
  associated with voice disorders, 68
  causing swallowing disorders, 124
Neuromuscular impairment. *See* Voice disorders, associated with neuromuscular impairment
Nortriptyline, use in tinnitus treatment, 46–48
Nursing homes
  consumer guide for, 28
  statistics for use of, 23
  treatment of swallowing disorders, 122

O

Olfaction
  anatomy, 92–93
  disorders affecting, 95
    treatment, 96
  pathology, 94
  physiology, 93
  See also Aging, and smell
Oncology. *See* Cancer
Organ of Corti, 42
Otolaryngology. *See* Gustation; Hearing disorders; Olfaction
Otosclerosis, 116–117, 119

P

Palatolaryngopharyngeal myoclnis, 76
Parkinson's disease, 73–74
  affecting olfaction, 100–101, 102
Perineurium, thickening with age, 141
Pharynx. *See* Voice disorders
Phorbol myristic acetate (PMA), and immune deficiency, 110

Photoglottography, 72, 73, 74, 75, 76, 77
Physicians
  statistics for use of, 23
Placebo, use in tinnitus treatment, 46–48
Plants, and death, 17
Plastic surgery, 168–183, 186–188
  reconstruction after cancer, 169–173
Presbyastasis, 54–57
Presbycusis, 40–44
  cochlear conductive, 43, 44
  neural, 40–42
  sensory, 40
  strial, 42, 43
Presbyphagia. *See* Dysphagia
Prescription drugs
  statistics for use of, 23
  for swallowing disorders, 126
Prosthetic devices, for hearing, 31
Protein kinase C (PK-C), and immune deficiency, 109–110
Psychiatric disorders, tinnitus related to, 46
Purkinje's cells, 56–57

R

Reconstructive surgery. *See* Plastic surgery
Reinke's space, 70
Rheumatoid arthritis, 115
Rhinoplasty, 186–187
  See also Plastic surgery
Rhytidectomy, 187–188
  See also Plastic surgery

S

Scarpa's ganglion, 55
Schwann cells, in aging human nerves, 139
Senescence. *See* Aging
Sensorineural hearing loss. *See* Hearing disorders
Shaw hemostatic scalpel, 174–176
Sjögren's syndrome, 29, 118
Skin
  and aging, 184–185
  and cancer. *See* Cancer

Small Business Innovative Research (SBIR), 30
Smell. *See* Olfaction
Somatic mutation, 14–15
Speech disorders, 32–35
  language and cognition related to, 34–35
  noisy and degraded speech, 34
  sensory aids to improve, 35
  See also Voice disorders
Squamous cell carcinoma. *See* Cancer
Streptomycin, and presbyastasis, 54
Stria vascularis, 42, 43, 44
Superoxide dismutase, 113–114
Surgery, 36–37
Swallowing disorders, 29–31, 122–123, 124–133
  electrical pacing used for, 131
  evaluating, 125–126
  head and neck related, 138–143
    blood vessel changes, 139, 141
    microtubules and neurofilaments, 141
    nerve fiber loss, 138–139
    nerve size changes, 139, 140
    oxidative metabolism, 141
    perineurium thickening, 141
    Schwann cell changes, 139
  nerve grafting used for, 130–131
  pharyngeal, examining techniques, 134–137
    electromyography, 135, 136
    manometry, 134–135
    videoradiography, 134
  related to neurologic disorders, 124
  and reversing neural degeneration, 131
  therapy for, 126–127
Systemic lupus erythematosis, 119

T

Taste. *See* Gustation
T cells. *See* Immune deficiency
Teflon, use in vocal cord augmentation, 128
Thymus gland, and immune deficiency, 107
Tinnitus, 45–48
Tinnitus Research Clinic, 45
Tracheotomy, to avoid aspiration, 128

U

Ultrasonography, in study of swallowing, 126
University of Pennsylvania Smell Identification Test (UPSIT), 95, 98
  and Parkinson's disease, 101, 102
Upper respiratory infections (URI), 25, 26, 27

V

Vagus, 127
Vestibular system, and aging, 58–61
Videoradiography, in examining pharyngeal swallowing, 134
Vocal cord. *See* Aspiration, and laryngeal dysfunction, vocal cord augmentation to correct; Voice disorders
Voice disorders, 29–31, 64–70
  associated with neurologic disorders, 68
  associated with neuromuscular impairment, 71–78
  case studies, 72–77
  compensating for, 67
  laryngeal trauma, 68–69
  laryngoscopic features of, 65–67
  psychogenic, 67–68
  treatment of, 69–70
  versus normal elderly voice, 79–89
    acoustic spectrum, 85–86
    fundamental frequency, 82–85
    intraoral breath pressure, 87
    laryngoscopic observations, 88
    rate of speaking, 86–87
    vital capacity, 87
    vocal intensity, 85
Voice onset time (VOT), 87

W

Weismann, A., on cell biology, 8–9
WI-38 cells, 12–13

X

Xerostomia, 103
  See also Gustation

NO LONGER THE PROPERTY
OF THE
UNIVERSITY OF R. I. LIBRARY